Colour Atlas of

CLINICAL ORTHOPAEDICS

Second Edition

W Anthony Jones

MCh (Orth.), FRCS, FRCS Ed.
Consultant Orthopaedic Surgeon,
Broadgreen Hospital, Liverpool,
UK

Robert Owen

OBE, DL, MCh (Orth.), FRIS
Emeritus Professor of Orthopaedic
Surgery, Liverpool University,
UK

Foreword
by
Alan Graham Apley
MB, BS, FRCS, FRCS Ed (Hon.)

Mosby-Wolfe

London Baltimore Bogotá Boston Buenos Aires Caracas Carlsbad, CA Chicago Madrid Mexico City Milan Naples, FL New York Philadelphia St. Louis Sydney Tokyo Toronto Wiesbaden

Published in 1995 by Mosby-Wolfe, an imprint of Times Mirror International Publishers Limited

Printed by Grafos S.A. Arte sobre Papel, Barcelona

ISBN 0 7234 2058 0 (UK edition)
ISBN 0 7234 2215 X (US edition)

For full details of all Times Mirror International Publishers Limited titles, please write to Times Mirror International Publishers Limited, Lynton House, 7–12 Tavistock Square, London WC1H 9LB, England.

A CIP catalogue record for this book is available from the British Library.

Library of Congress Cataloging-in-Publication Data applied for

Project Manager: Peter Harrison

Developmental Editor: Claire Hooper

Designer/Layout Artist: Hollock Waine

Cover Design: Lara Last

Illustration: Lee Smith

Production: Mike Heath

Index: Jill Halliday BSc

Publisher: Geoff Greenwood

Contents

Foreword

The distinction between a preface and a foreword can be a matter for linguistic debate. What cannot be denied is that the authors of this present book have themselves provided such a good preface that a foreword hardly seems necessary. They pay graceful tribute to the late Professor Kessel who compiled the first edition and acknowledge that, while they have retained much of his work, they have enlarged some sections, especially that on the spine, where Professor Owen has made such notable advances. They have also cleverly tailored the work to suit those studying for examinations.

The authors list those for whom the book will be valuable, indicating when and how it might be used. Little therefore remains for the writer of a preface other than to congratulate the authors and the publishers on a splendid production, a most worthy successor to Professor Kessel's work. The book is a joy to skim through, to browse through, and to handle.

Alan Graham Apley MB BS FRCS FRCSEd (Hon)

Preface

This second edition of *Color Atlas of Clinical Orthopedics* is long overdue. In editing this edition we have heavily relied upon the material originally compiled by the late Professor Lipmann Kessel for the first edition; his work remains at the core of this book.

The format of a General and a Regional section is retained. In this new edition the General section has been more structured into subsections covering bone dysplasias, malformation syndromes, disorders of joints and soft tissues, metabolic and endocrine diseases, orthopaedic neurology and tumours. It is hoped that this more organised layout will improve understanding by putting some of the rarer conditions into context.

In the Regional section most sections have been enlarged, particularly those on the spine, wrist and hand, reflecting the expansion in knowledge, particularly in diagnosis and imaging, that has occurred over the last ten years.

This atlas is not a comprehensive orthopaedic textbook, but sets out to illustrate the clinical features of the commoner conditions met in orthopaedic practice by means of clinical photographs, radiographs and other modern imaging techniques. Clinical signs are demonstrated where appropriate, management and treatment are mentioned where pertinent points need to be made, although treatment of the conditions described is not the purpose of this book. Pictures are supported by captions and text to provide a useful 'pen picture' of the conditions described.

Some less common conditions are included where completion and maintenance of a balance demands. It is hoped that the contents will serve to stimulate the reader to further study.

This edition should continue to prove useful to senior medical students and GP practices who seldom have the time to consult larger textbooks in orthopaedics. Accident and Emergency departments will find this book a useful and easy reference, and even the postgraduate studying for Fellowship examinations will find this book a helpful and relaxing browse before clinicals. Physiotherapy and Occupational Therapy departments will also, it is hoped, find value in the contents.

Acknowledgements

We are grateful to the late Professor Lipmann Kessel and his photographer Uta Boundy for the pictures retained from the first edition. The Departments of Medical Photography at the Royal Liverpool University Hospital and Alder Hey Children's Hospital have produced a large number of additional pictures not taken by the editors themselves or Mr Aaron Lim.

Thanks are extended to the following for providing assistance with clinical pictures: Mr R. Evans for Figures 8 and 9; Mary Evans Picture Library/Explorer for Figure 21; Dr T. Yuille for Figure 57; Dr J. Verbov for Figure 186; Dr H. Carty for Figures 201 and 417; Mr M.S. Ghorbal for Figures 370 and 371; Mr R. Mulholland for Figures 407 and 408 and Mr A. Simison for Figure 703.

We are grateful to Dr Barbara Ansell for permitting the use of Figures 16, 24 and 170 from her *Colour Atlas of Paediatric Rheumatology*, and to Dr Victor Parsons for similar permission to reproduce Figures 40, 100, 192, 205, 294, 470, 471, 473 and 474 from his *Color Atlas of Bone Disease*.

1 Generalised disorders

One of the fascinations of clinical orthopaedic practice is to detect the patient who presents with an obvious local deformity or disability, which in the event turns out to be an expression of some generalised disease process. It is important that the clinician's attention is not overwhelmed by the local presenting disorder but that he remains aware of the fact that he may be seeing only the tip of an iceberg. Sometimes the generalised nature of the disease is obvious. At other times, e.g. a child presents with knock knees who is, in fact, suffering from some form of rickets; or a child in whom the spinal curvature turns out to be the local manifestation of generalised neurofibromatosis.

The clinician should be on his guard lest the part that the patient presents to him obscures the whole picture.

There is little known of the basic pathology of the generalised developmental disorders of the skeleton but they can usefully be classified by grouping similar clinical types. The bone dysplasias have in common an abnormality of bone and cartilage growth and may be divided into those that give rise to dwarfism and those which do not. Malformation syndromes are not easily differentiated from the bone dysplasias but have in common multi-system abnormalities as well as structural musculoskeletal disorders and can be divided into those with chromosome anomalies and those without.

Bone dysplasias with dwarfism

Dwarfs may be subdivided into those with short limbs, those with short trunks and proportionate dwarfs. Some of these conditions will be considered.

- Short-limbed dwarfism: achondroplasia, chondro-ectodermal dysplasia, diastrophic dwarfism.
- Short trunk dwarfism: spondylo-epiphyseal dysplasia.
- Proportionate dwarfism: mucopolysaccharidoses, pyknodysostosis.

Achondroplasia

Classical achondroplasia is of autosomal dominant inheritance. The condition is either apparent at birth or soon after. The abnormal skull and short limbs are characteristic. Physical strength and intelligence are not impaired.

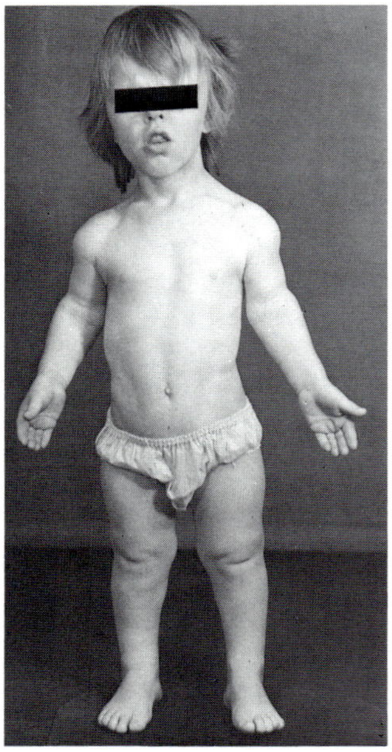

1

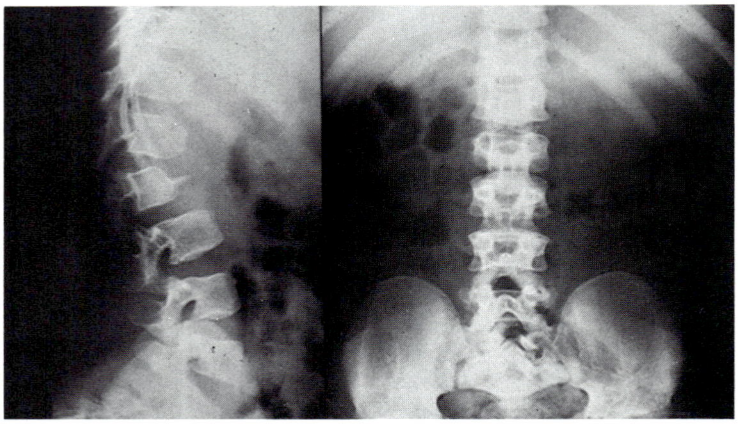

2

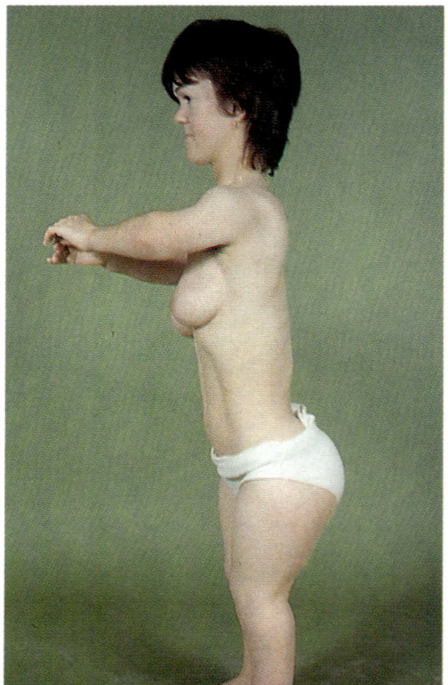

3

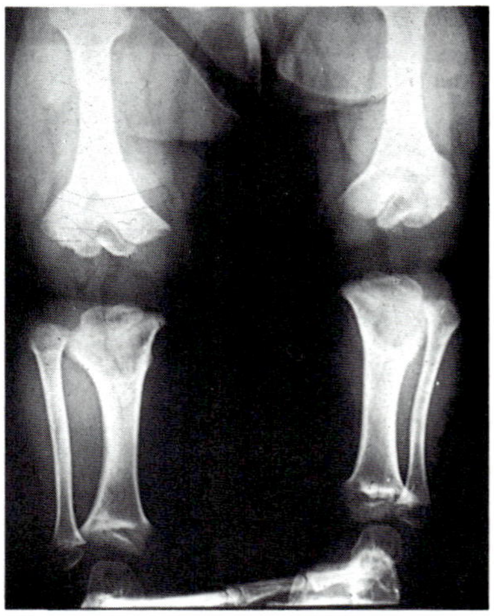

4

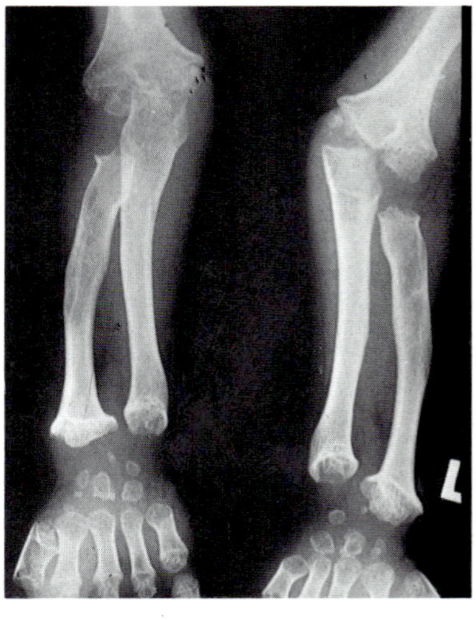

5

1–5 These strong little dwarfs are of typical appearance. Radiographs of the spine show flattening of the antero-superior aspect of the lumbar vertebrae and widening of the intervertebral spaces in the lateral view. In the antero-posterior view there is a progressive decrease in the interpedicular distances. Radiographs of the extremities show the characteristic 'ball and socket' epiphyses and flared metaphyses. The bones are short, giving an impression of diaphysial thickness.

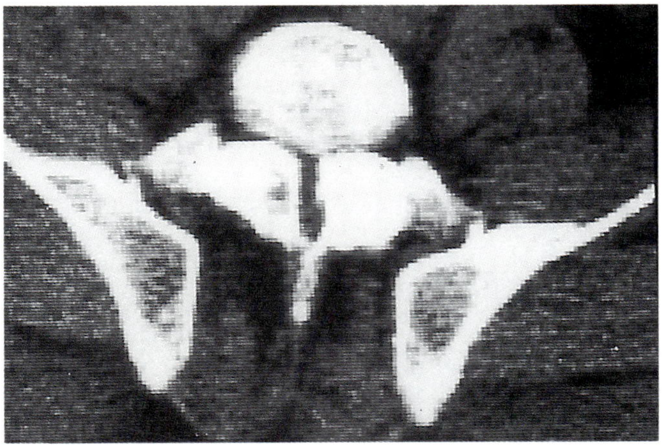

6 In adult life the development of symptoms of spinal stenosis is not uncommon. This CT scan shows severe narrowing of the spinal canal at the lumbo-sacral level. (See also **584** & **585**)

Chondro-ectodermal dysplasia

The Ellis–Van Creveld syndrome is of autosomal recessive inheritance. The condition is apparent at birth and is characterised by polydactyly, dysplastic finger nails and congenital heart disease is often a feature (60%), most frequently an atrial septal defect. Prognosis depends upon congenital heart disease. If there is none, expectation of life is normal.

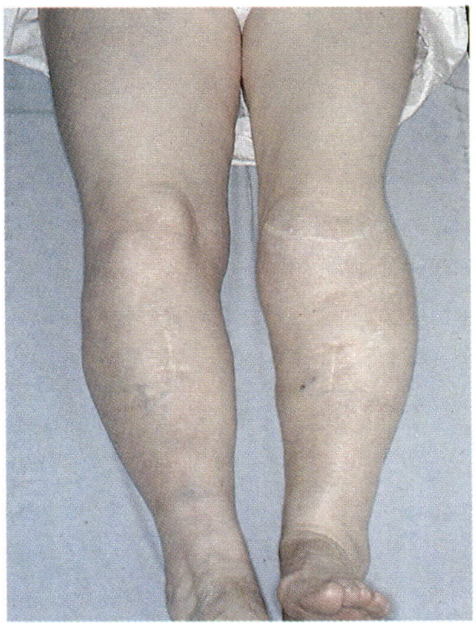

7 Short-limbed dwarfing results due to shortening of the distal segments of the limbs. The relative shortening of tibial to femoral segments in this middle-aged lady can be seen. Surgical scars from procedures to correct deformity are present.

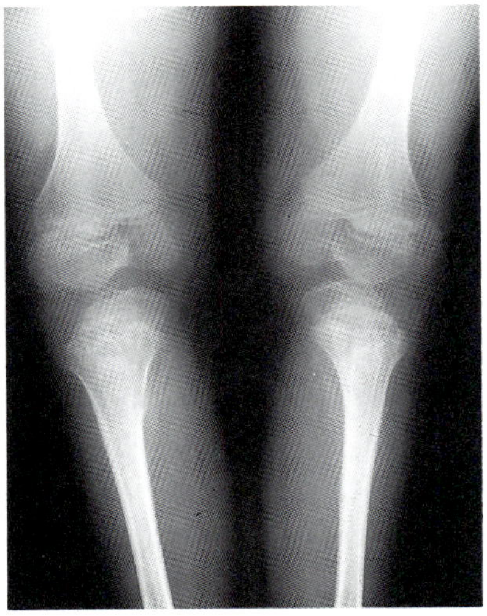

8 In the lower limb defective growth of the upper lateral portion of the tibia results in genu valgum.

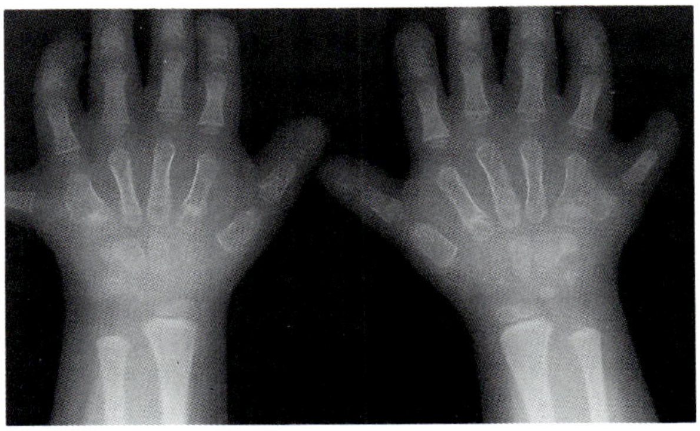

9 Polydactyly is post-axial and results in either an extra digit or a sixth metacarpal fused to the fifth. A capitate-hamate coalition sometimes exists. Distal phalanges are disproprtionately short compared to the proximal phalanges.

Diastrophic dwarfism

This condition is of autosomal recessive inheritance and is characterised by short-limbed dwarfism accompanied by joint contractures, severe talipes equino varus, deformed ears and the later development of scoliosis. The condition is apparent at birth. 'Cauliflower ears' develop shortly after birth and later calcification of the pinna occurs. Deafness may be a feature.

Long bones are short and broad with flared metaphyses. Flexion contractures involve hips, knees and elbows. A particularly refractory club foot is a characteristic feature.

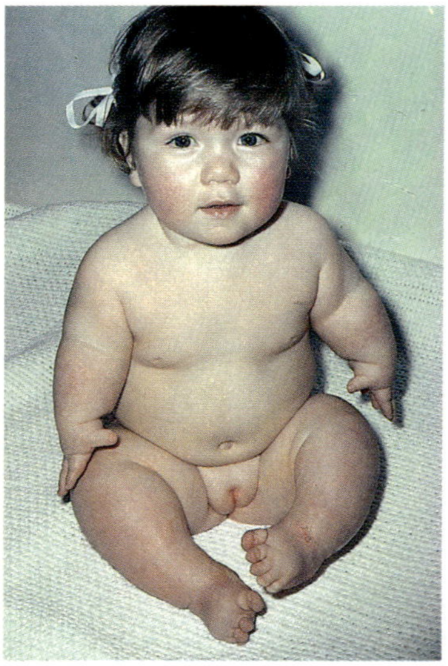

10 General appearance.

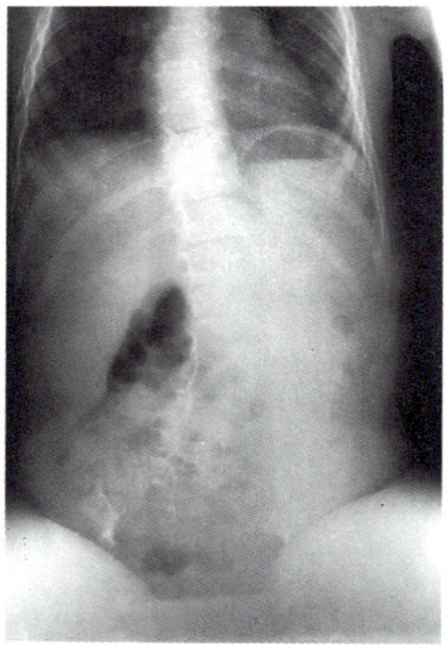

11 The vertebral column is normal at birth but structural scoliosis develops in childhood.

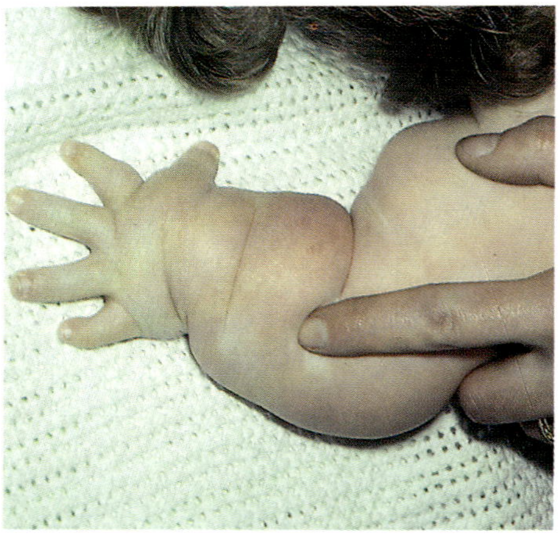

12 In the hand a short first metacarpal with proximal placement of the thumb results in a typical 'hitch-hikers' thumb posture.

Spondylo-epiphyseal dysplasia

A comparatively rare type of generalised developmental disorder with a variety of autosomal patterns of inheritance. Characteristically, the trunk is short with scoliosis. Only the large proximal joints (hips and shoulders) are affected. Progressive scoliosis usually develops and premature degenerative arthritis of the hips and shoulders may occur, but the expectation of life is unaffected.

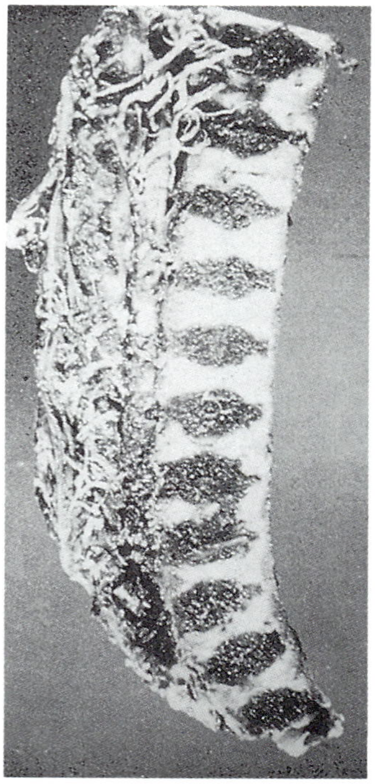

13 This pathological specimen shows an excess of spinal cartilage owing to the failure of proper ossification.

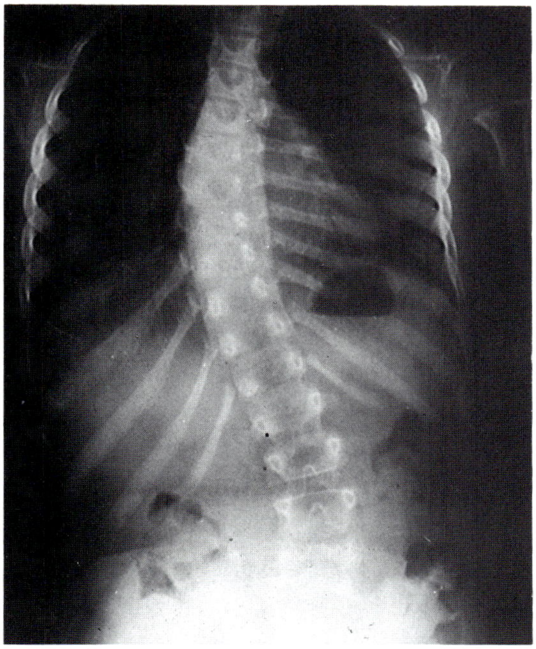

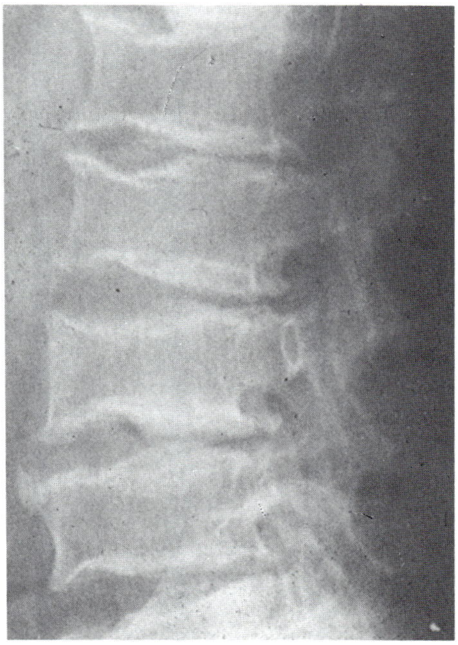

14 (left) & **15** (right) The vertebral end plates are deformed and the vertebral bodies consequently distorted and typically flattened (platyspondyly) causing scoliosis to develop.

Mucopolysaccharide disorders

This group of conditions have in common an inborn error of mucopolysaccharide (MPS) metabolism. Not all give rise to dwarfism but for completeness are best considered together.

They are differentiated by their clinical features, the presence of a characteristic urinary MPS and their mode of inheritance (**Tables 1** & **2**).

Table 1. Mucopolysaccharide disorders (a)

Type of syndrome	*Inheritance*	*Urinary MPS*	*Age of onset*
I Hurler's	Autosomal recessive	Dermatan Heparan sulphate	Months
II Hunter's	X-linked recessive	Dermatan Heparan sulphate	6–12 months
III Sanfilippo	Autosomal recessive	Heparan sulphate	Early childhood
IV Morquio Brailsford	Autosomal recessive	Keratan sulphate	2–4 years
V Scheie	Autosomal recessive	Dermatan sulphate	Late childhood
VI Maroteaux Lamy	Autosomal recessive	Dermatan sulphate	early to late childhood

Table 2. Mucopolysaccharide disorders (b)

Type of disorder	*Mental retardation*	*Bone changes*	*Prognosis*
MPS I	Severe	Moderate, kyphosis	Death 10–15 years
MPS II	Late onset less severe than MPS I	Moderate, no kyphosis	Survival to third decade
MPS III	Severe	Minimal	Survival to third or fourth decade
MPS IV	Absent	Severe and characteristic	Normal longevity
MPS V	Absent	Moderate	Survival to adulthood
MPS VI	Absent	Severe	No data

Hunter's syndrome has features similar to Hurler's disease but less severe and all individuals with this condition are male owing to the X-linked mode of inheritance.

Maroteaux Lamy syndrome again is similar to Hurler's disease, but less severe and intelligence is normal.

Morquio Brailsford's syndrome

The best known of the group is Morquio Brailsford's syndrome (MPS IV) which exhibits characteristic skeletal features. Intelligence is normal but marked skeletal changes result in dwarfism. The skull and facial appearance is normal.

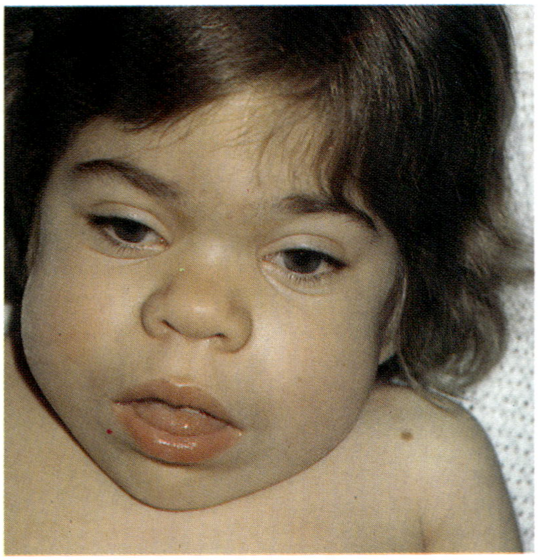

16 Hurler's syndrome is characterised by short stature and progressive mental retardation. The coarse facies and enlarged tongue led to the synonymous term Gargoylism.

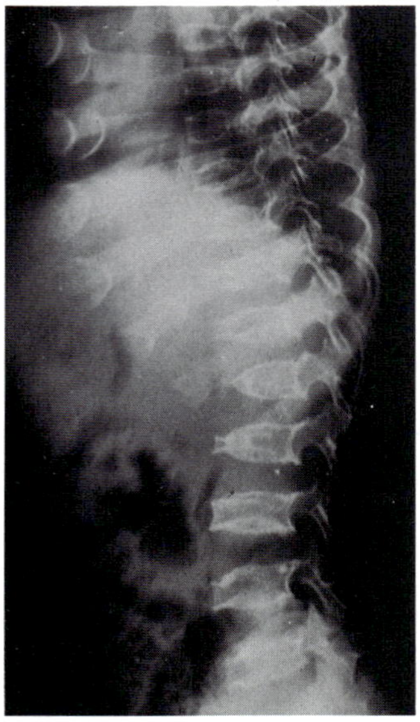

17 The axial skeleton exhibits marked platyspondyly with anterior beaking of vertebrae resulting in a relative shortness of the trunk.

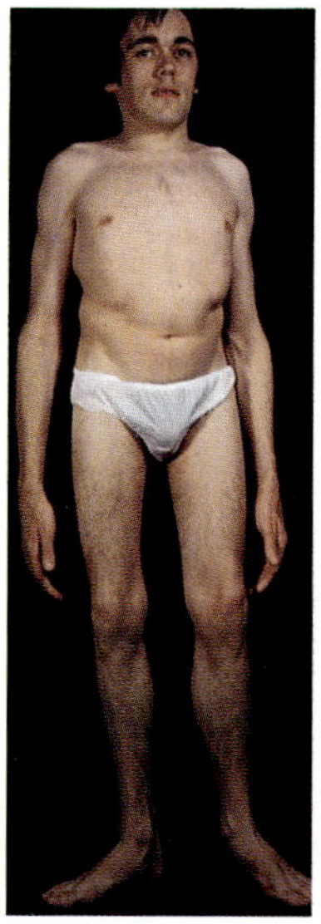

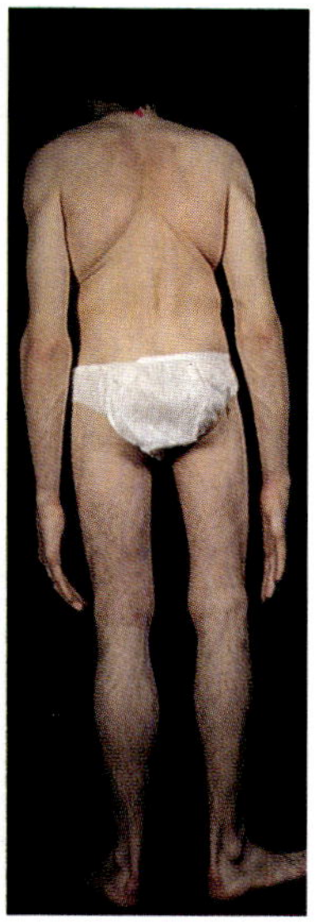

18 (left)&
19 (right) There is flaring of the rib cage and a pronounced 90° angulation of the manubrio-sternal joint is characteristic of the condition.

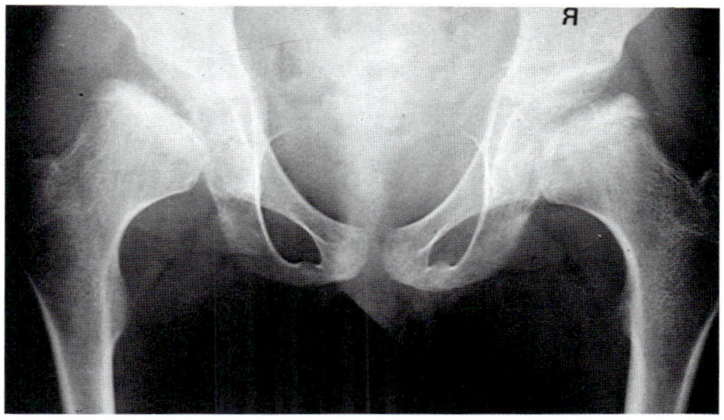

20 Laxity of joints is a common feature with epiphyseal dysplasia of the hips.

Pyknodysostosis

This is a rare generalised developmental disorder of autosomal recessive inheritance which results in a proportionate type of dwarfism; affected individuals rarely achieve an adult height of 1.52 m. It is said that the artist Henri de Toulouse-Lautrec was afflicted by this condition.

There is a generalised increased density and fragility of bone. There are shared features resembling both osteopetrosis and cranio-cleido dysostosis. Radiologically there is increased bone density and pathological fractures are common.

In the skull there is delayed closure of sutures and Wormian bones are present. The vault bulges, the face is small and the jaw recedes. Dental abnormalities are frequent.

The distal end of the clavicle may be dysplastic or absent. In the hand the digits are short with hypoplastic terminal phalanges.

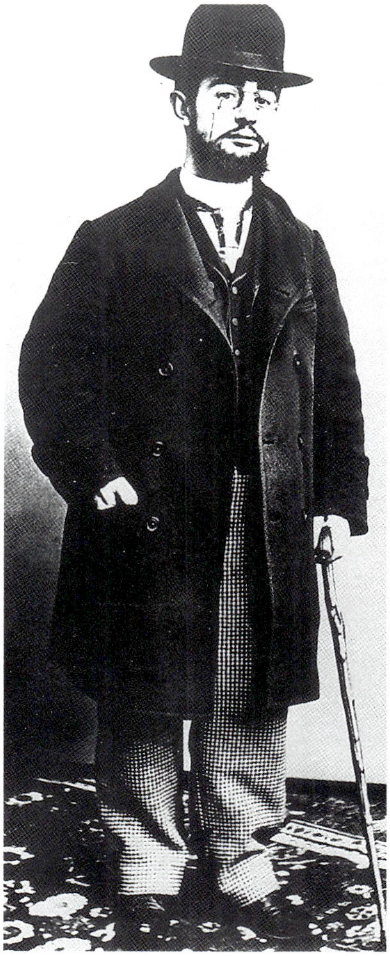

21 Henri de Toulouse-Lautrec (1864–1901), famous for his paintings, drawings and prints of late 19th century Parisian night life.

Bone dysplasias without dwarfing

Affecting epiphyses

Multiple epiphyseal dysplasia

A heterogeneous group of conditions of variable inheritance in which the epiphyses of long bones are affected by a growth disorder. The disorder is confined to the skeleton and there tends to be a similarity of distribution of lesions within any given family, e.g. confined to the lower limbs or principally affecting the hips.

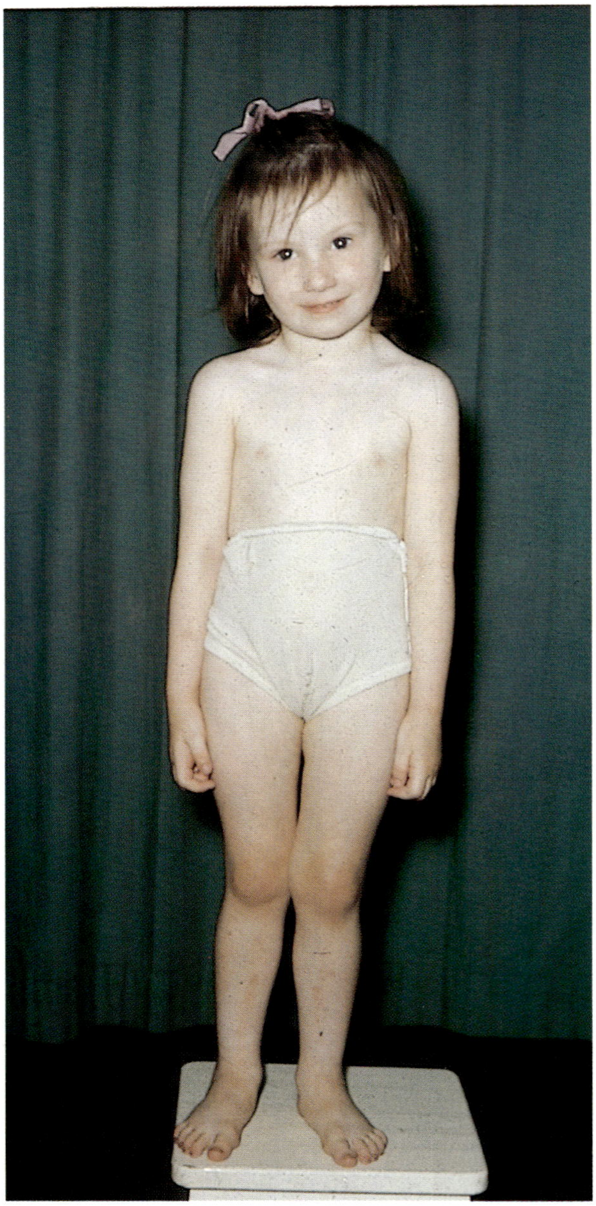

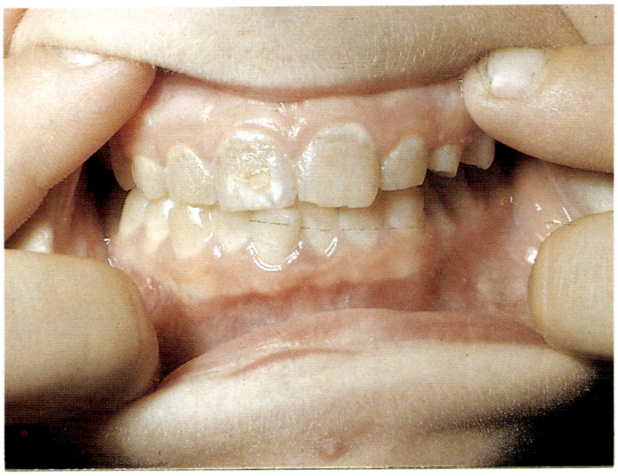

22 & **23** General appearance of a child with a strong familial incidence of the disease. The skull and axial skeleton are normal. She is of short stature for her age but not a dwarf. Anomalies of dentition were also present.

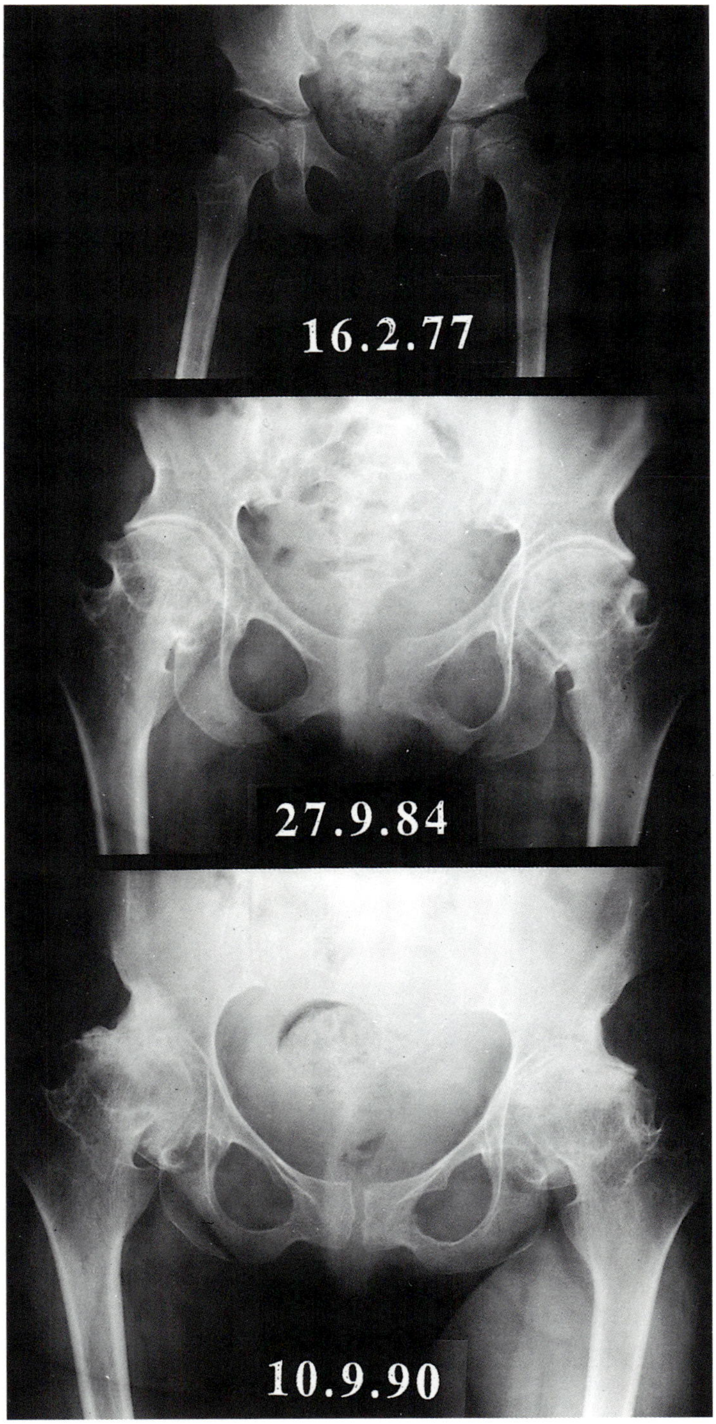

24 The epiphyses of long bones are typically small and sometimes mottled. Ossification occurs late and irregularly. This series of radiographs shows progression of premature degenerative changes to age 18 years.

Dysplasia epiphysialis hemimelica (Trevor's disease)

A sporadically occurring dysplasia in which osteo-cartilaginous exostoses are found arising from the medial or lateral half of the epiphysis of a single limb. The lower limb is more commonly affected than the upper and there is a male preponderance of 3:1.

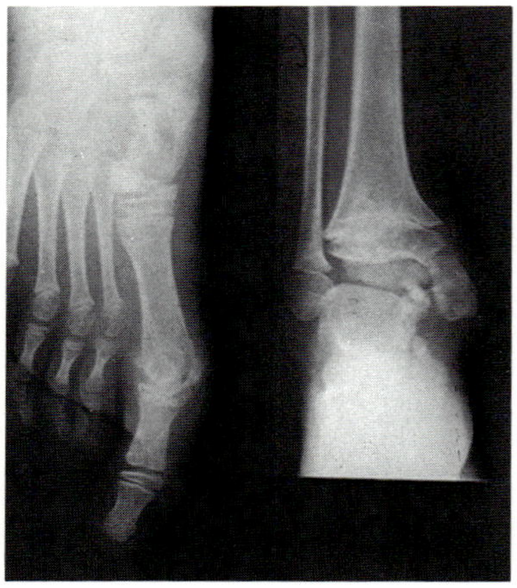

25 A calcified mass shown in radiographs of the ankle simulating a cartilage-capped exostosis, hypertrophied medial malleolus and medial cuneiform, and the whole of the first metatarsal ray. The disease presents with limitation of movement and some pain.

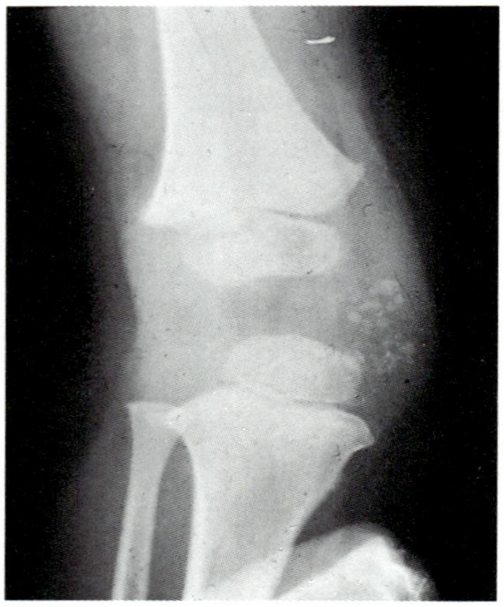

26 Speckled calcification within a mass arising from the upper medial tibial epiphysis giving rise to a valgus deformity at the knee.

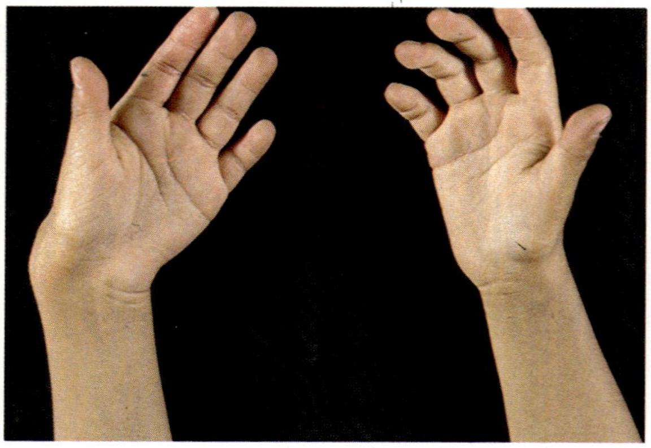

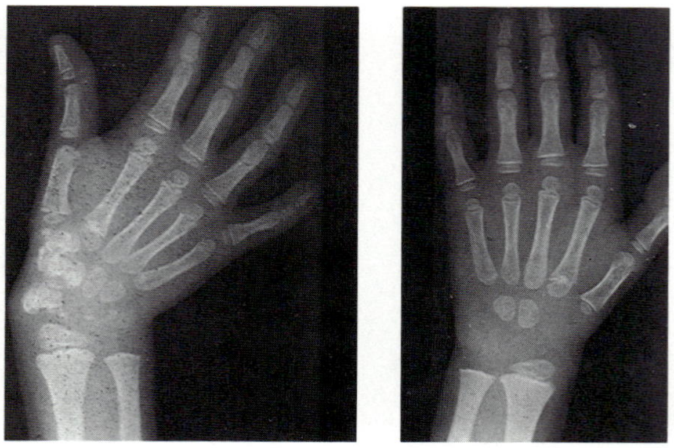

27 & **28** Radial enlargement and ulnar deviation of the left wrist of this ten-year-old boy is clinically obvious. The radiographs show considerable precocity of maturation of the carpus as well as the development of bosses of new bone simulating ossified chondromata.

Juxta epiphyseal dysplasia – Diaphyseal aclasis (multiple hereditary exostoses)

Although called 'diaphyseal' this is a juxta epiphyseal disorder of bone growth giving rise to cartilage-capped exostoses that point away from the joint. This is of autosomal dominant inheritance.

Malignant change is extremely rare but more likely in proximal lesions affecting the flat bones of the pelvis or scapula.

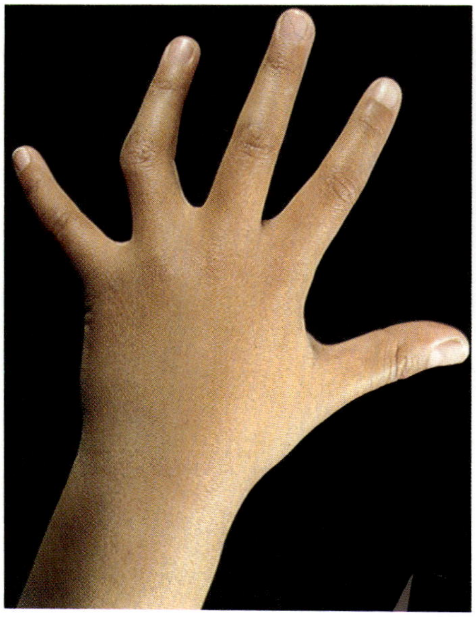

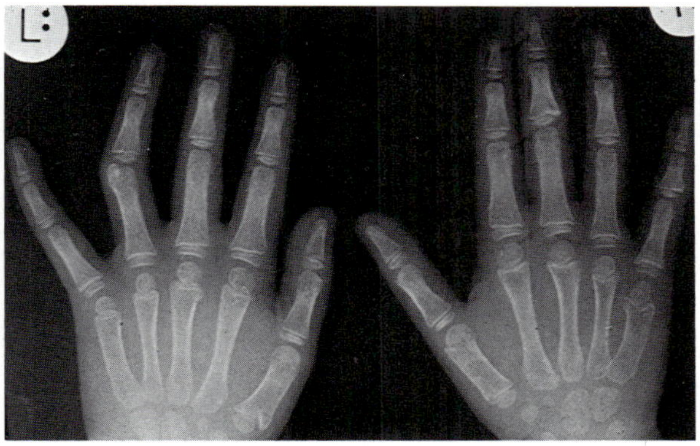

29 & **30** Stature is rarely affected but deformity of affected bones and associated joints occurs. Angulation of the left ring finger has been caused by a cartilage-capped exostosis at the distal end of the proximal phalanx.

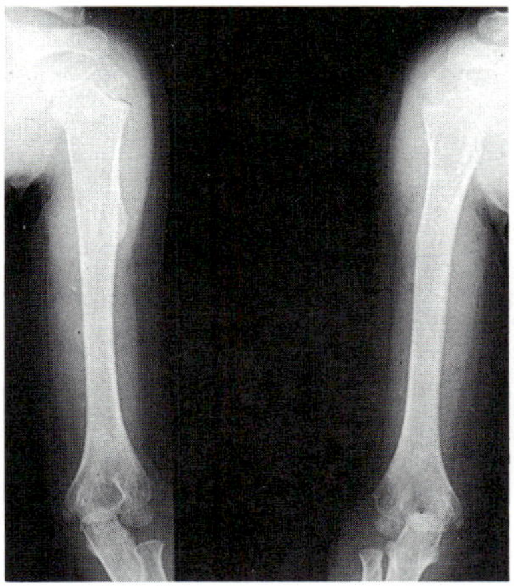

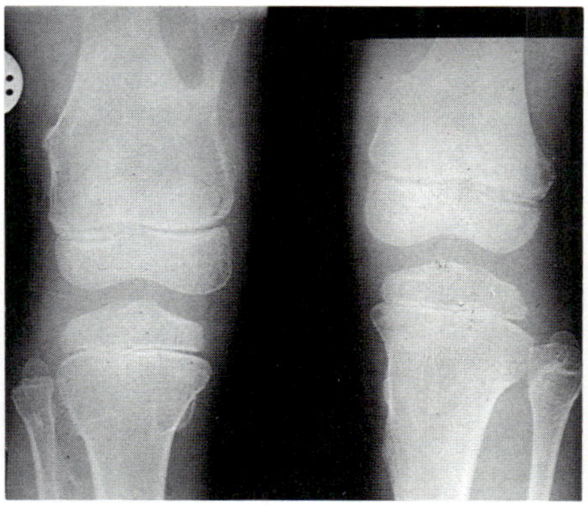

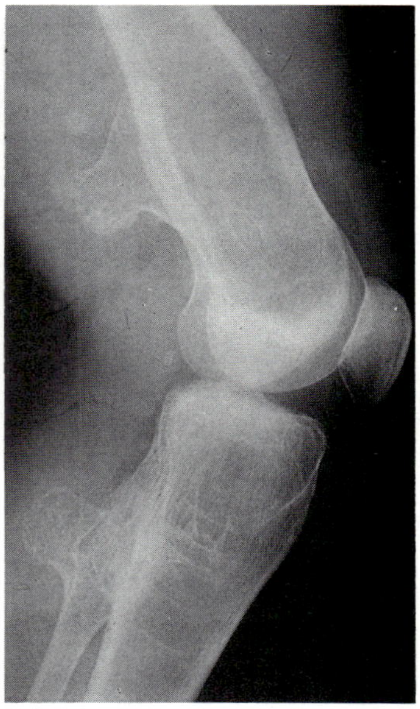

31–33 The exostosis always projects away from the adjacent joint. The exostosis is always capped by cartilage and is therefore actually larger than seen on the radiographs.

Metaphyseal dysostosis

A rare disorder of autosomal dominant inheritance. There is severe growth disturbance of the metaphyses of the long bones, obvious deformity and joint dysfunction. Two types are described here.

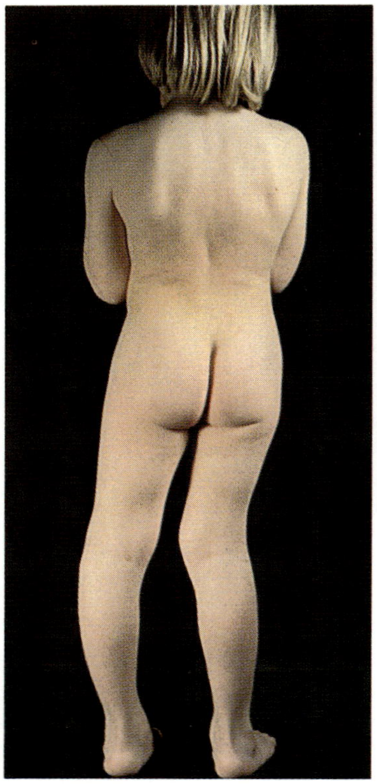

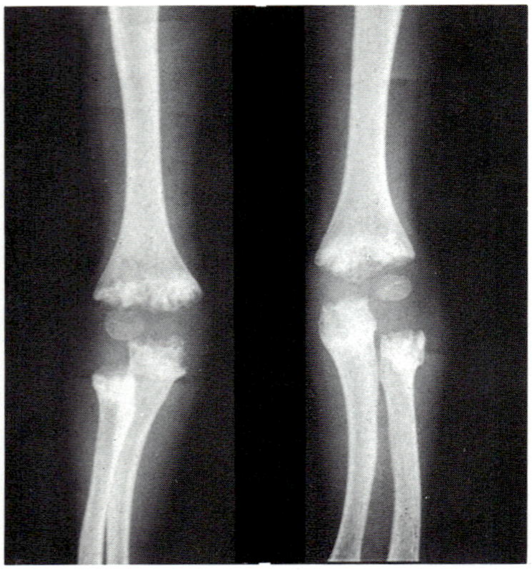

34 & **35** The Schmid type is relatively benign and occurs during infancy.

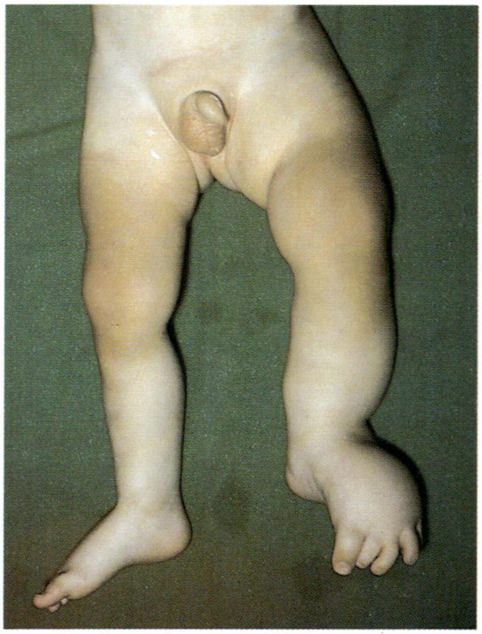

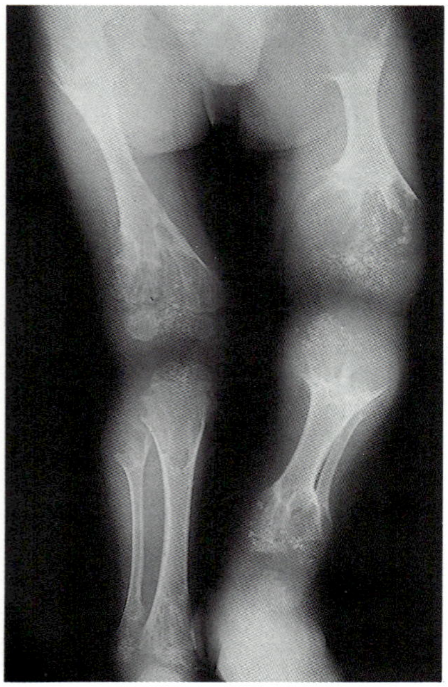

36 & **37** The Jansen type is apparent at birth and more severe with shortness of stature.

Dysplasias of membrane bone – Cranio-cleido-dysostosis

This condition is of autosomal dominant inheritance, although up to one-third of cases occur as new mutations. It is the only condition in which the growth of membrane bones alone is affected.

The skull shows bulging frontal regions, there is delayed closure of sutures and Wormian bones are present. Late eruption of teeth and supernumary teeth are common.

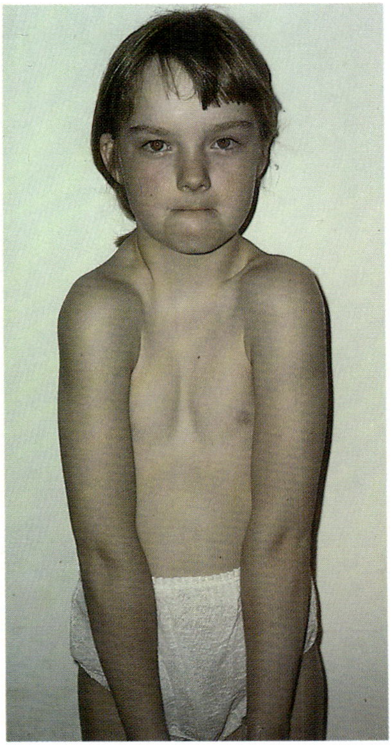

38 The characteristic feature is hypoplasia or complete absence of clavicles and associated muscles, permitting the shoulders to be anteriorly opposed.

Dysplasias of enchondral bone – Osteogenesis imperfecta

The severe congenital type generally occurs sporadically, although there is a possibility of autosomal recessive inheritance. The 'tarda' form is the more common in clinical practice and is of autosomal dominant inheritance.

Both conditions are characterised by a generalised connective tissue disturbance, most particularly of bone.

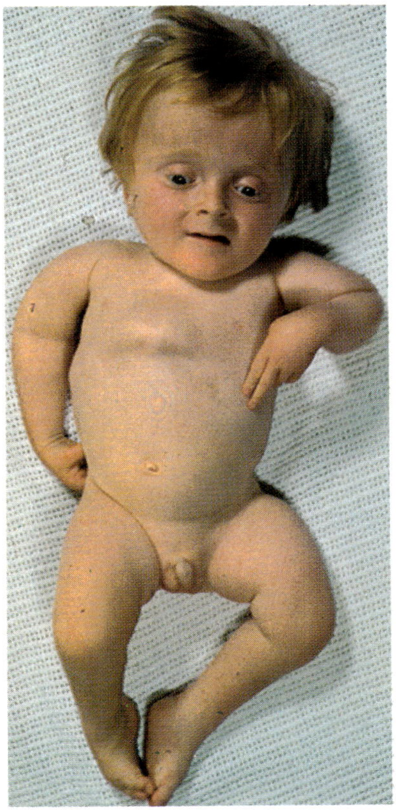

40

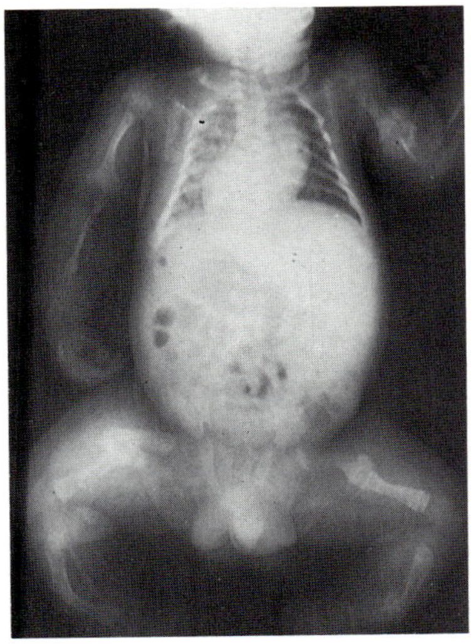

39

39 & **40** Osteogenesis imperfecta congenita presents with multiple fractures at birth.

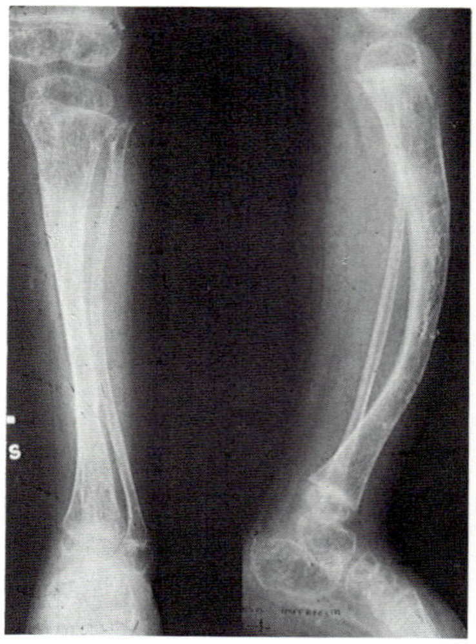

41

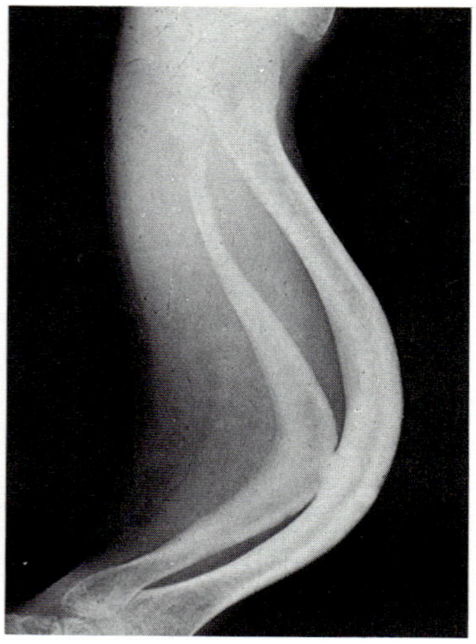

42

41 & **42** If the child shown in **39** & **40** survives, dwarfing is severe with gross distortion of long bones.

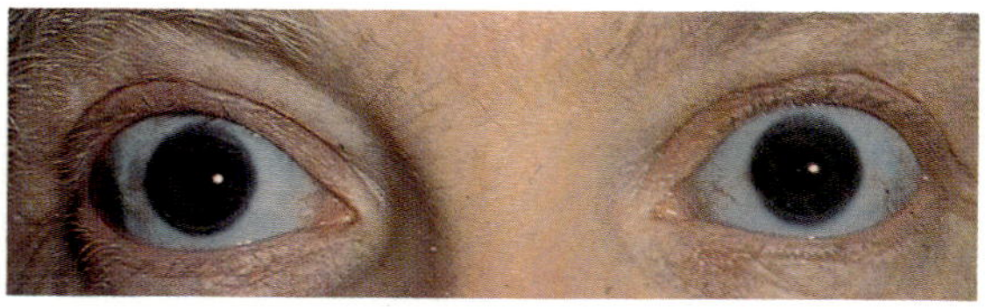

43 & **44** The 'tarda' type presents in childhood, with the number of fractures decreasing towards puberty. Both types exhibit other manifestations of connective tissue disturbance, e.g. blue sclera, imperfect dentition, joint laxity and poor wound healing.

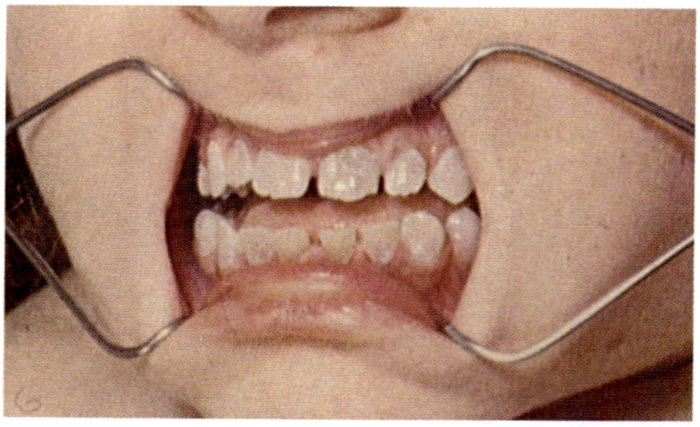

Enchondromatosis: Ollier's disease and Maffucci's syndrome

Characteristically Ollier's disease is unilateral with multiple enchondromata of bone. Cases tend to be sporadic with no known hereditary background. Affected limbs show considerable deformity and are frequently short. The condition is compatible with long life. Chondrosarcomatous change within lesions can occur in middle and old age.

46

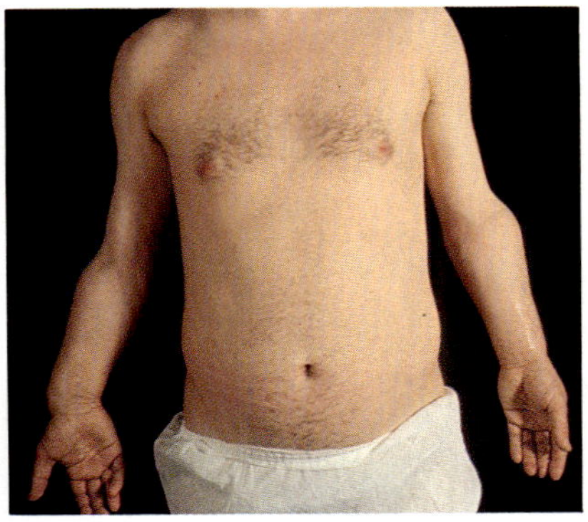

45

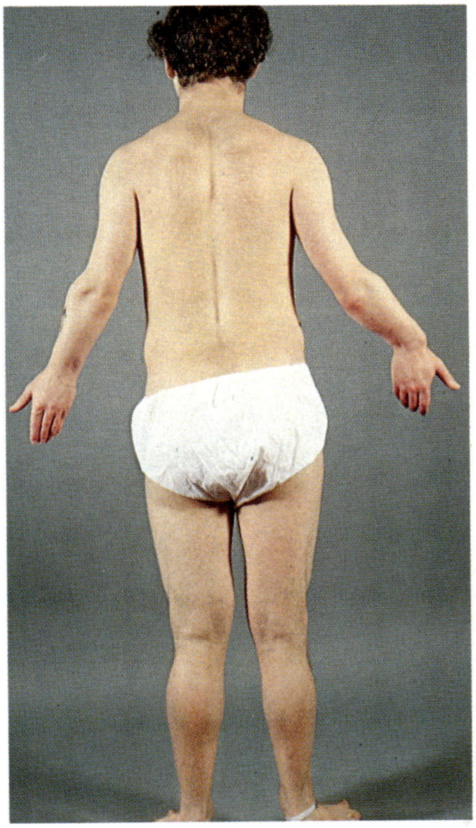

47

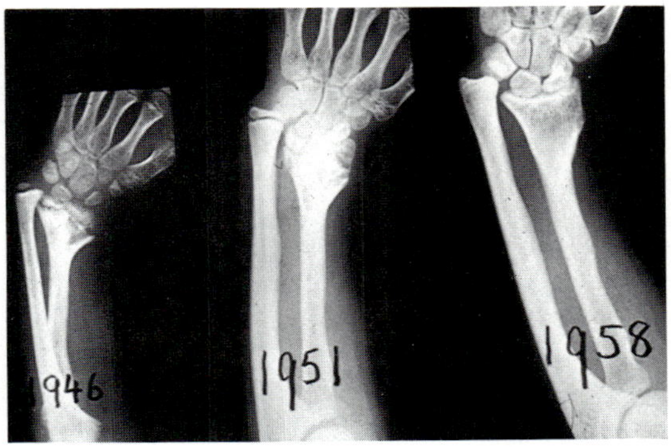

48

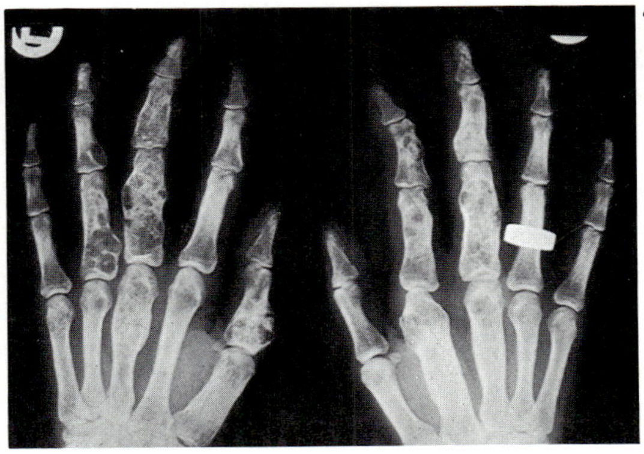

45–48 This patient shows the typical disparity of growth of the arms. The radiographs show multiple enchondromata of the hands and disturbance of growth leading to deformity at the lower end of the radius.

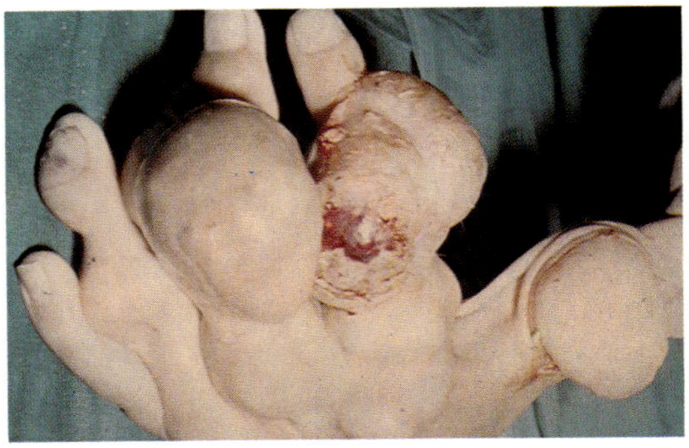

49 When multiple soft tissue haemangiomata are associated with multiple enchondromatosis the condition is called Maffucci's syndrome. Malignant change of lesions is again not uncommon.

Fibrous dysplasia of bone

There are three clinical presentations of fibrous dysplasia of bone: monostotic, polyostotic and Albright's syndrome. The disease is of unknown origin and presents during the first two decades of life.

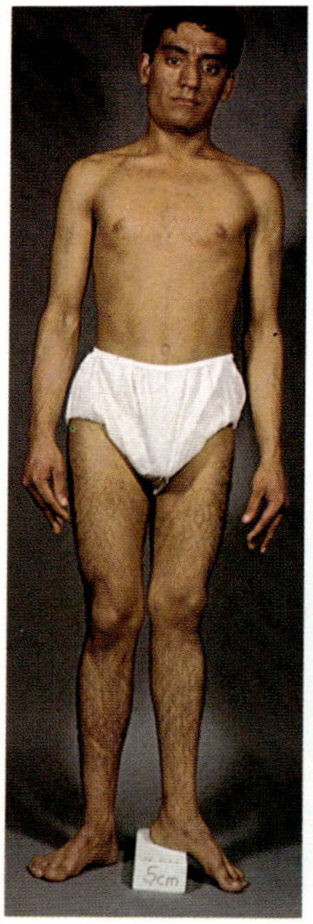

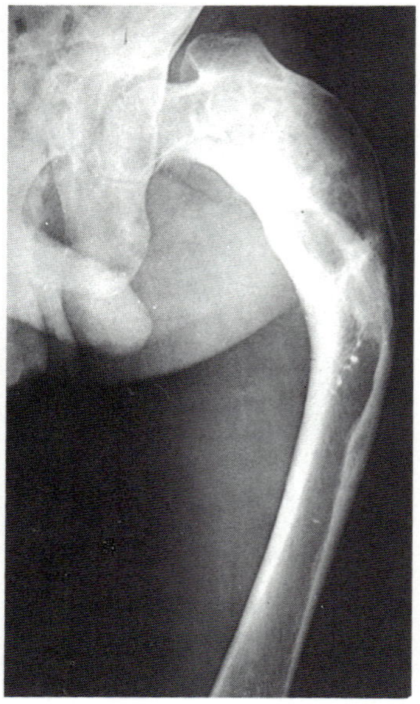

50 & **51** Monostotic fibrous dysplasia affecting the femur in a 20-year-old man. The condition was symptomless until a pathological fracture occurred and healed with bowing.

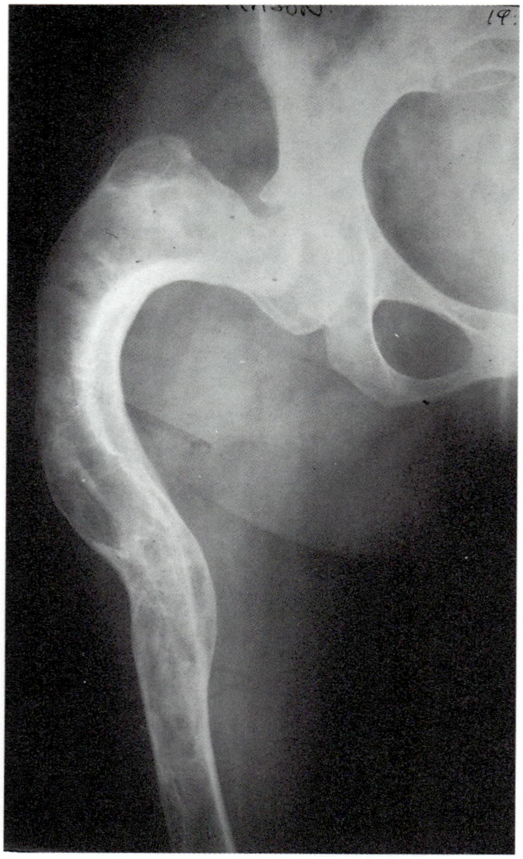

52 The radiograph shows the characteristic 'shepherd's crook' appearance of the upper femur, which develops as the diseased bone deforms.

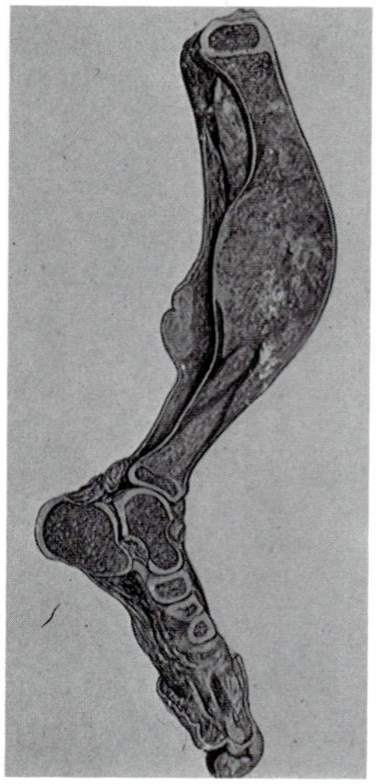

53 When the tibia is involved an indolent pathological fracture can result, usually within the first three years of life. This is one cause of congenital pseudoarthrosis of the tibia.

Polyostotic fibrous dysplasia

There is a widespread distribution of lesions without systemic endocrine disturbance.

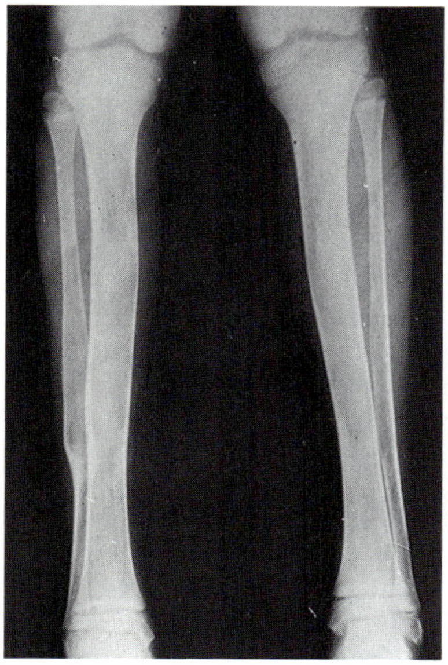

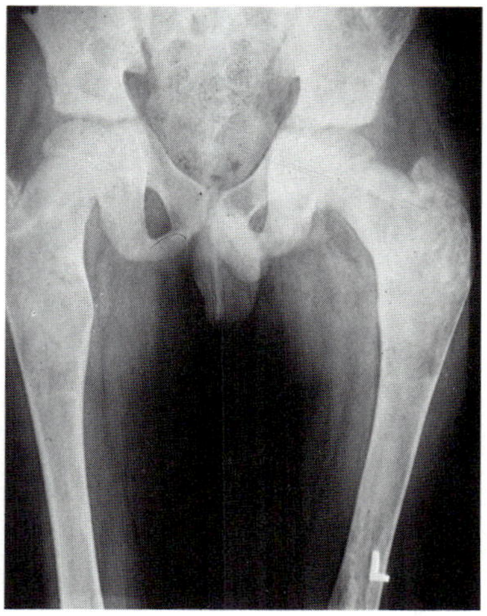

54 & **55** Fibrotic areas in the bone appear as scattered patches of rarefaction. The epiphyses are not affected. The lower extremities are most frequently and extensively involved.

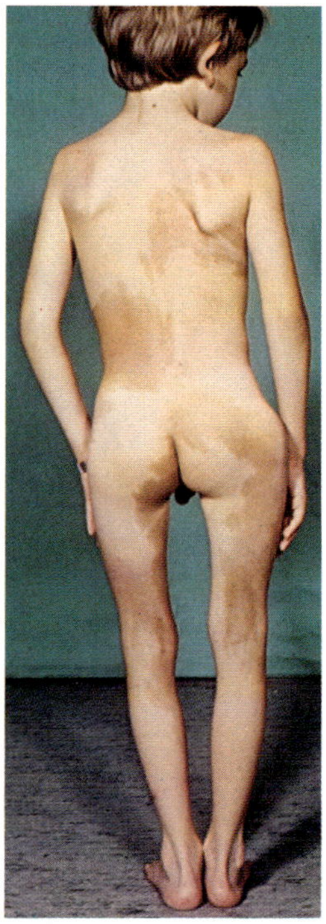

56 Albright's Syndrome. Polyostotic fibrous dysplasia associated with irregular brown cutaneous pigmentation and precocious puberty in girls.

Malformation syndromes with chromosomal abnormalities

Down's syndrome

The commonest of the chromosomal anomalies affecting 1:660 births with a female:male ratio of 3:1. Over 90% are true trisomies, occur sporadically and are associated with advanced maternal age. Others are due to chromosome translocations with no relationship to maternal age and a risk of subsequent pregnancies being affected.

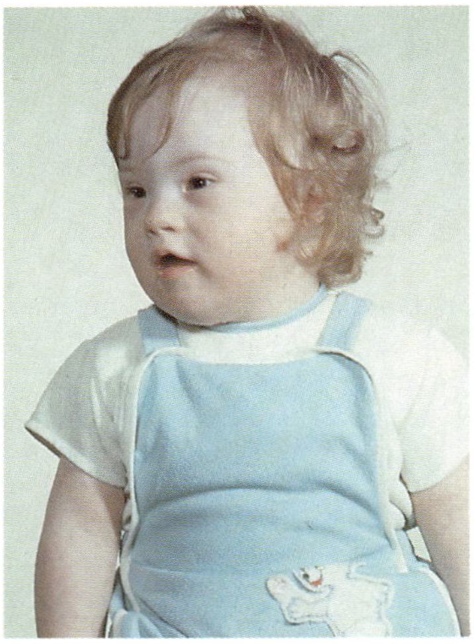

57 Affected individuals are of short stature and mentally retarded with typical facies. Metacarpals are short leading to a trident hand usually with an incurved little finger. There is a wide space between the first and second toes. In the pelvis there is lateral flaring of the ilium and a shallow acetabulum. Muscular hypotonia and joint laxity are common features. Congenital heart disease is present in about a third of cases and may lead to death in infancy.

Turner's syndrome

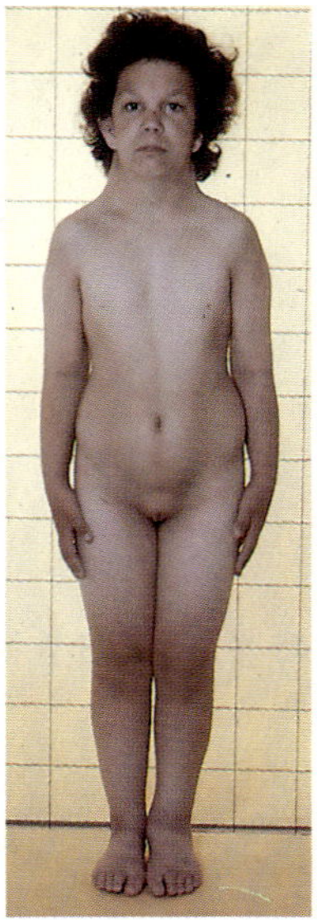

58 This is a rare chromosomal anomaly affecting females in whom one X chromosome is missing. The features, which become noticeable in childhood, include short stature and webbing of the neck. The chest is broad with wide spacing of the nipples. Coarctation of the aorta, cubitus valgus and vertebral anomalies with scoliosis or kyphosis may also occur.

Malformation syndromes without chromosomal abnormality

Radial club hand

Congenital absence or hypoplasia of the radius though uncommon is not rare and is one of the commoner skeletal limb deficiencies. The radial portion of the carpus is usually absent and the thumb either absent or rudimentary. The ulna is short and curved, with the forearm being some two-thirds of its normal length and the hand forming an angle of 90 degrees or more with the forearm. The condition is bilateral in 50% of cases.

It is one of the commoner thalidomide deformities, occurs as a sporadic isolated defect and not infrequently forms part of a syndrome.

Syndromes associated with radial club hand:

- Heart/hand syndromes: Holt Oram syndrome with associated CHD, usually septal defect.
- Fanconi's anaemia: pancytopenia.
- Erythrogenesis imperfecta: red cell dyscrasia.
- Thrombocytopenia/absent radius: platelet deficiency.
- Head/hand syndromes: mandibular facial dysostosis.

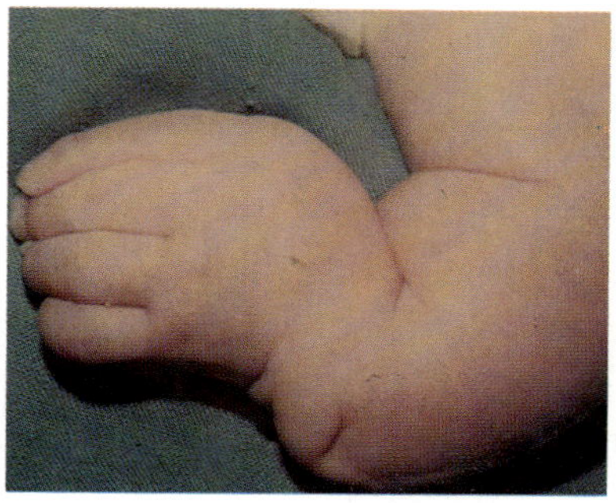

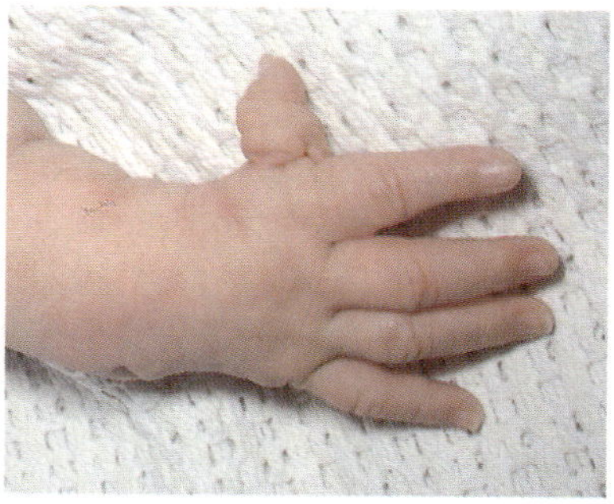

59 & **60** The whole of the pre-axial (radial) side of the forearm is under-developed or absent. The thumb is usually absent or hypoplastic.

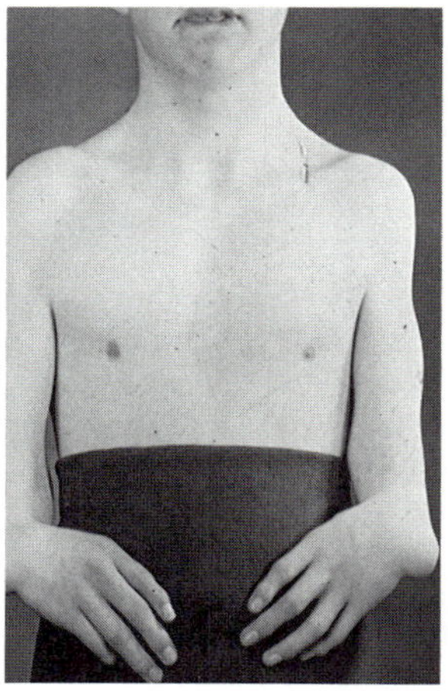

61 Bilateral radial club hand showing the considerable underdevelopment of the forearm between the elbow and hand.

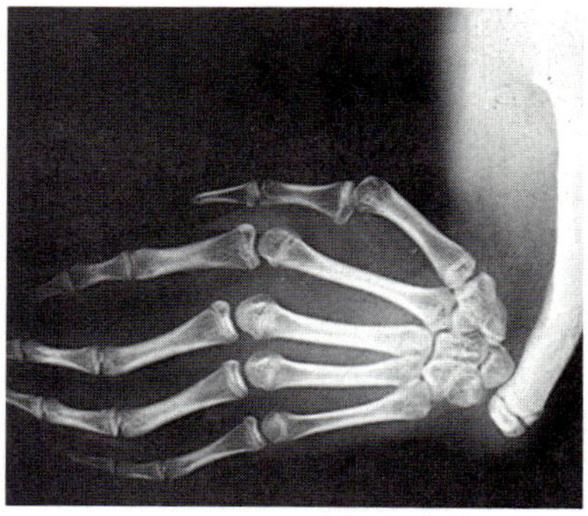

62 Radial club hand in which, uncommonly, the thumb element remains.

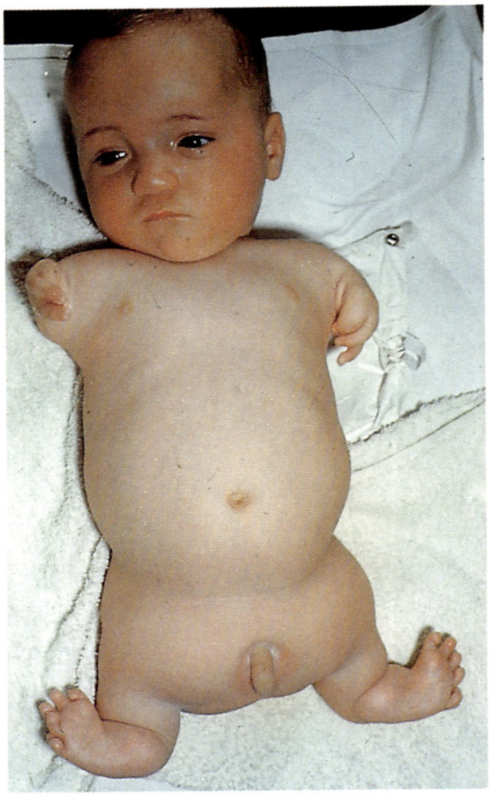

Phocomelia

The thalidomide disaster has drawn attention to the possible serious consequences of noxious intra-uterine influences on the foetus. Maternal infection by rubella as well as the use of thalidomide during pregnancy are probably only the most obvious and serious examples.

63–65 The boy shown in **64** and **65** is of normal intelligence and well developed in all respects except that his upper limbs have failed to develop. He has no left arm and his right arm consists of a little flipper (Greek *phoke*, seal; *melos*, limb). The infant shown in **63** shows severe deformities with failure of development of all four limbs.

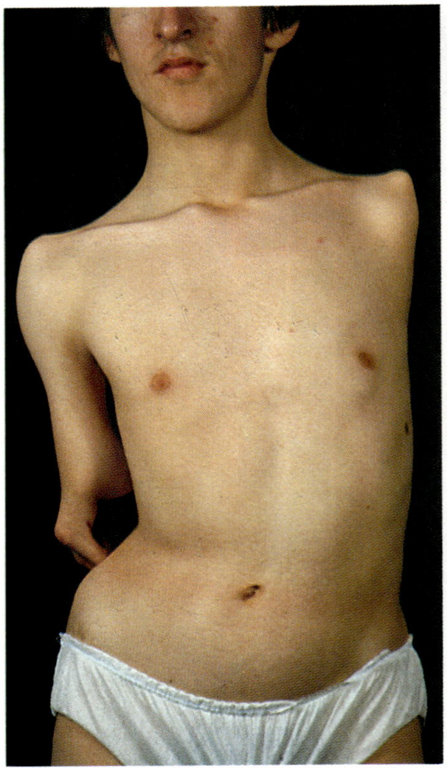

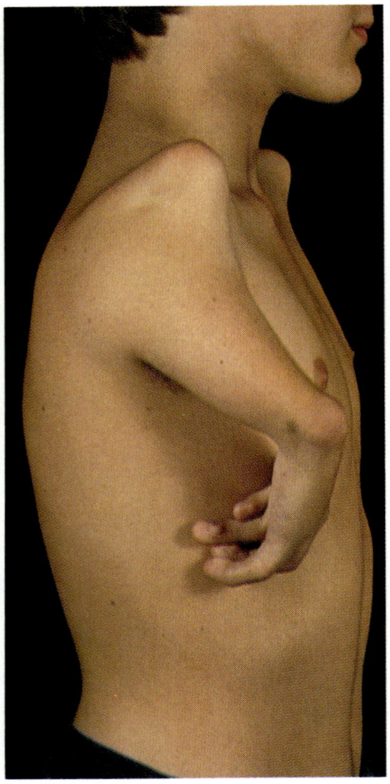

Neurofibromatosis (von Recklinghausen's disease)

This is a syndrome of autosomal dominant inheritance that varies considerably in the extent to which its features are manifest. The syndrome is characterised by café-au-lait patches, tumours of nerve trunks, overgrowth of tissues and various skeletal deformities.

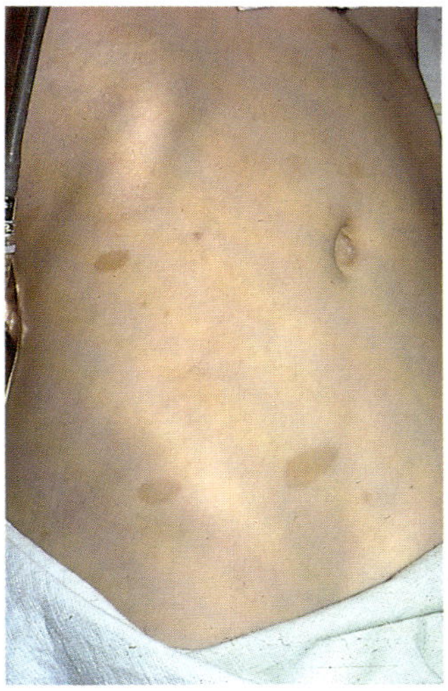

66 Cutaneous manifestations. Café-au-lait patches are pathognomonic of neurofibromatosis if there are at least four patches of 1.5 cm diameter or greater. These pigmented patches, however, are not always present from birth and can appear at any time up to adolescence.

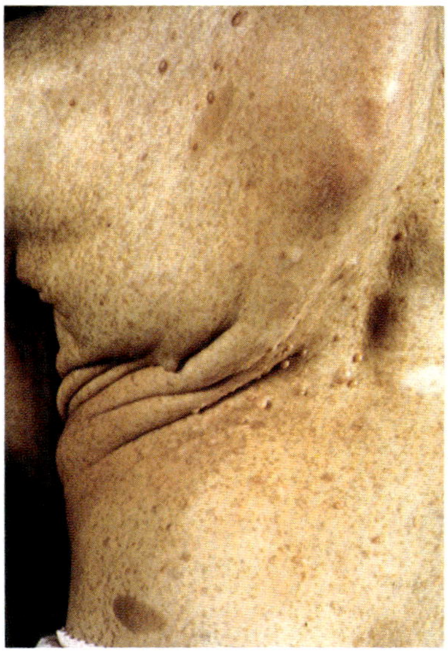

67 Multiple subcutaneous neurofibromata are another feature of the condition.

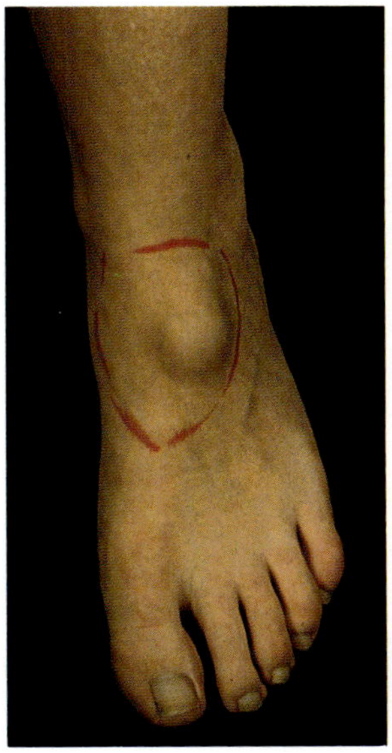

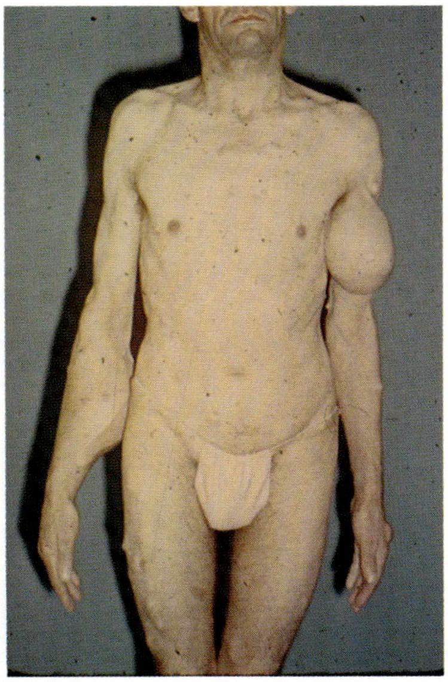

68 & **69 Tumours of nerve trunks.** Neurofibromata may develop along the course of peripheral nerve trunks.

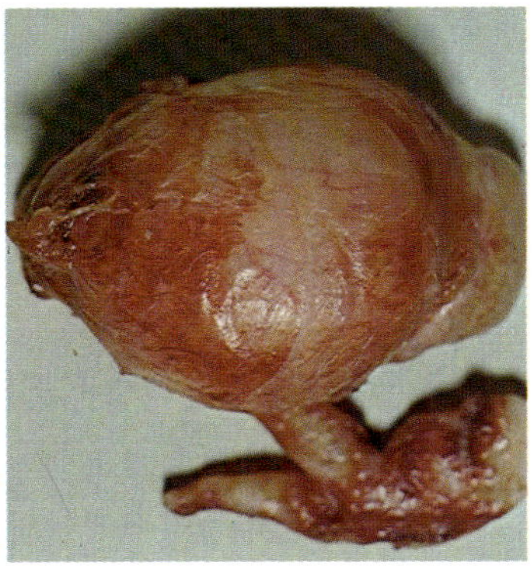

70 Tumour removed from patient's arm shown in **69**.

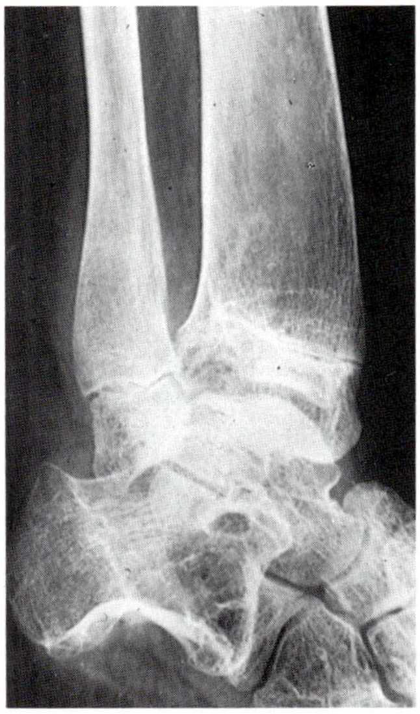

71 Erosion of the plantar aspect of the calcaneus owing to an adjacent neurofibroma.

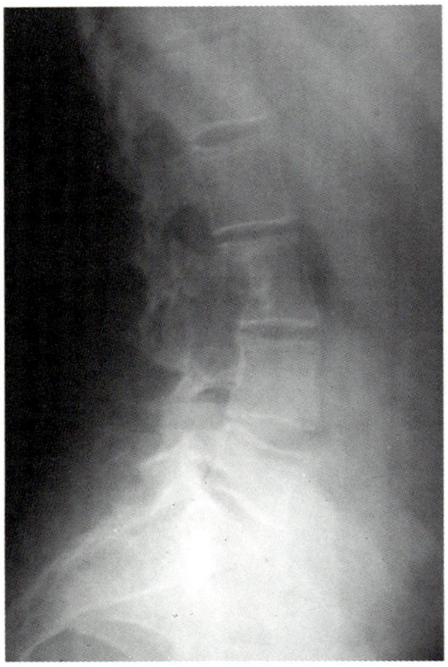

72 When spinal nerve roots are involved the margins of the exit foramina may be eroded and enlarged.

73

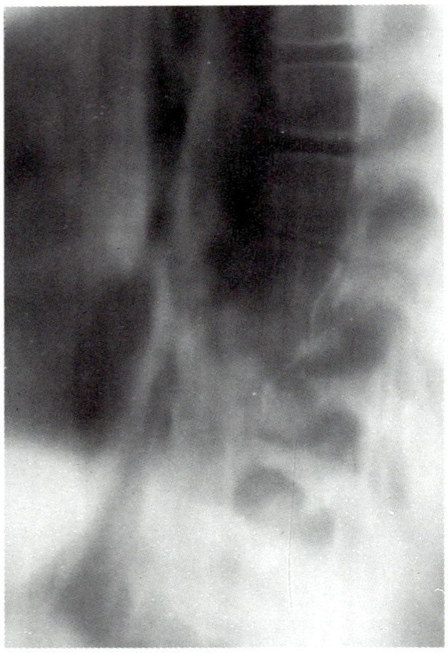

74

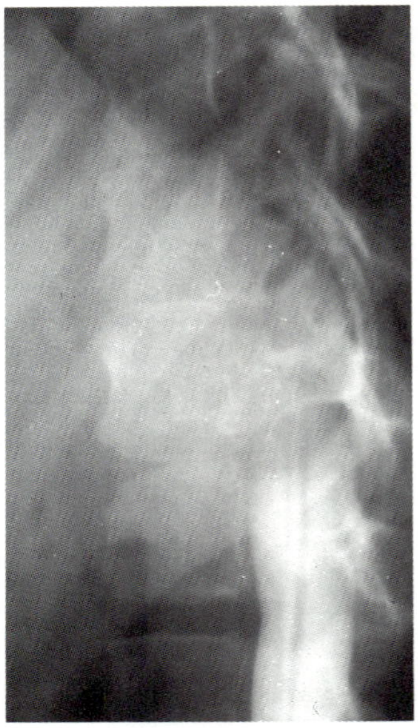

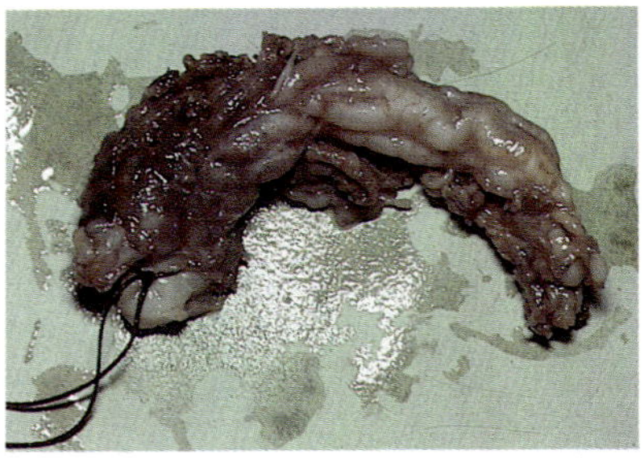

75

73–75 Similar widening of intercostal nerve exit foramen. A radiculogram in the same patient shows a block caused by the intraspinal extension of the lesion, sometimes called a 'dumbell' tumour. The excised intercostal nerve neuroma is shown.

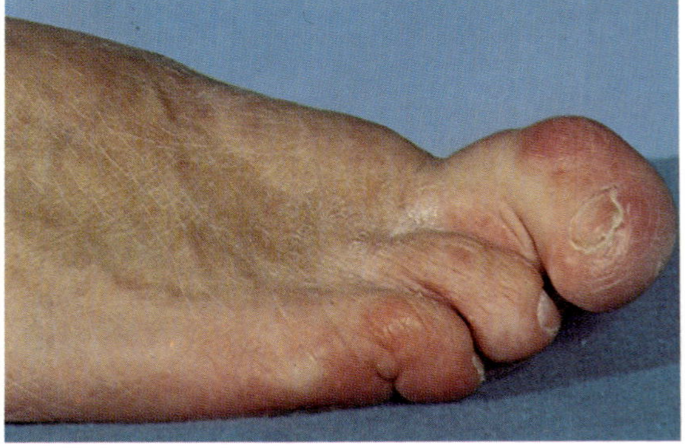

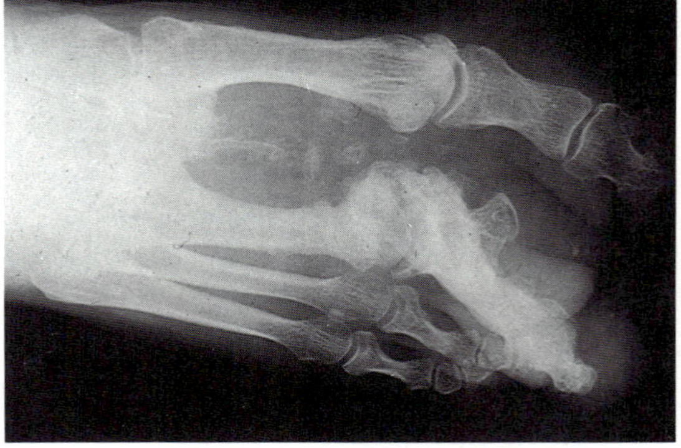

76 & **77 Overgrowth of tissues**. There may be a diffuse hypertrophy of all tissues in a particular site giving rise to macrodactyly or in some instances enlargement of the entire limb.

Skeletal manifestations. These may be present in as many as 50% of affected individuals. Scoliosis, overgrowth of bones as part of a more generalised hypertrophy and tibial bowing or pseudarthrosis are the commonest lesions.

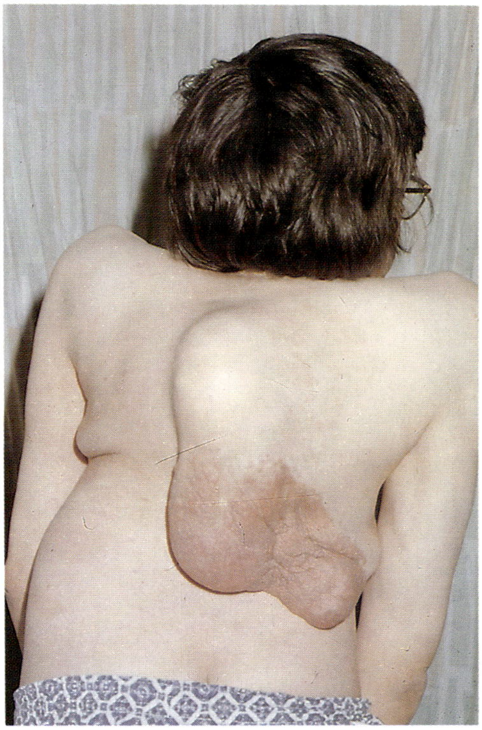

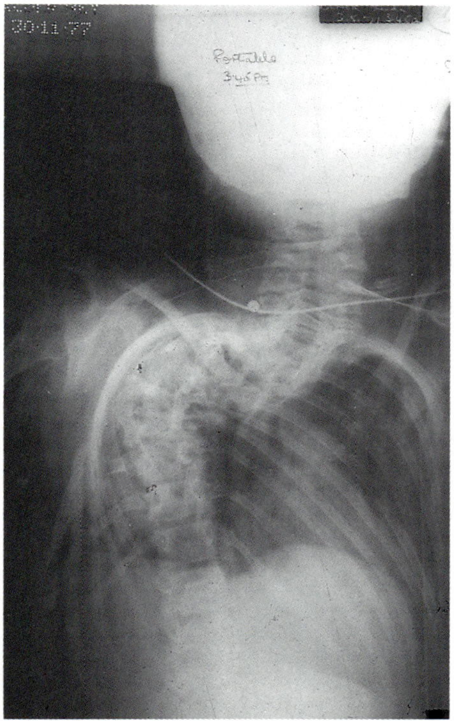

78 & **79** Scoliosis has been variably reported in 15%–40% of all cases. It may appear in infancy or childhood. Typically, the curvature involves a short spinal segment and is progressive and severe, with the curvature frequently approaching 90°. The scoliosis is not caused by any vertebral anomalies nor is it due to spinal neurofibromata.

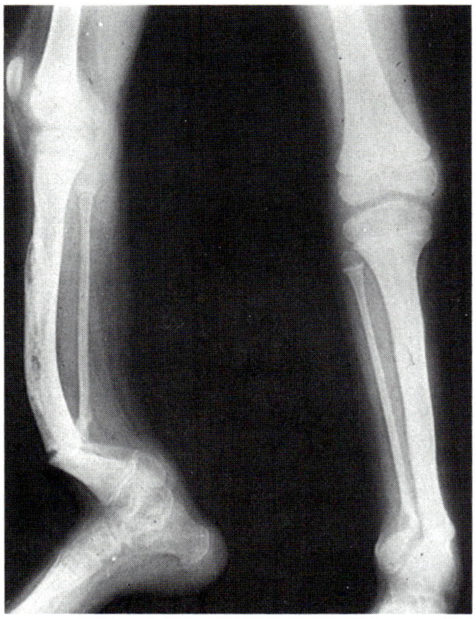

80 Pseudarthrosis of the tibia. A pathological fracture has occurred through a bowed and dysplastic tibia in a child with neurofibromatosis.

Congenital pseudarthrosis of the tibia

This is a rare condition resulting from a pathological fracture through a congenitally dysplastic and anteriorly bowed tibia during the first few years of life. In affected individuals pseudarthrosis is established by 5 years in 95% of cases; in most of these cases the lesion is present by 2 years of age. Five per cent of pseudarthroses are present at birth and a further 5% occur after the age of 5.

The dysplasia is associated with neurofibromatosis in 50–60% of cases, a small proportion are associated with fibrous dysplasia and the remainder occur following osteotomy, trauma or spontaneous fracture through a congenital anterolaterally bowed tibia with no evidence of the above two conditions.

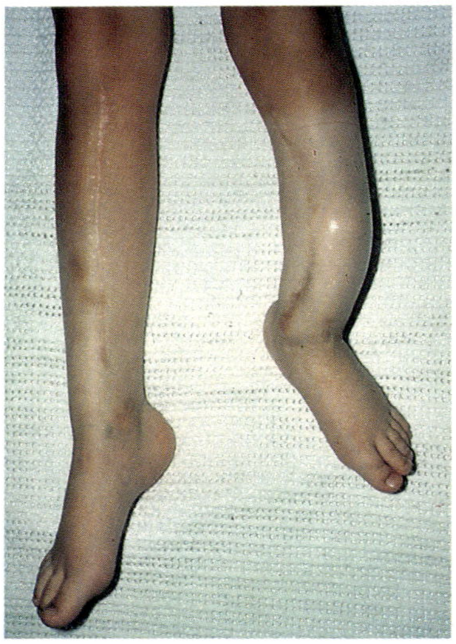

81 Bilateral pseudarthrosis. This child developed bilateral pseudarthroses associated with neurofibromatosis. The severe and typical deformity is shown on the left side where the pseudarthrosis was present from birth.

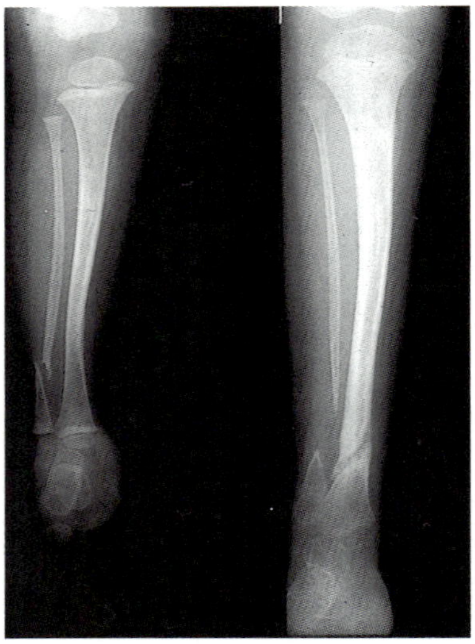

82 Radiographs of the right tibia of the patient shown in **81**. At 18 months of age a fibular pseudarthrosis was present. The tibia, although intact shows a characteristic bowing with a double tibial curve and 'middle segment dissociation' typical of the dysplasia in neurofibromatosis. Spontaneous fracture progressing to pseudarthrosis occurred at 3 years 10 months.

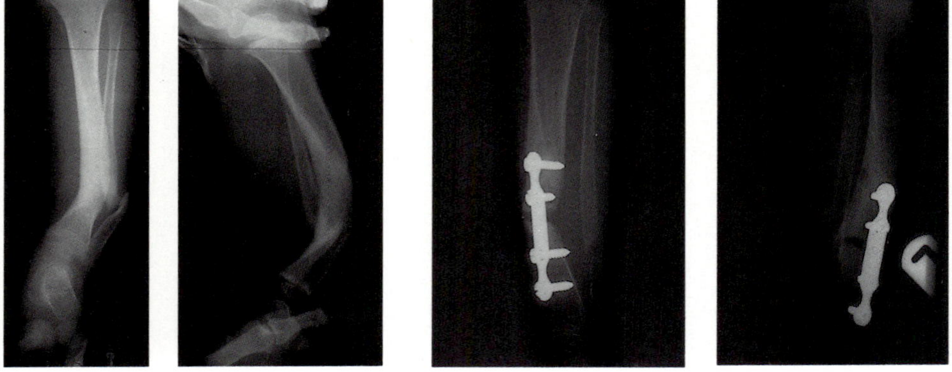

83 & **84** Congenital antero-lateral bowing of the tibia with no evidence of neurofibromatosis. There is a smooth single antero-lateral curve. Pseudarthrosis followed attempted corrective osteotomy.

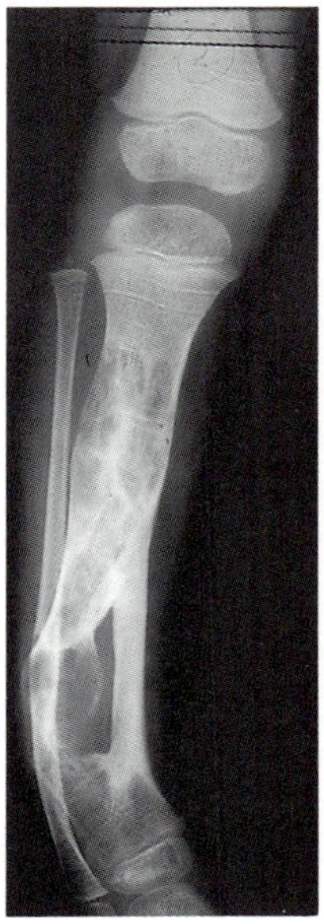

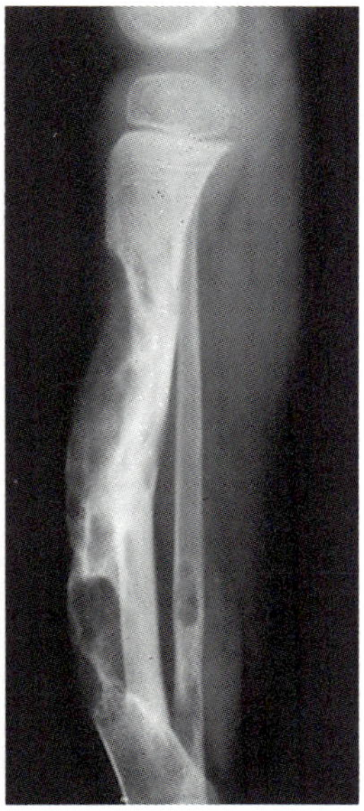

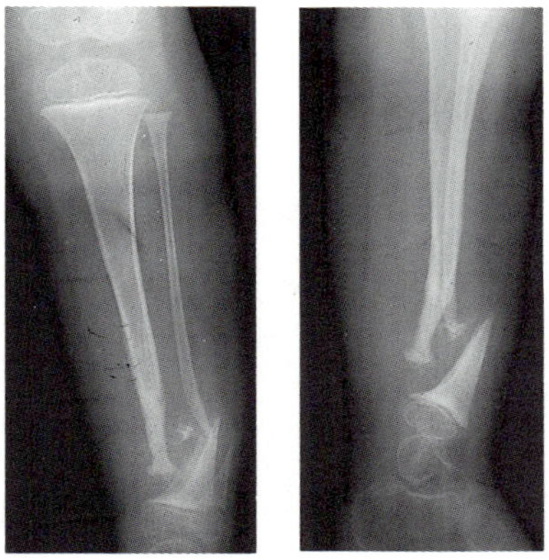

87 Dysplastic pseudarthrosis. Some pseudarthroses can develop an extremely 'dysplastic' radiographic appearance. The bone ends having the appearance of 'sucked candy'.

85 & **86** Pseudarthrosis through a tibia affected by fibrous dysplasia. This patient was successfully treated with a McFarland bypass graft.

88

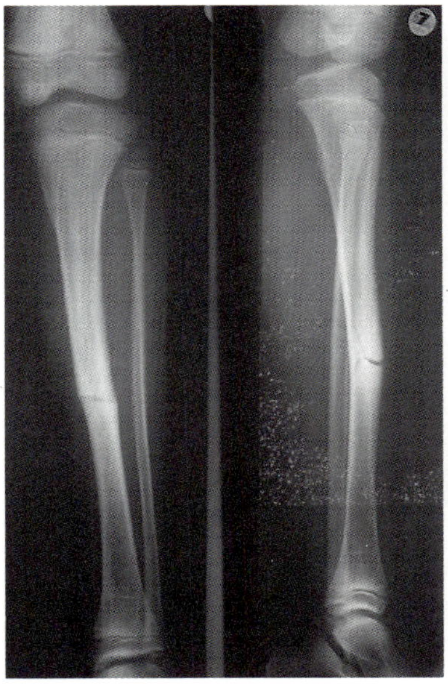

89

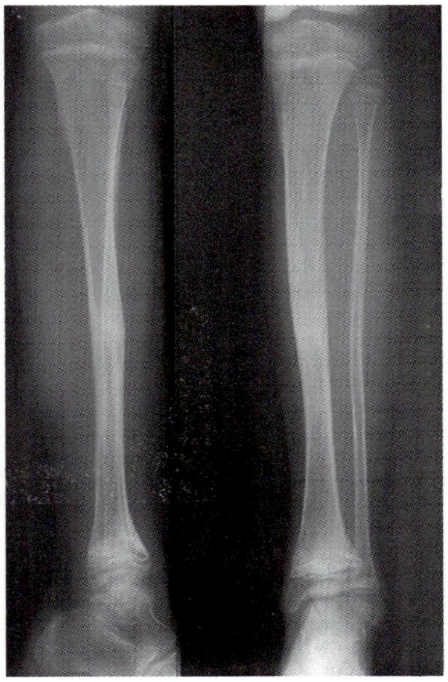

90

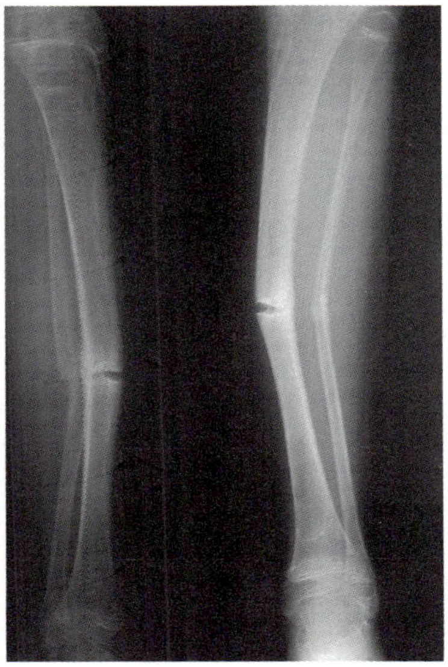

88–92 'Late' pseudarthrosis of childhood. This series of radiographs are of a girl who developed a fracture of the left tibia after trivial trauma at the age of 9 years (**88**). Union ultimately occurred 8 months after fracture (**89**). At the age of twelve a further fracture occurred, again with minor trauma (**90**). It united only after bone grafting (**91**) to refracture again at the age of 17 years (**92**). Cutaneous stigmata of neurofibromatosis developed in adolescence.

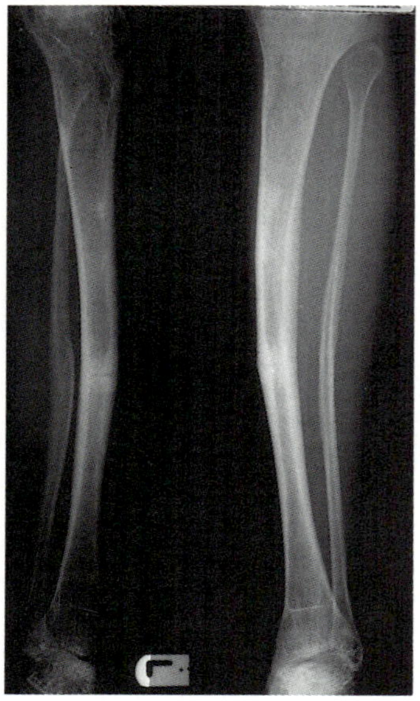
91

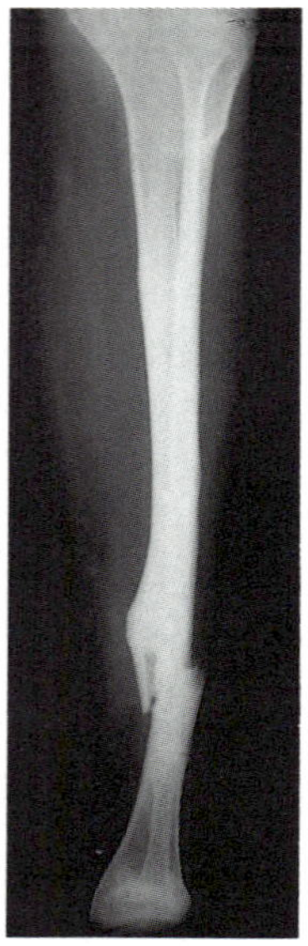
92

Bowed or bent tibiae

Congenital
- Antero-lateral bowing:
  - Neurofibromatosis }
  - Fibrous dysplasia } pre-pseudarthrotic
  - with neither of above }
- Congenital absence of fibula
- Congenital postero-medial angulation
- Infantile tibia vara (Blount's disease)
- Osteogenesis imperfecta

Traumatic
- Fracture malunion
- Adolescent tibia vara

Infective
- Syphilis

Metabolic
- Rickets
- Paget's disease

93
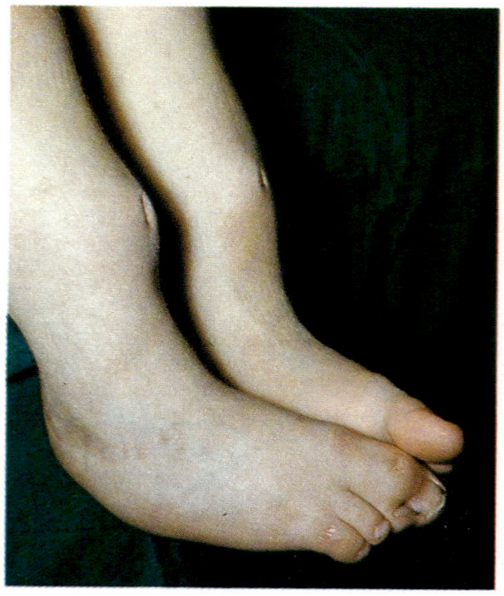

94
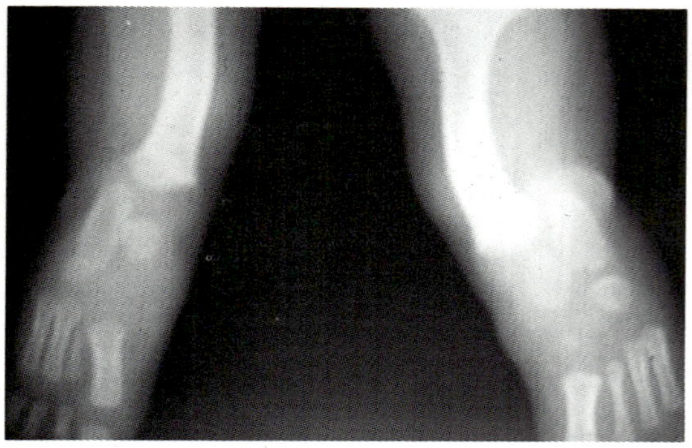

93–95 Congenital absence of the fibula (**93**). A child with bilateral fibular aplasia showing the tibial bowing with skin dimpling over the apex of the angulation. The radiographs (**94**) show complete absence of the fibulae in this case although frequently a fibular anlague remains. Lateral ray deficiencies of the foot frequently accompany the condition (**95**).

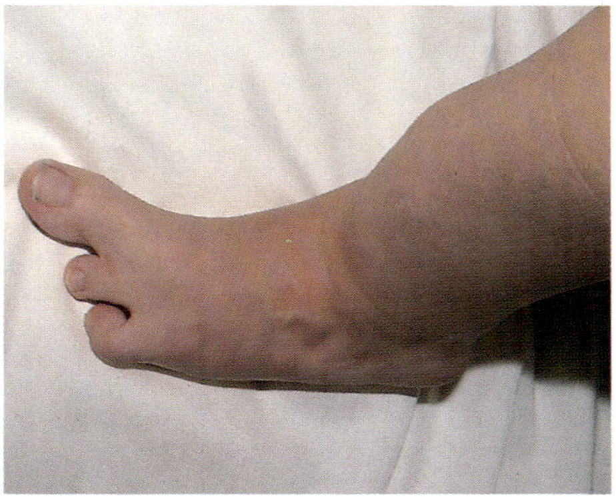

95

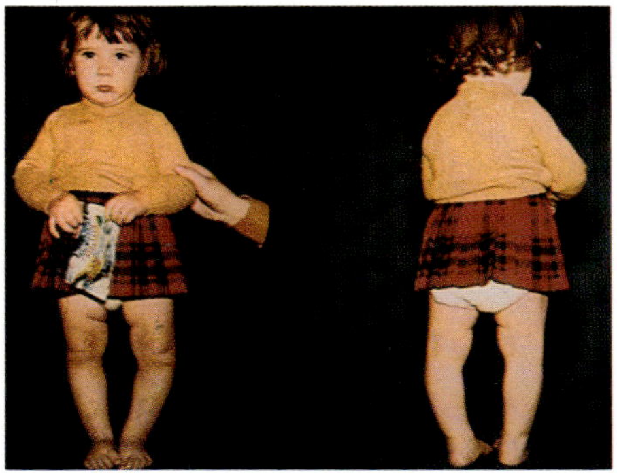

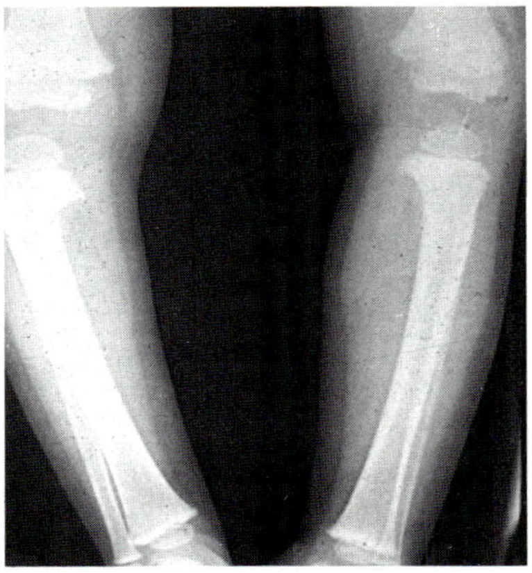

96 & **97** Infantile tibia vara, Blount's disease. This condition presents as a persistent infantile bow leg. It may be uni- or bilateral and is caused by failure of growth and early closure of the upper medial tibial growth plate. The radiograph shows typical beaking of the medial metaphysis. The exact aetiology is unknown but the condition tends to be commoner in West Indian races.

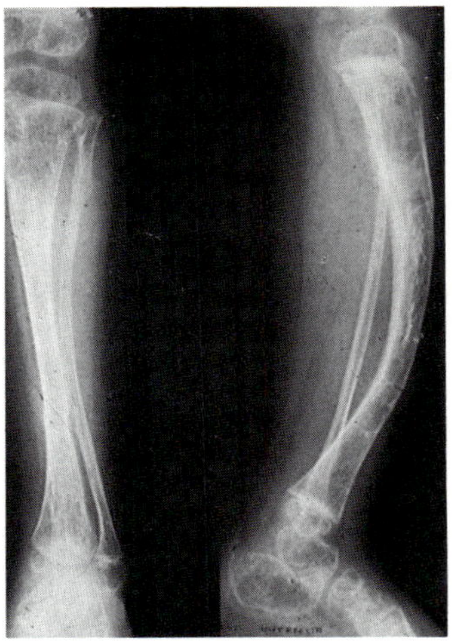

98 Bowing of the tibia in severe osteogenesis imperfecta.

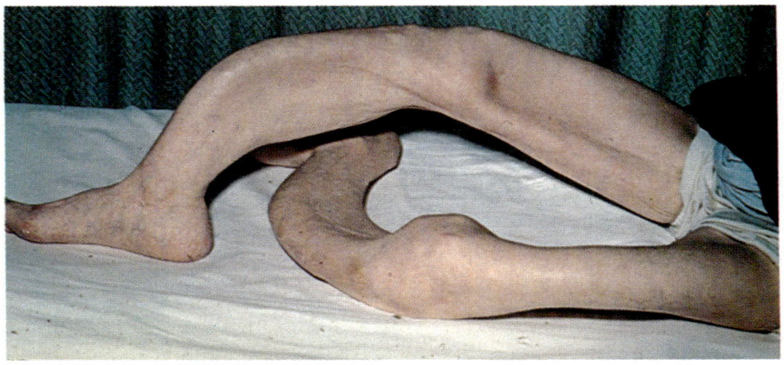

99 Severe tibial bowing owing to bone softening which occurs in advanced Paget's disease.

Disorders of joints and soft tissues: Joints

Gout and pseudogout

Gout is caused by a disorder of purine metabolism, resulting in elevated levels of serum uric acid and the concomitant deposition of crystals of sodium urate monohydrate in synovial and periarticular tissues.

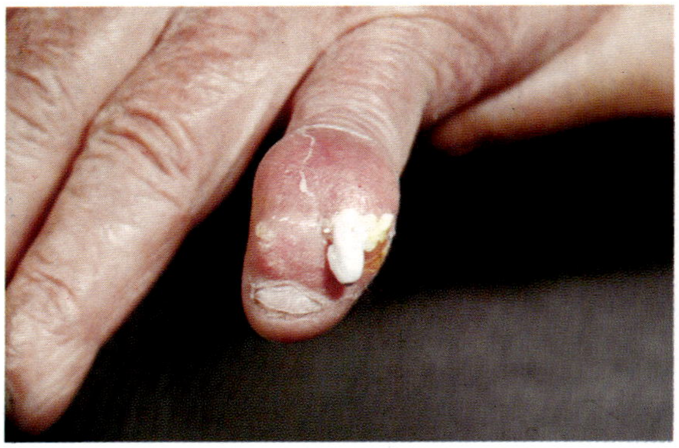

100 Repeated deposition of crystals in the joints of the fingers may ultimately lead to a destructive arthropathy.

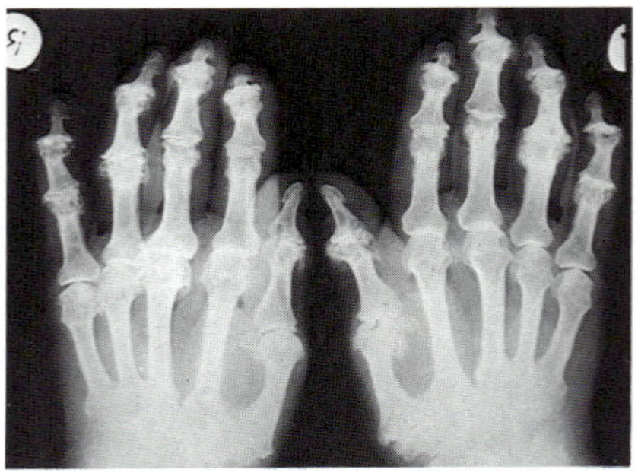

101 Radiographs of the hands in gouty arthritis.

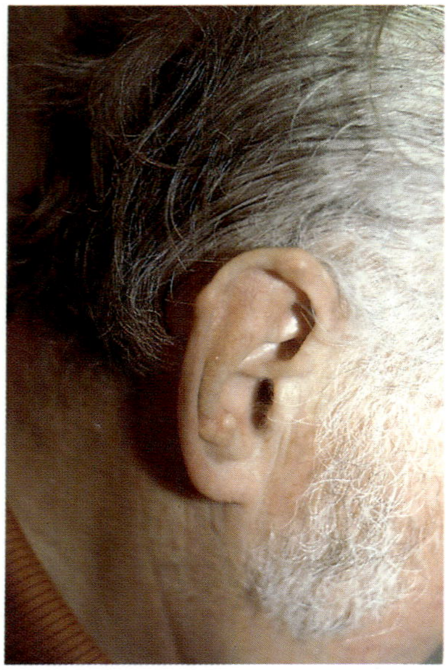

102 Gouty tophi in the perichondrium of the ear lobe.

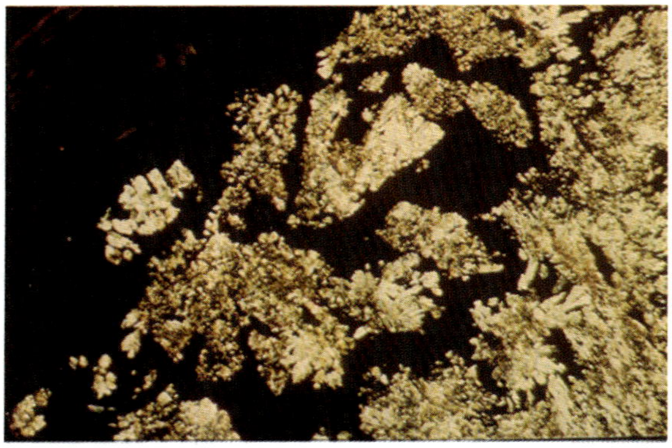

103 The crystals of sodium urate monohydrate are seen best by polarised light microscopy. (*x 400*)

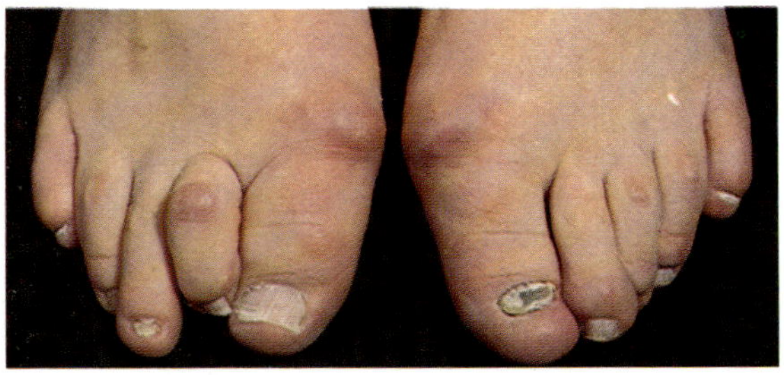

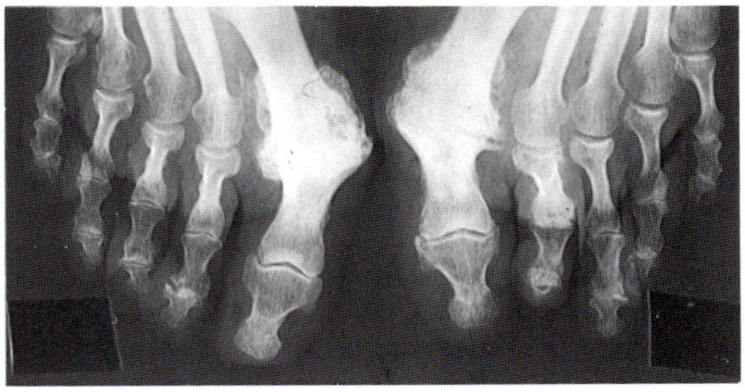

104 & **105** Gout affecting the 'typical' site at the MP joint of the great toe.

Pseudogout or chondrocalcinosis is also an arthropathy caused by microcrystalline deposits in the synovium. Crystals of calcium pyrophosphate dihydrate give rise to an inflammatory reaction and, in addition, cause calcification in articular cartilage, intervertebral discs and the menisci of the knee.

Monoarticular involvement (pseudogout) is the commonest presentation, the knee being most frequently involved. A symmetrical polyarthritis (pseudo rheumatoid arthritis) or a chronic progressive arthritis can also occur.

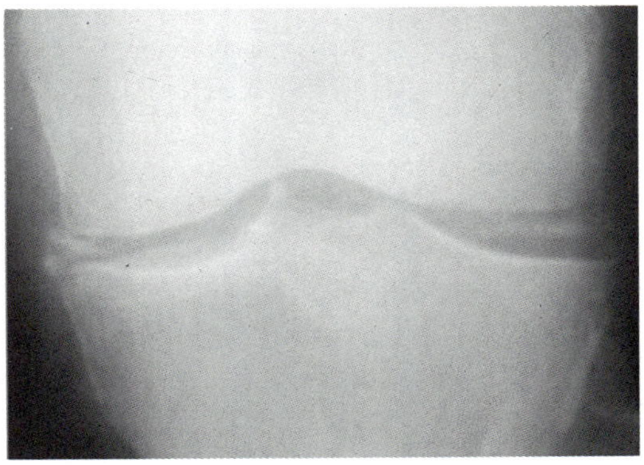

106 Calcification within the menisci and articular cartilage of the knee in pseudogout or chondrocalcinosis.

Haemophilia

Classical haemophilia is transmitted by the female and becomes manifest in the male. It is therefore of X-linked recessive inheritance. In addition to its obvious manifestations of excessive bleeding owing to impairment of clotting factors in the blood, it may give rise to haemorrhagic tumours in muscle. Joints are damaged by repeated haemarthroses from trivial injuries.

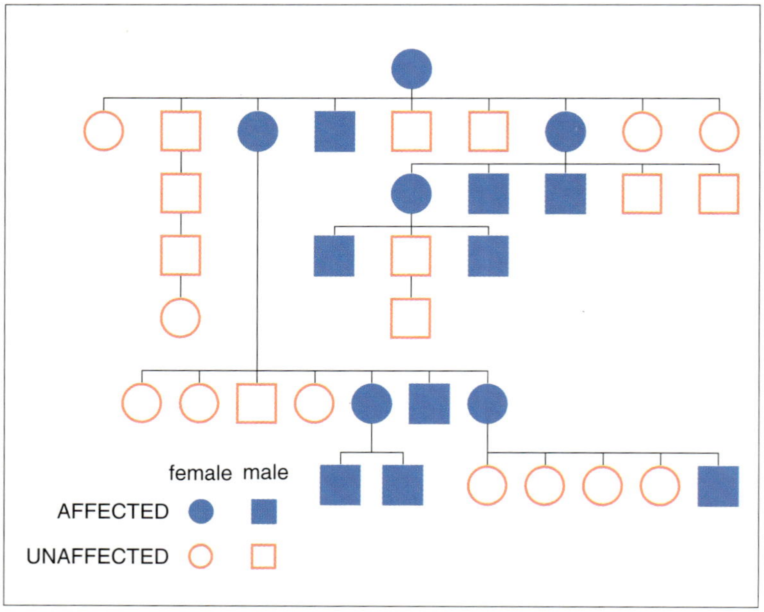

107 Queen Victoria's family tree.

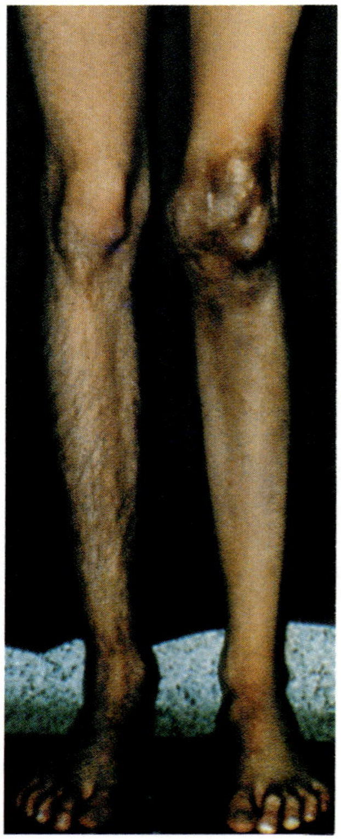

108 Discolouration and swelling of the left knee caused by repeated minor haemorrhagic incidents.

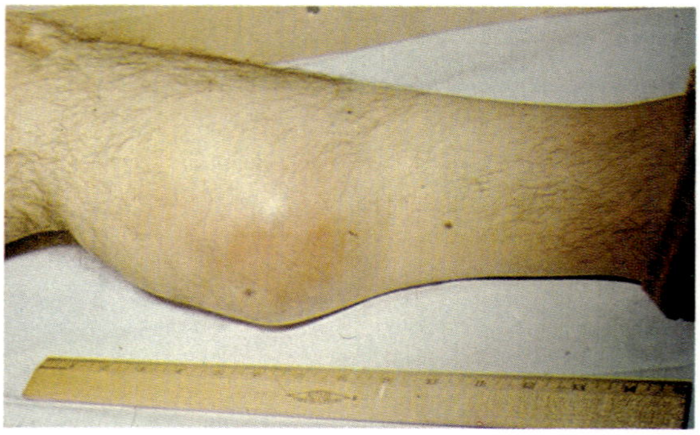

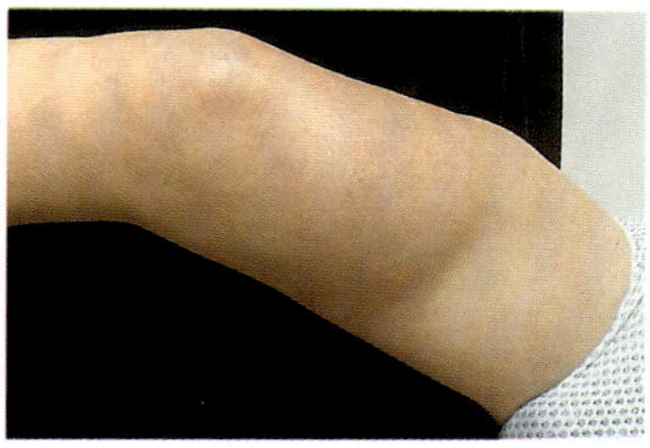

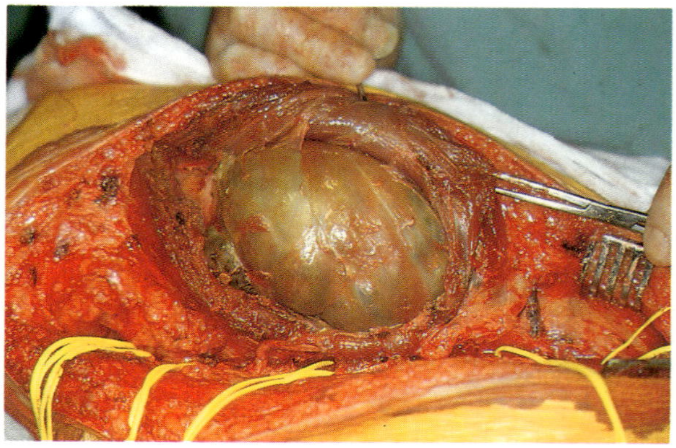

109–111 Haemorrhagic pseudotumour in the calf muscle and within the thigh. The operative picture shows the thigh lesion exposed.

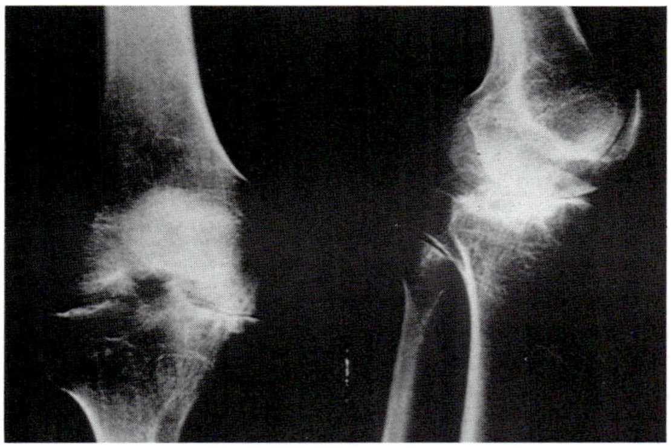

112 & **113** One or several joints become damaged by repeated haemarthroses. Ultimately a destructive arthropathy becomes manifest.

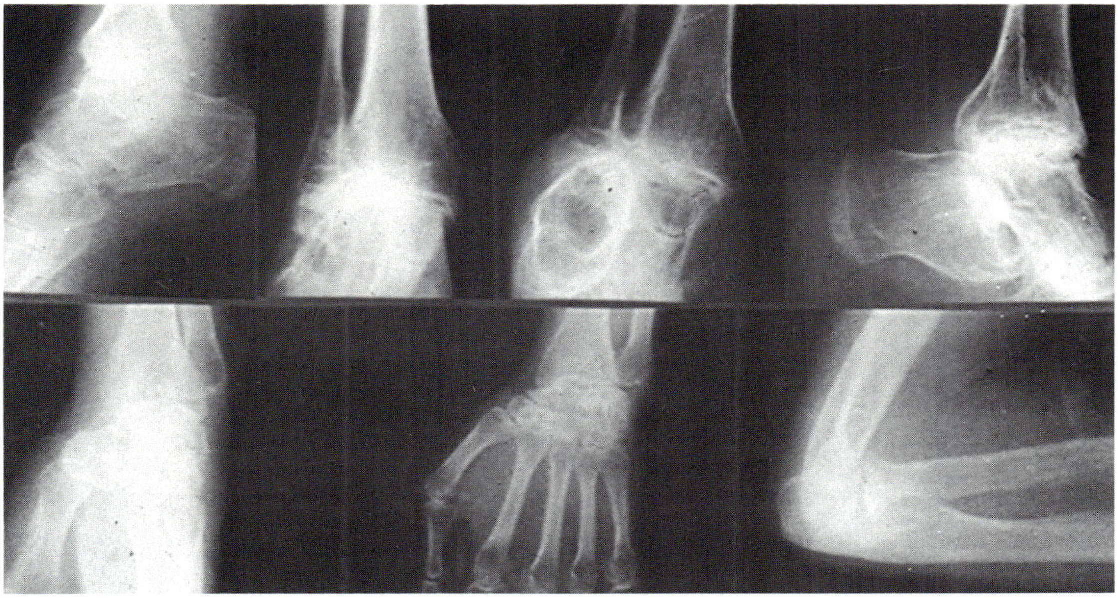

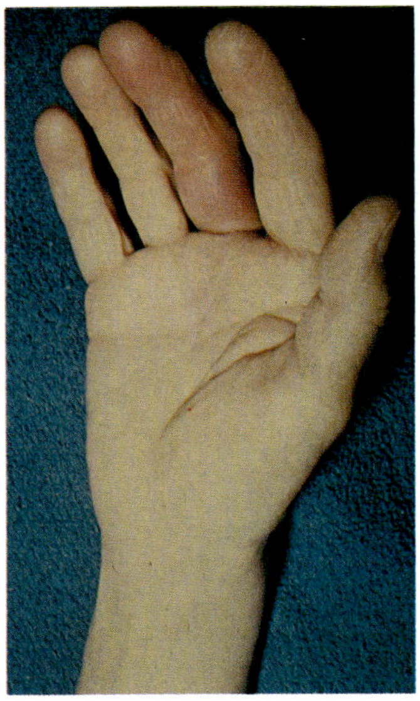

114 Von Willebrand's disease. Although by definition classical haemophilia cannot occur in women, there is a rare dyscrasia that does affect women. Von Willebrand's disease is much less severe, and unlike haemophilia, petechiae of the skin do occur in this disease.

Alkaptonuria (ochronosis)

This is a condition of autosomal recessive inheritance in which there is a defect of the metabolism of phenylalanine and tyrosine, resulting in the appearance of homogentisic acid in the urine, which darkens on standing.

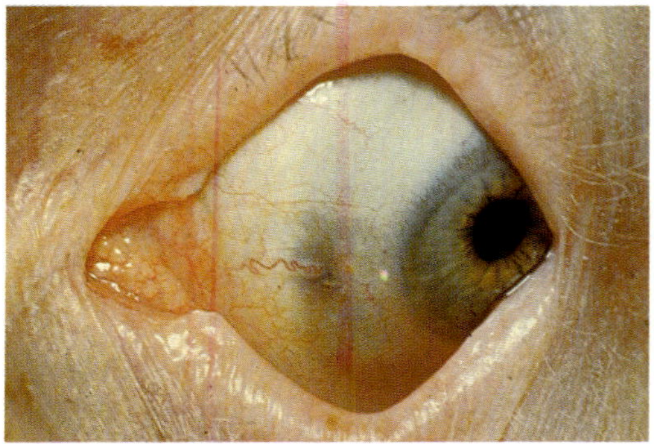

115 The sclera. Dark blue melanin-like products deposited in the eyes.

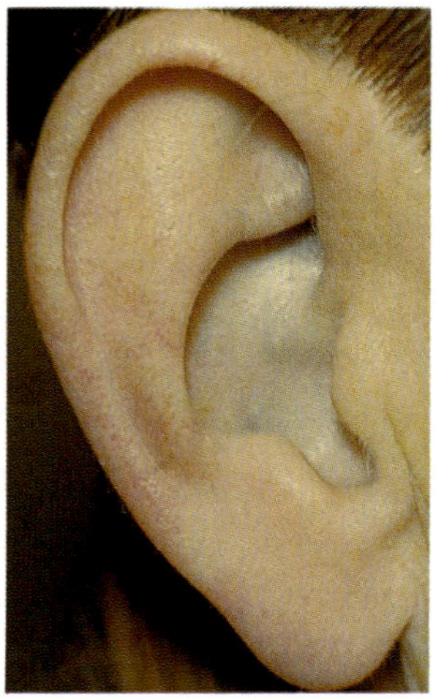

116 Ear lobes containing deposits in the cartilage.

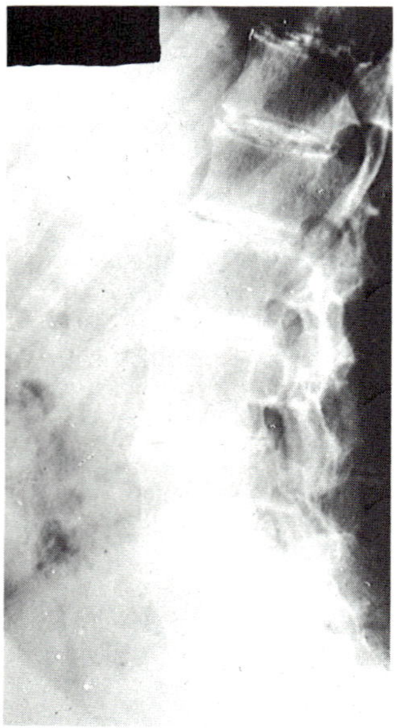

117 The intervertebral discs are affected early in ochronosis leading to a typical radiographic appearance.

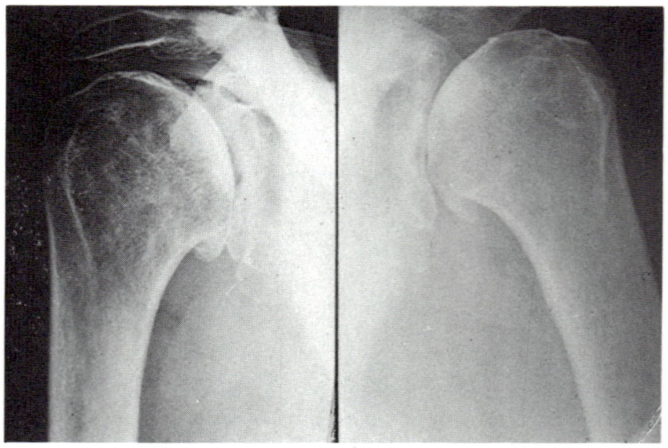

118 Ochronosis is one of the rare causes of osteoarthritis of the shoulder joint.

Generalised osteoarthritis

Osteoarthritis is a degenerative process beginning in the articular cartilage and eventually involving the whole joint. Osteoarthritis should be regarded as secondary to a cause which careful search should disclose.

All the cases of 'primary' generalised osteoarthritis as depicted here are probably secondary, although at present their cause or causes are unknown.

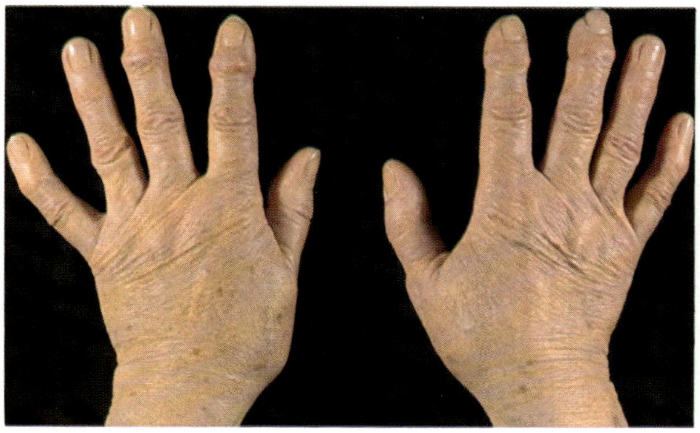

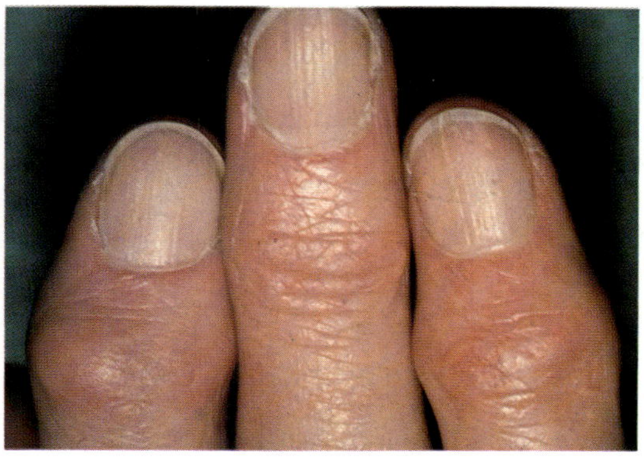

119 & **120** Primary generalised osteoarthritis is typified by the involvement of the terminal interphalangeal joints of the fingers in which Heberden's nodes can be seen on the dorsum of the joints.

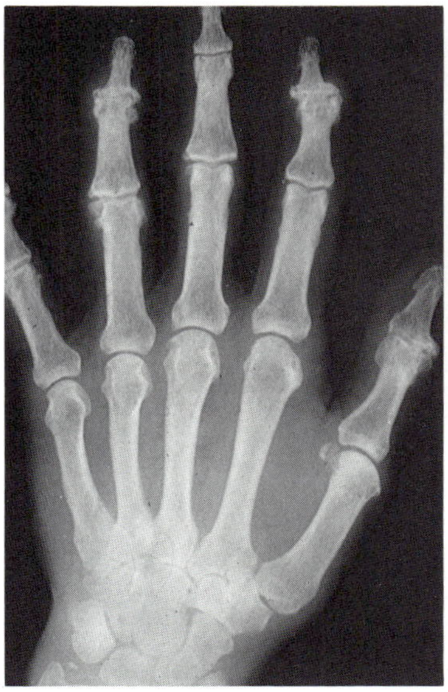

121 The terminal phalangeal joints are primarily affected.

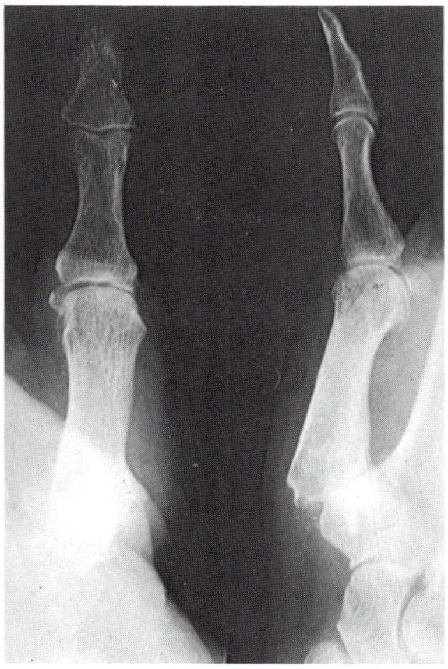

122 The carpometacarpal joint of the thumb is commonly affected.

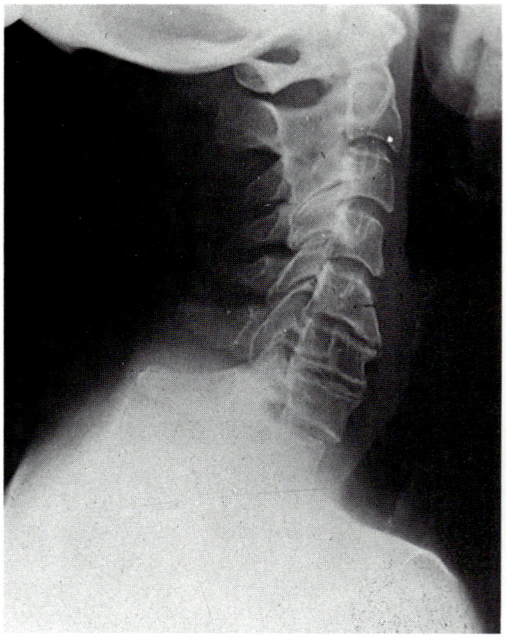

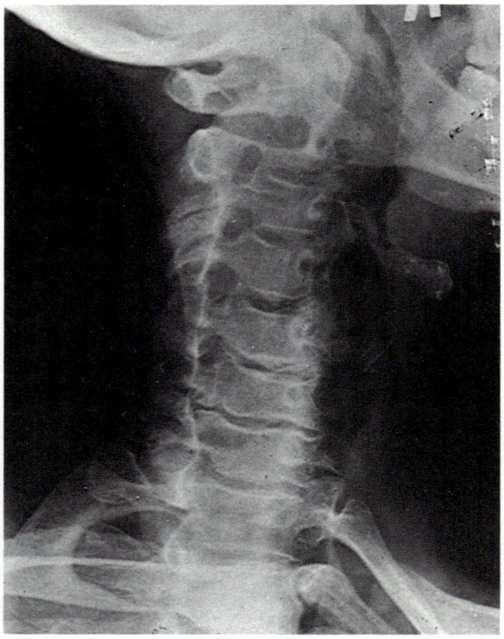

123 & **124** Cervical spondylosis: the complex of joints of the cervical spine are commonly affected.

There are a variety of causes of painful neck including aprolapsed cervical intervertebral disk, tuberculous or pyogenic infection, or tumours involving the vertebral column. By far the commonest, however, is osteoarthritis of the cervical spine (cervical spondylosis).

Although primary degenerative arthritis of the cervical spine can be initiated by injury, it is often simply a manifestation of generalised degenerative changes which occur with increasing age (see diagram **516**).

Degenerative osteoarthritis usually commences at the most mobile section of the neck, starting at C5/6 and moving downwards to involve the lowest three cervical joints. The changes effect first the intervertebral joints with accompanying disc degeneration, and later the postero-lateral facet joints. Osteophytes developing at the margin of the facet joints encroach upon the intervertebral foramina and irritate the emerging cervical nerve roots by direct pressure.

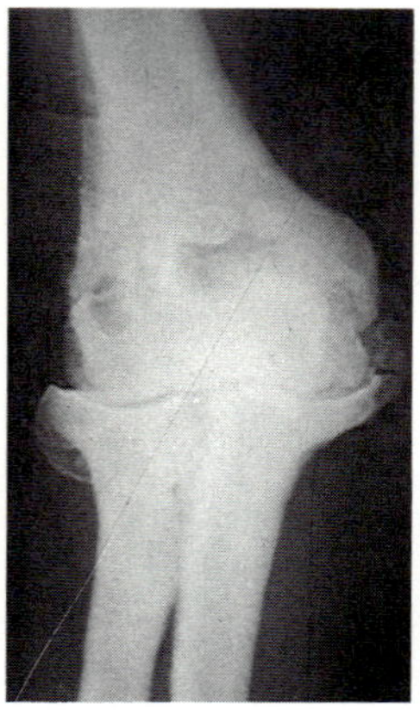

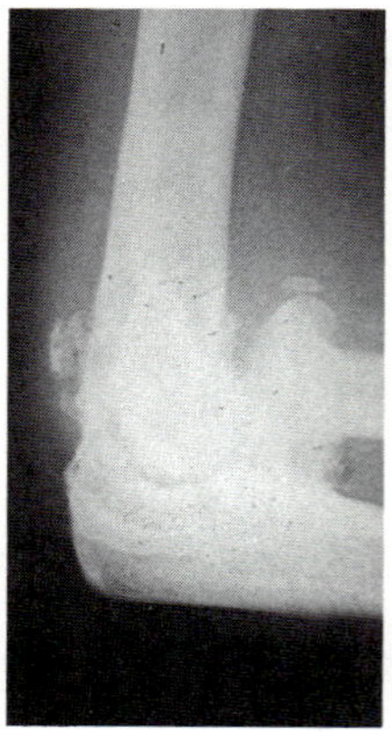

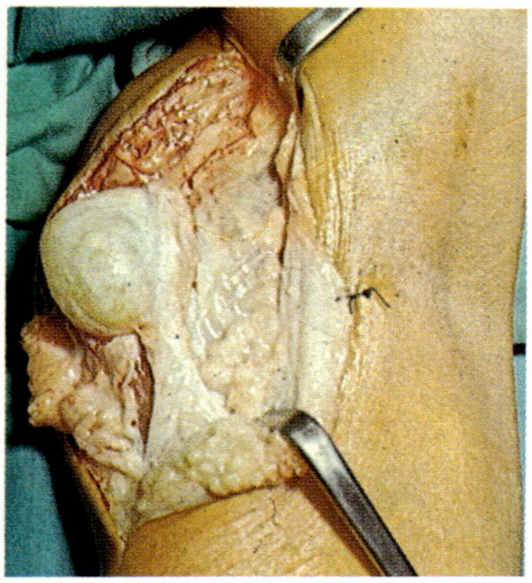

125–127 The elbow joints are less commonly affected by osteoarthritis. Synovial protrusions may develop, particularly from affected elbows (**127**) and knees. In the knee these arise in the popliteal fossa: a so-called Baker's cyst.

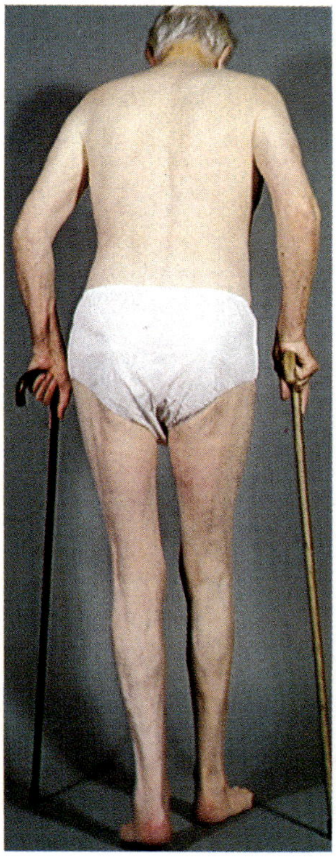

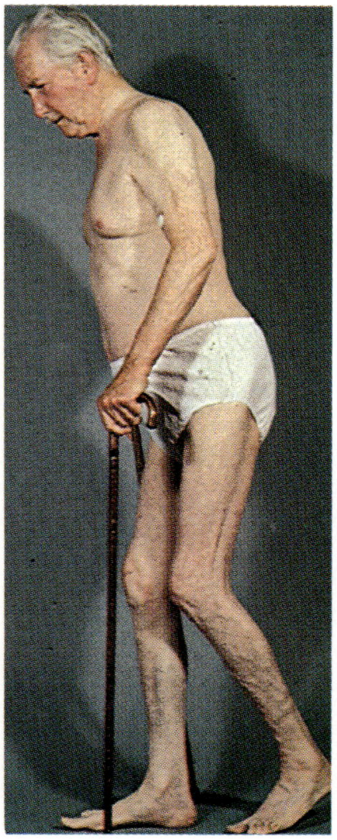

128–130 Degenerative osteoarthritis. This elderly gentleman requires two walking sticks to overcome the disability of painful, stiff and flexed hip joints. Radiographs show the typical appearances of degenerative osteoarthritis. There is loss of joint space due to loss of articular cartilage, sub-articular sclerosis of the bone on either side of the joint with sub-articular cyst formation and marginal and central osteophyte formation has occurred.

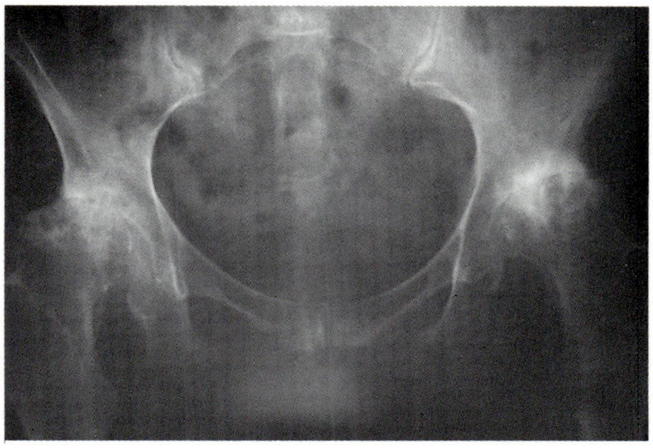

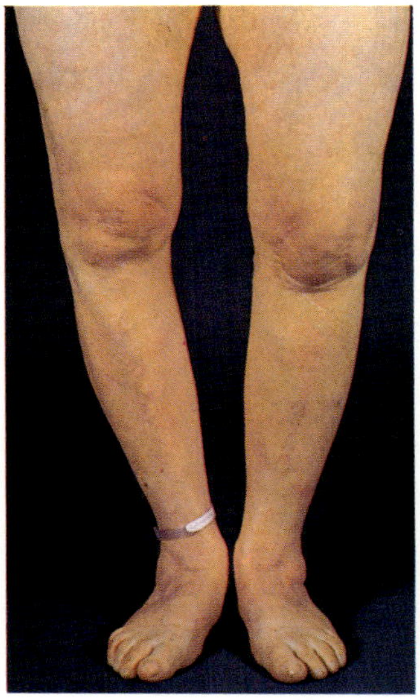

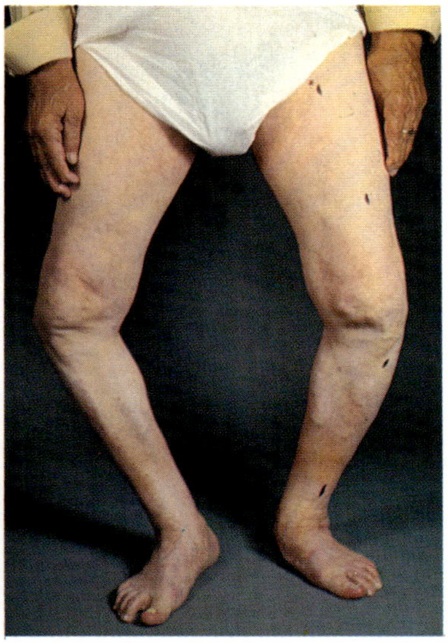

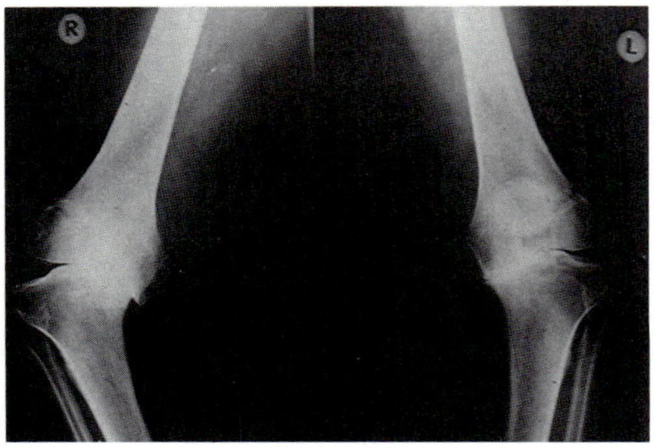

131–133 Osteoarthritis of the knee is only slightly less common. Genu varum gradually develops and may become very severe.

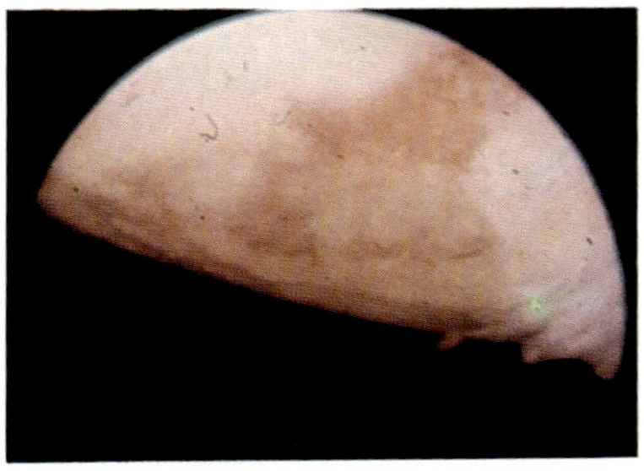

134 Arthroscopic view illustrates how the disease starts in the articular cartilage.

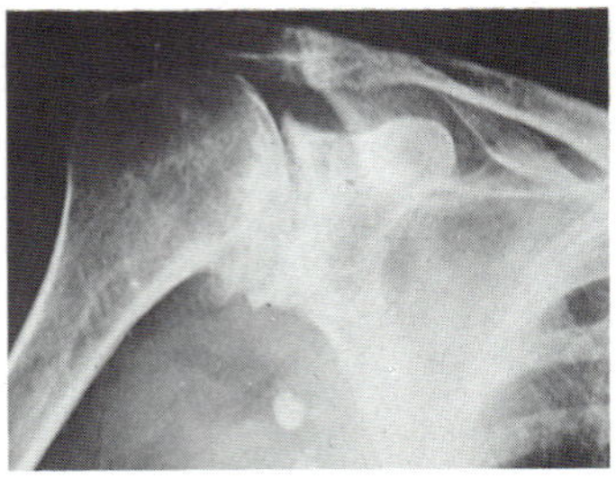

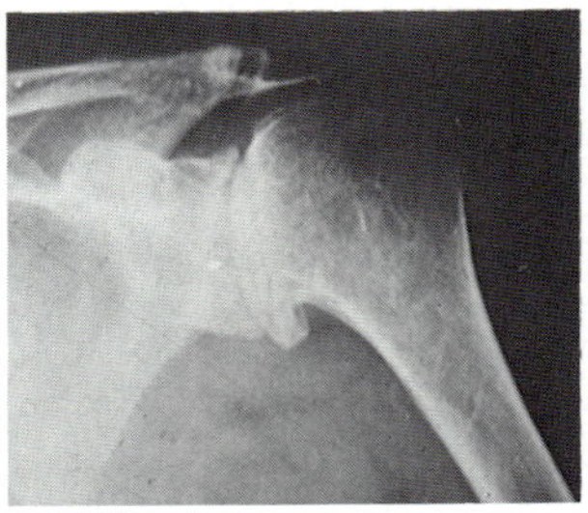

135 & **136** Severe degenerative osteoarthritis: in the shoulder of a 70-year-old lady, affecting both glenohumeral and acromio-clavicular joints. The cause of this osteoarthritis certainly can be guessed: it is calculated that she rowed some 1.5 million strokes during 50 years rowing as a member of a ladies' rowing club!

Rheumatoid arthritis and related disease

Rheumatoid arthritis is merely the most obvious effect of general systemic rheumatoid disease and is probably caused by a number of factors that are, at present, obscure. Current knowledge suggests that it may be due to an autoimmune response in a genetically susceptible individual. One of its more obvious orthopaedic manifestations is the enlargement of synovial lined tissues such as bursae, tendon sheaths and the synovial membrane of joints.

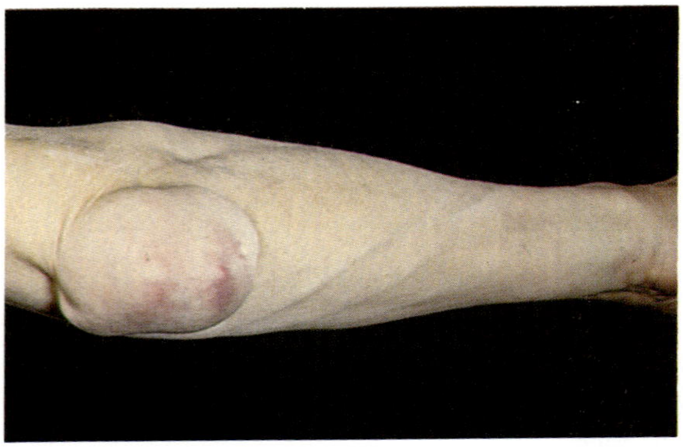

137 Olecranon bursitis.

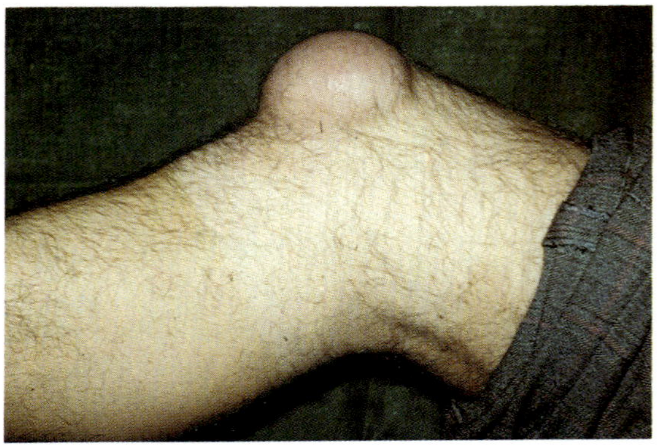

138 Prepatellar bursitis.

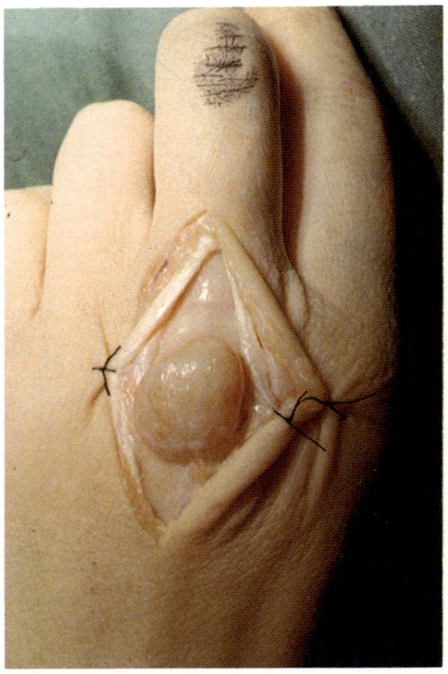

139 A single extensor sheath of a finger is involved.

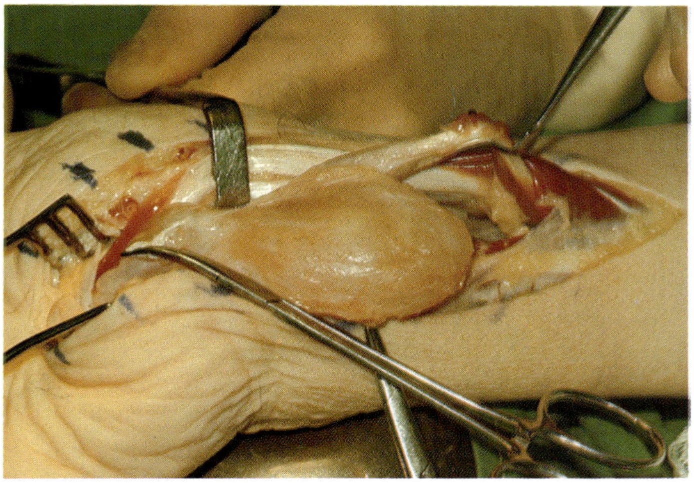

140 Ulnar bursa at the wrist, which is enlarged and inflamed.

Criteria for the diagnosis of rheumatoid arthritis

1. Morning stiffness
2. Pain on motion or tenderness in at least one joint.
3. Swelling (synovial or effusion) in at least one joint continuously for not less than 6 weeks.
4. Swelling of at least one other joint.
5. Symmetrical joint swelling.
6. Subcutaneous nodules.
7. Typical radiographic changes.
8. Positive RA latex.
9. Characteristic synovial histology.
10. Characteristic rheumatoid nodule histology.

- Classic: any seven criteria for at least 6 weeks.
- Definite: any five criteria for at least 6 weeks.
- Probable: any three criteria for at least 4 weeks.

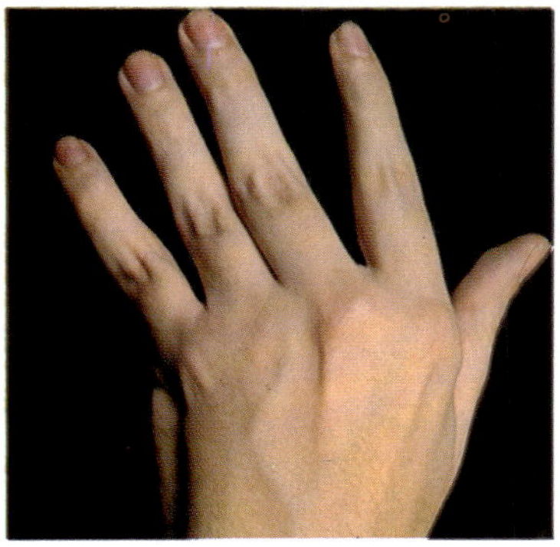

141 Ulnar deviation of the fingers is often an early and characteristic deformity of the hand in rheumatoid arthritis.

Factors contributing to ulnar drift

1. The normal approach from the ulnar side of long flexor and extensor tendons
2. Stretching of capsulo-ligamentous and tendon sheath structures by hypertrophy leading to further ulnar displacement of long flexors and extensors.
3. Radial deviation at the wrist.
4. Intrinsic contracture.
5. Gravity.

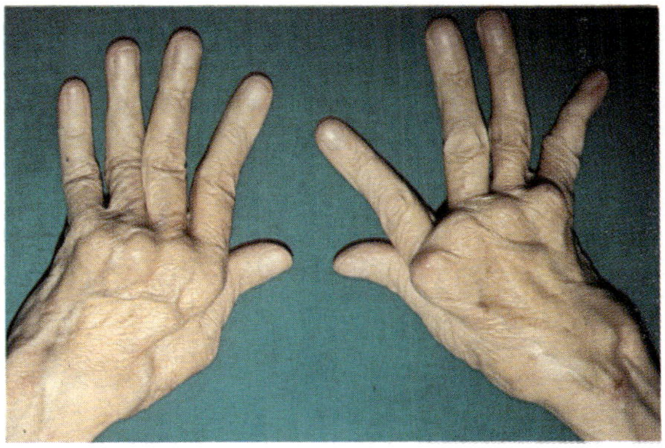

142 Disorganisation of all the joints of the hands. This affects principally the metacarpophalangeal joints and the proximal interphalangeal joints of the fingers in an advanced case.

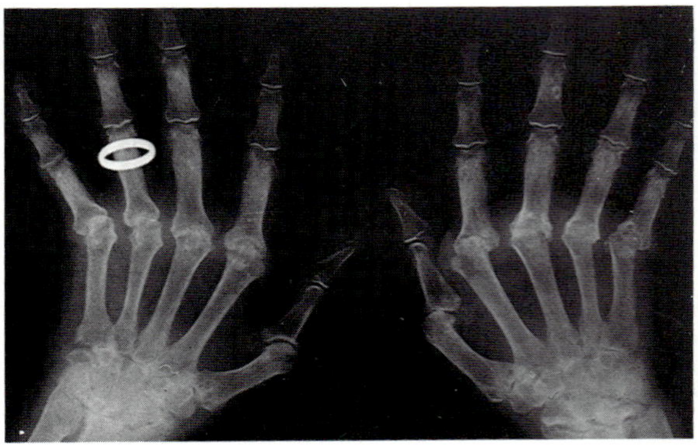

143 Disorganisation of all the joints of the hand.

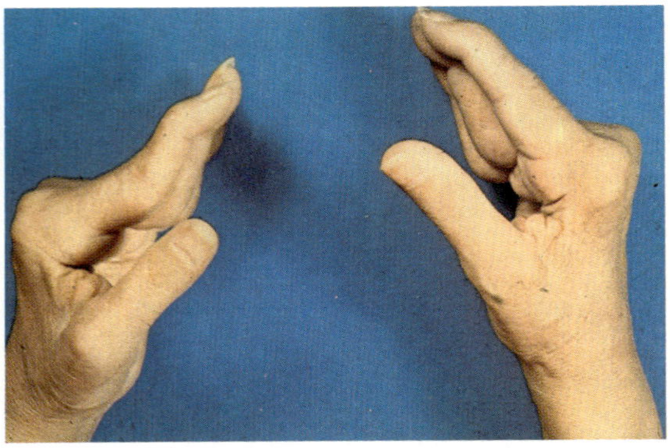

144 'Swan-neck' deformity of fingers due to rupture of the volar plate of PIP joints, or impediment of function of flexor sublimis.

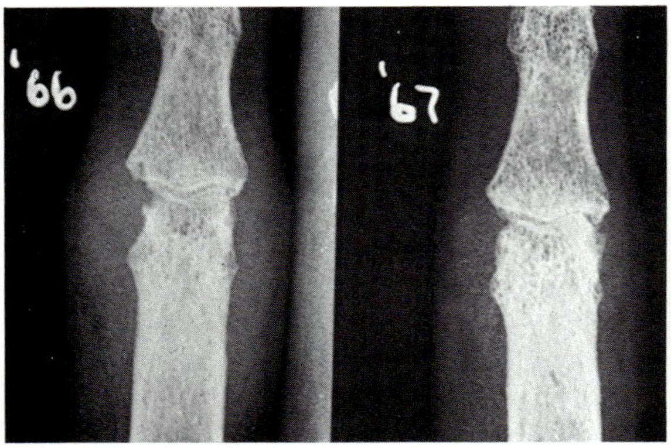

145 Erosive arthropathy of affected joints.

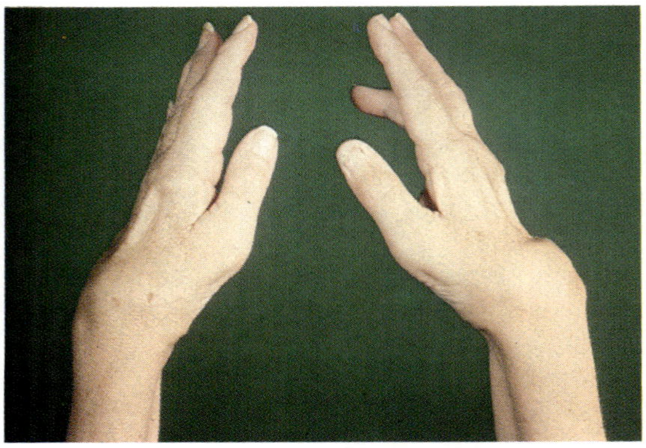

146 Diseased synovial membrane of the wrist showing hypertrophy.

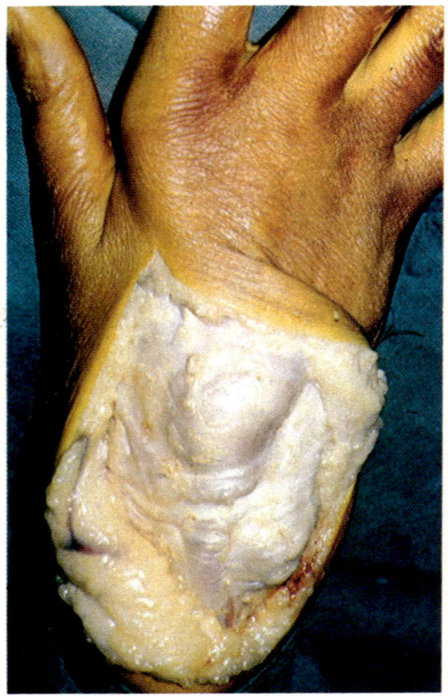

147 Inflamed synovial membrane of the extensor tendon sheaths at the wrist with hypertrophy.

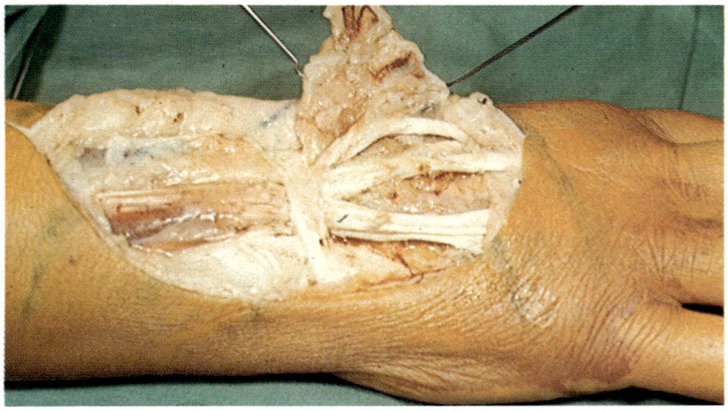

148 Surgical removal of the diseased synovial tissue.

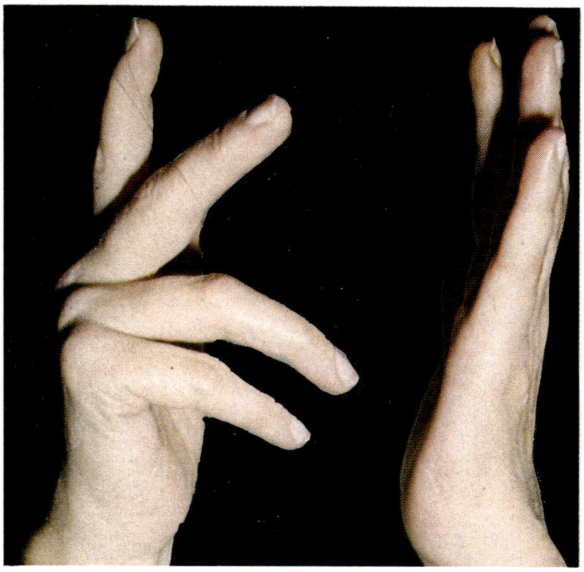

149 Rupture of extensor tendons due to synovial disease at the wrist, causing 'dropped fingers'.

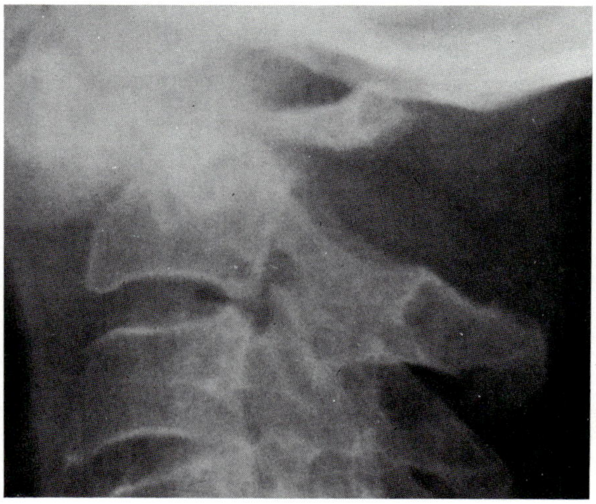

150 Subluxation of the atlas on the axis. Many patients with rheumatoid disease have lax ligaments of the joints of the cervical spine, leading to subluxation.

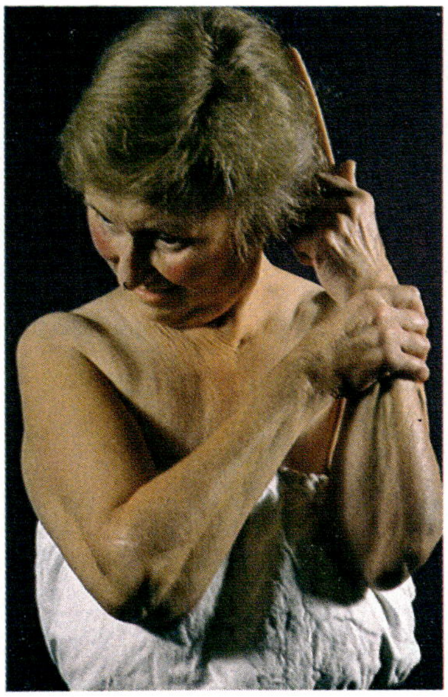

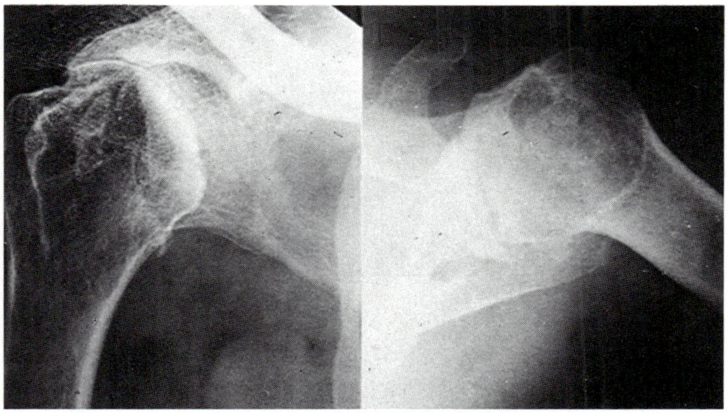

151 & **152** Rheumatoid arthritis of the shoulder joints. Rheumatoid disease is the only common cause of glenohumeral arthritis.

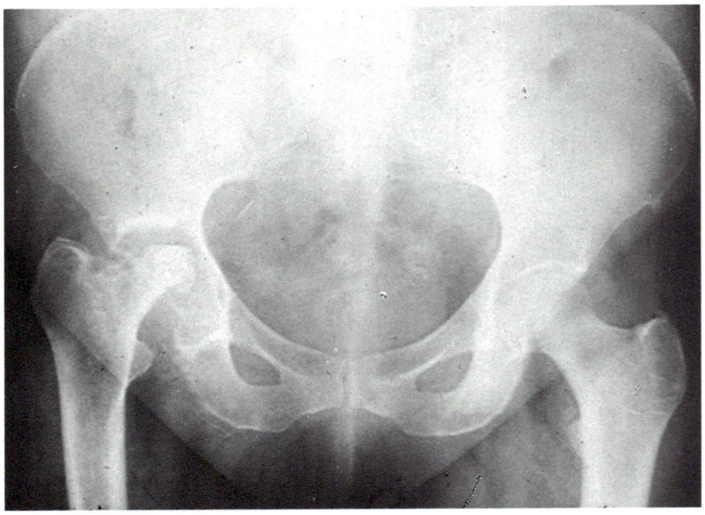

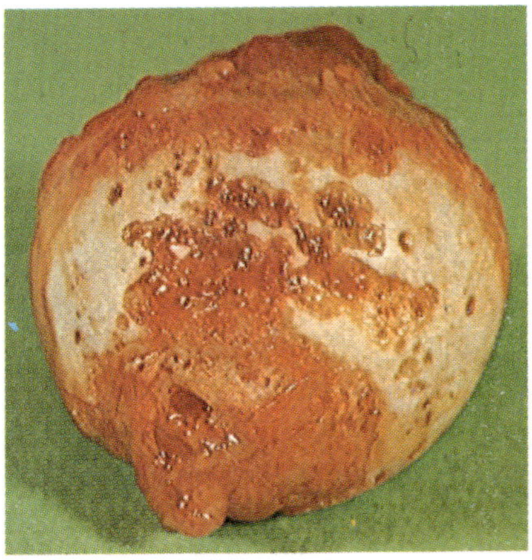

153 & **154** Destructive arthropathy of the hip joint produced by rheumatoid arthritis. This leads to erosions of the femoral head and acetabulum.

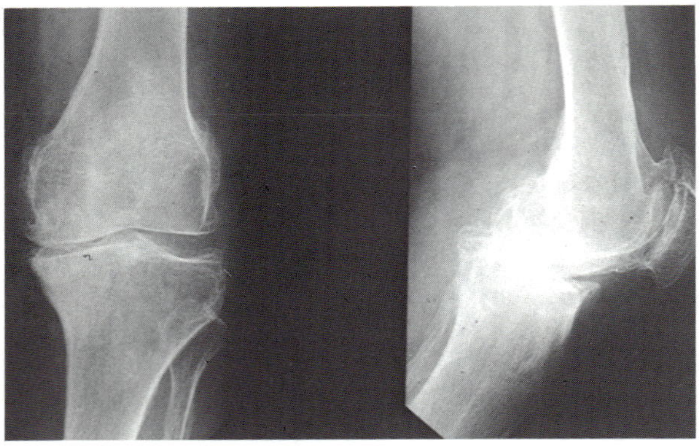

155 The knee joints are often affected.

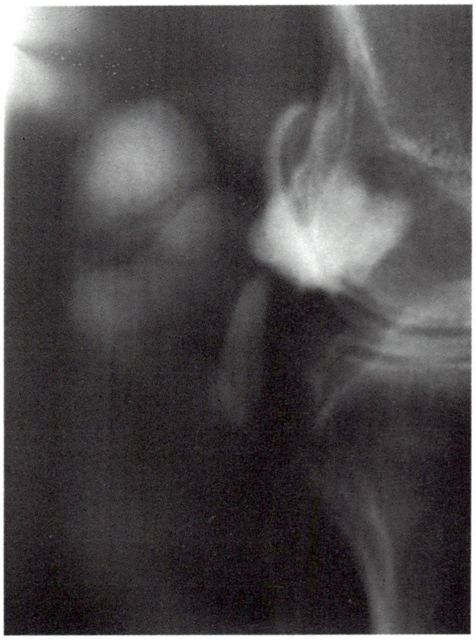

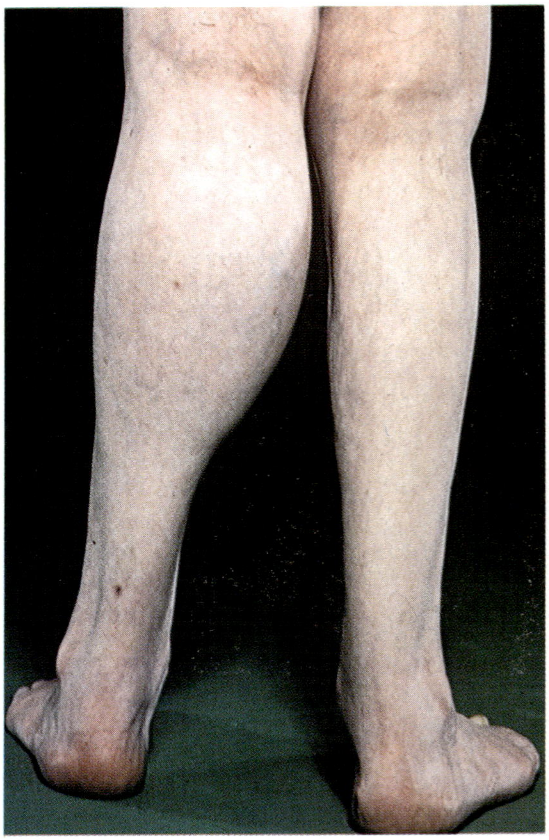

156 & **157** Baker's cyst. Enlargement of the calf in a patient following rupture of a Baker's cyst. Presentation is with acute pain and swelling making differential diagnosis with deep venous thrombosis difficult. An arthrogram showing contrast tracking into the calf confirms the diagnosis.

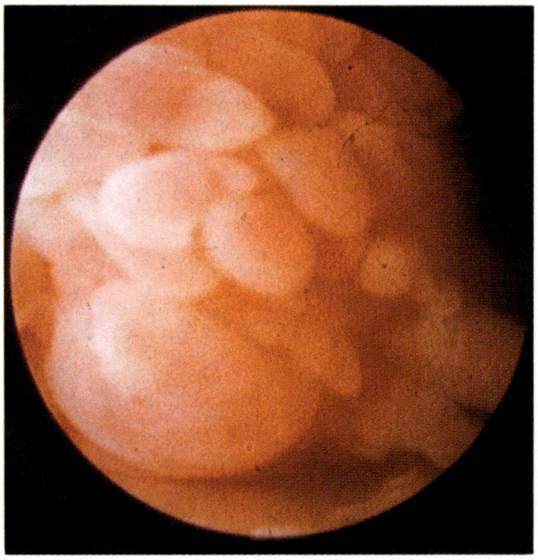

158 Multiple synovial villi in the knee of the same patient as in **156**, seen through an arthroscope.

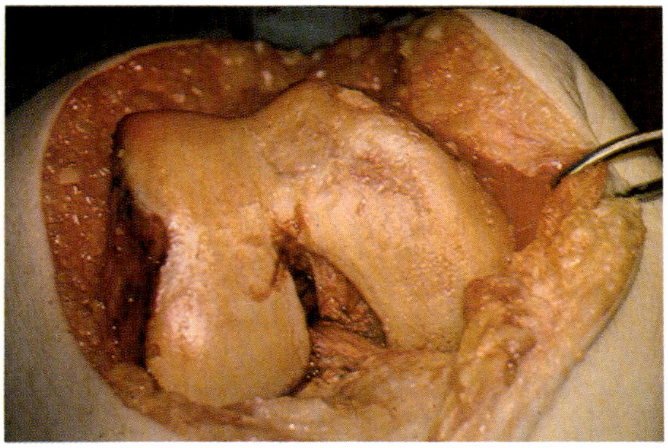

159 Loss of articular cartilage and general destructive arthropathy seen at operation in the same patient as in **156**.

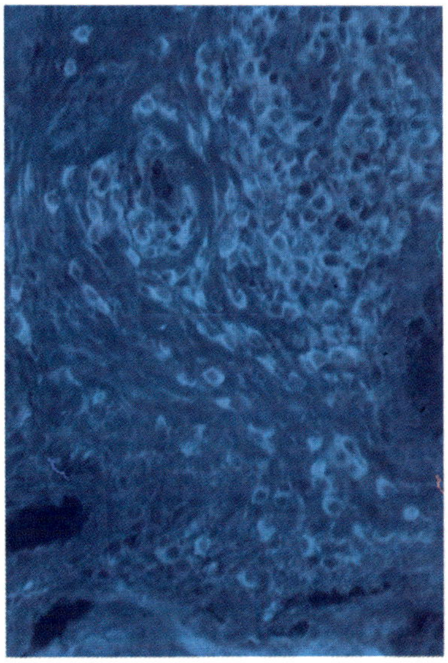

160 Rheumatoid synovial membrane prepared to show immunofluorescence in the plasma cells.

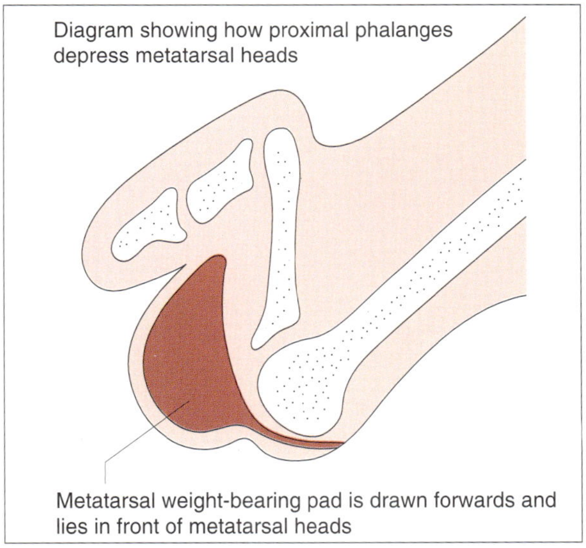

161 The metatarsal fat-pad is displaced forwards and the metatarsal heads become subcutaneous.

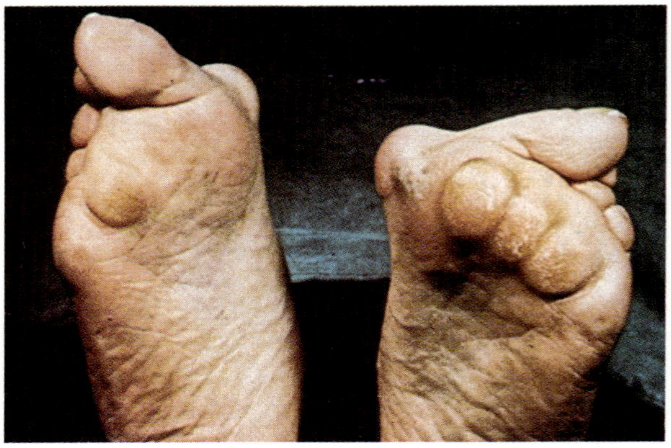

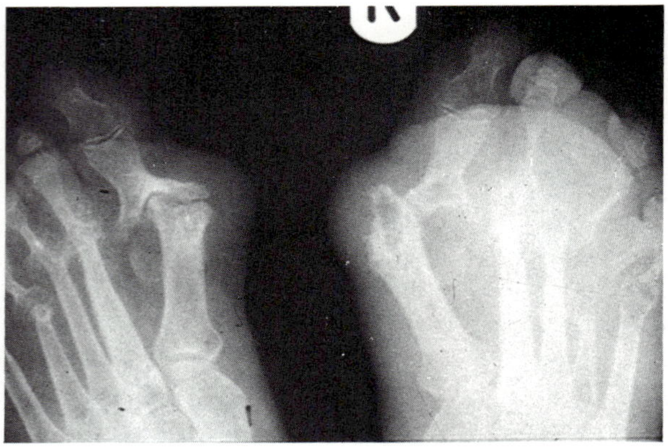

162 & **163** Rheumatoid arthritis may cause gross destructive arthropathy and distortion of the foot leading to painful callosities. Multiple subluxation and discolouration of the joints of the forefoot are present.

Juvenile rheumatoid disease (Still's disease)

This illness corresponds to rheumatoid disease in the adult. Various clinical subtypes have been defined varying from polyarticular to pauci-articular involvement to those with marked systemic features.

Adult pattern disease can occur in the child, but more frequently the childhood disease differs in many features. Systemic manifestations are common with rash, fever, leucocytosis, lymphadenopathy and splenomegaly; pericarditis may occur. The arthritis is usually less destructive and nodules and rheumatoid factor are frequently absent. There is an important relationship between iridocyclitis and the pauci-articular pattern of disease.

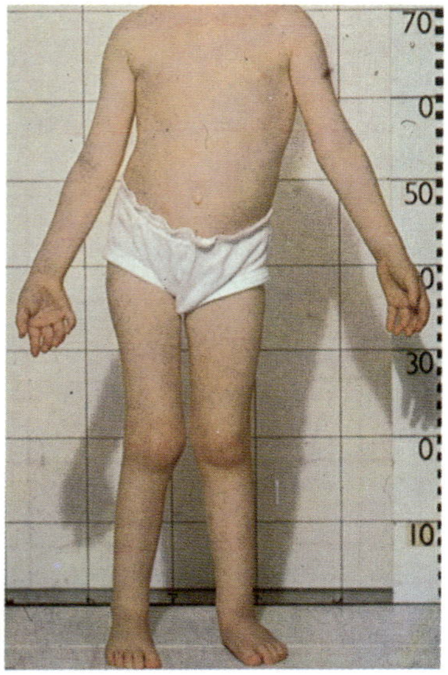

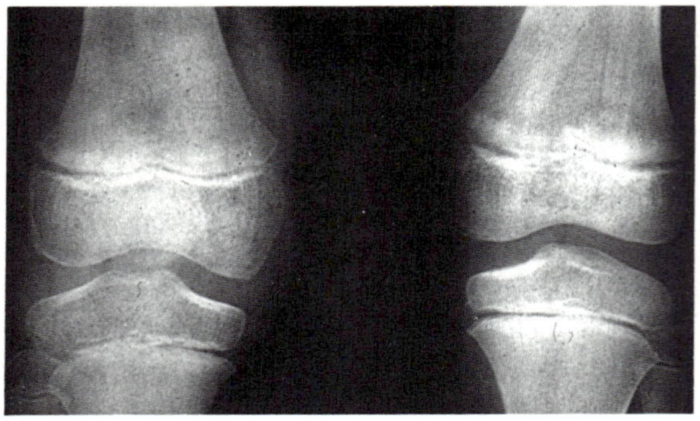

164 & **165** Early Still's disease in a child showing some swelling of the knee joints. The radiographs of the early stages show only soft tissue swelling with osteoporosis.

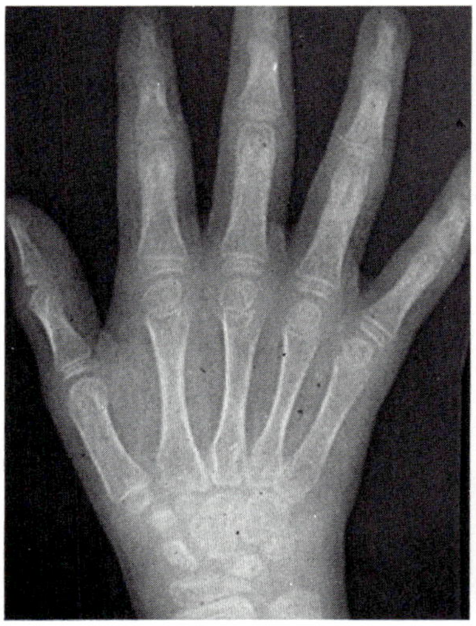
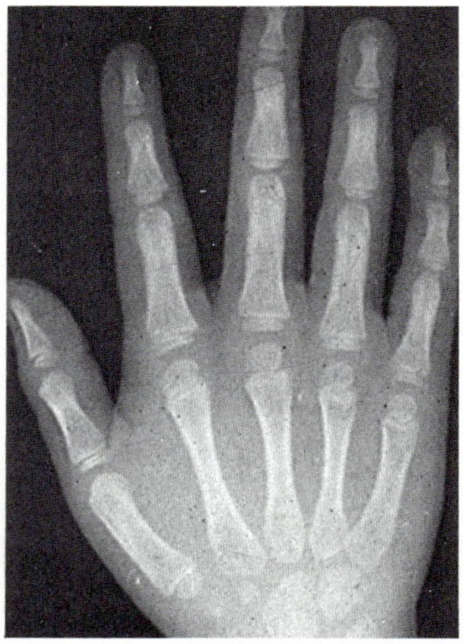

166 & **167** There is an enlargement of the growing ossific centres. Compare the radiographs of two children of the same age: on the left, a child with Still's disease; on the right, a normal child.

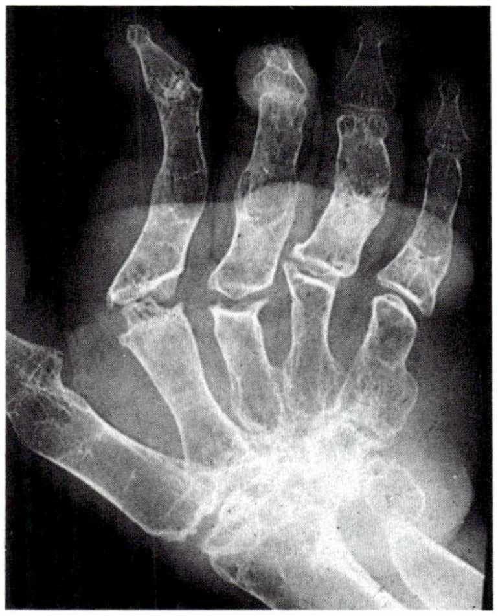

168 Enlargement of the shafts of the phalanges owing to repeated periosteal reaction may occur.

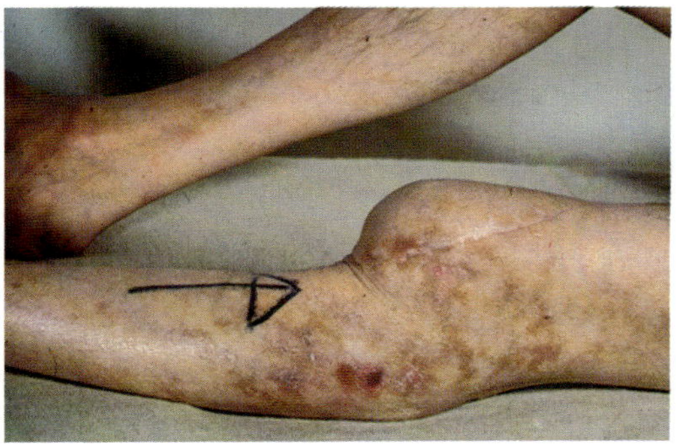

169 The end result of a severe case. Deformity and spontaneous ankylosis has occurred. Such a serious result is the exception rather than the rule.

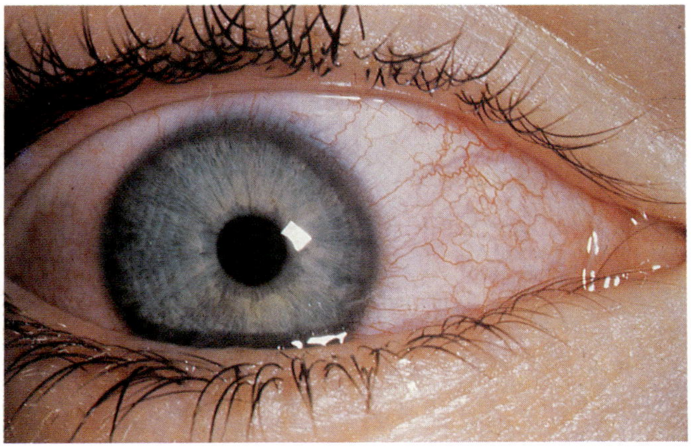

170 Pauci-articular juvenile rheumatoid arthritis is frequently punctuated by episodes of acute iridocyclitis, which can culminate in blindness. Frequent ophthalmological assessment is essential.

Ankylosing spondylitis

The condition is characterised by increasing pain and stiffness in the lumbar spine and buttocks, occasional vague pains elsewhere, e.g. in the heels, associated with general malaise and fatigue. The aetiology is unknown, but recent work suggests a genetic factor. Males are more often affected than females (8:1) and the histocompatibility antigen HLA-B27 is present in over 90% of patients but in less than 10% of the general population.

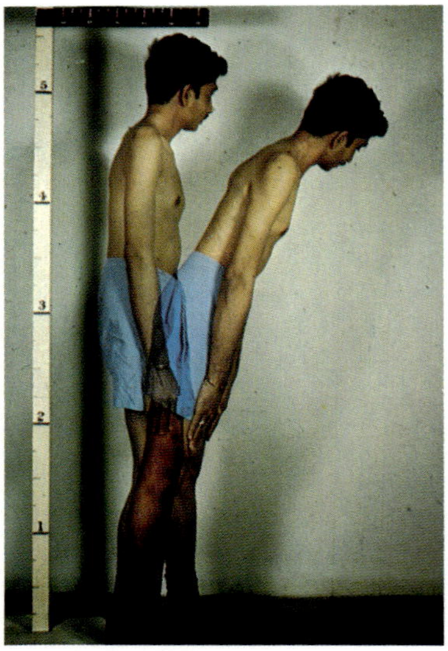

171 Gross loss of forward flexion on attempted toe-touching.

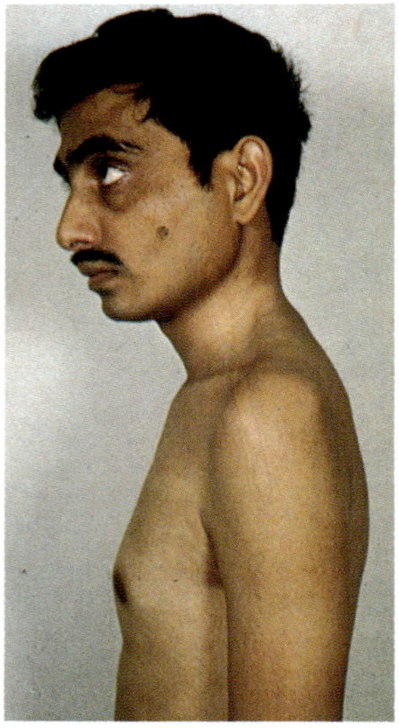

172 On attempting to turn his head the patient turns his eyes outwards, but his neck is held rigidly.

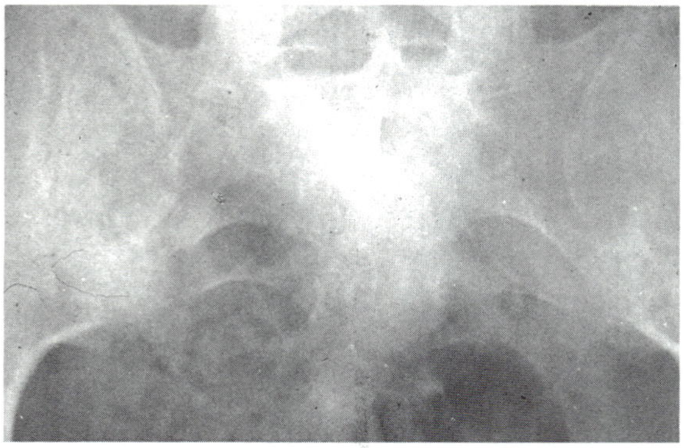

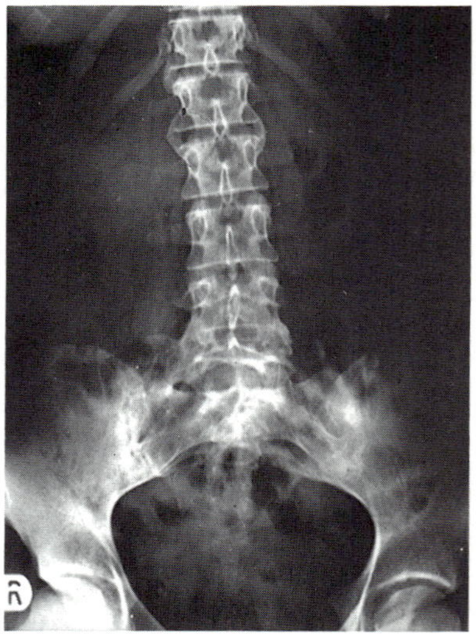

173 & **174** Apart from limited chest expansion and a raised ESR the earliest objective evidence is blurring and later, obliteration of the sacro-iliac joints.

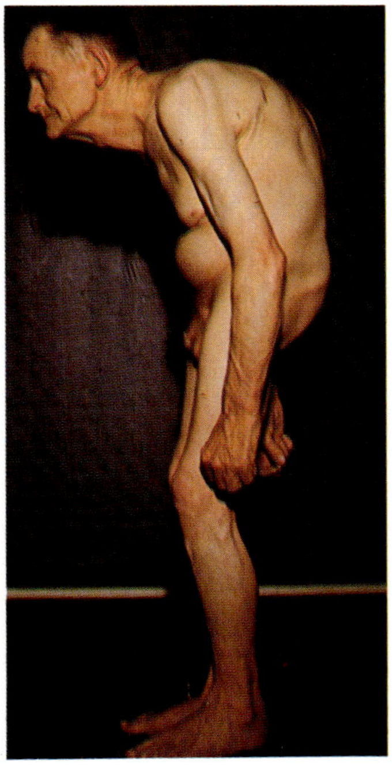

175 Eventually the trunk may become fixed in a fully bent position, so that the patient cannot see ahead.

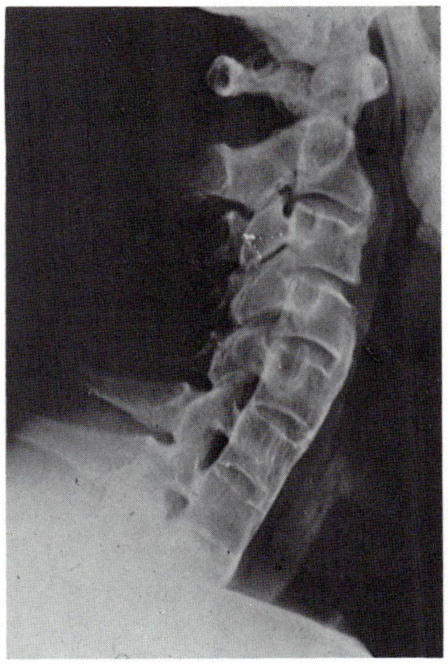

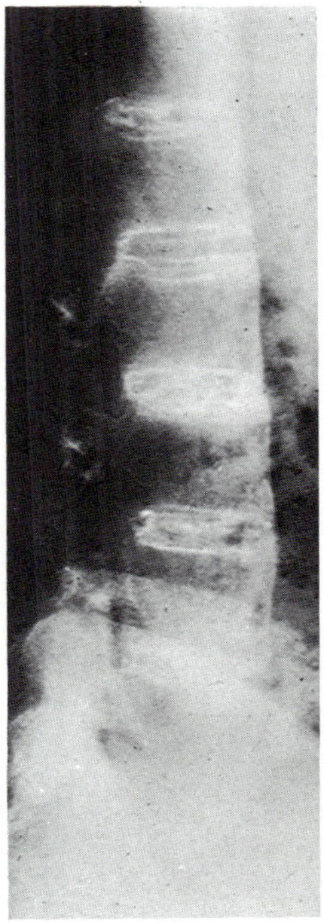

176 & **177** 'Bamboo spine'. Rigid bony ankylosis of all major spinal joints.

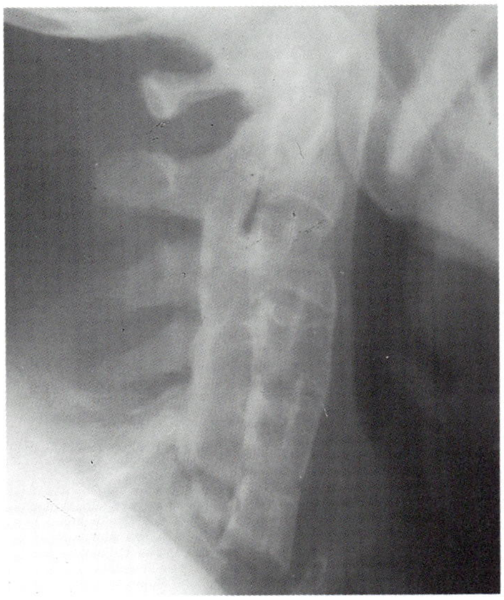

178 Minor injuries to the head and neck of patients with ankylosing spondylitis can have disastrous consequences. A fracture dislocation of C6 on C7 is seen here. In patients fortunate enough to escape immediate neurological injury who present to their casualty departments with neck pain, this sort of injury is all too frequently missed.

Psoriatic arthropathy

There is a peculiar association between psoriasis and arthropathy which affects principally the joints of the hands and feet and rarely the larger proximal joints. About 8% of psoriasis sufferers will develop arthritis. Although the arthropathy resembles rheumatoid disease, rheumatoid factor is negative (seronegative arthropathy) and nodules do not occur. Sex incidence is equal and the arthropathy is asymmetrical with a predilection for the terminal interphalangeal joints.

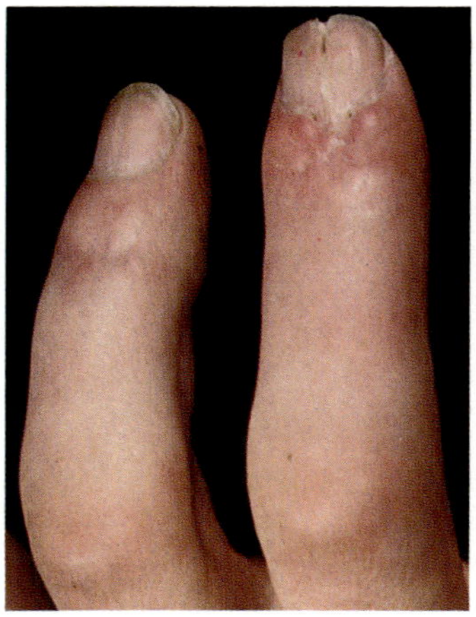

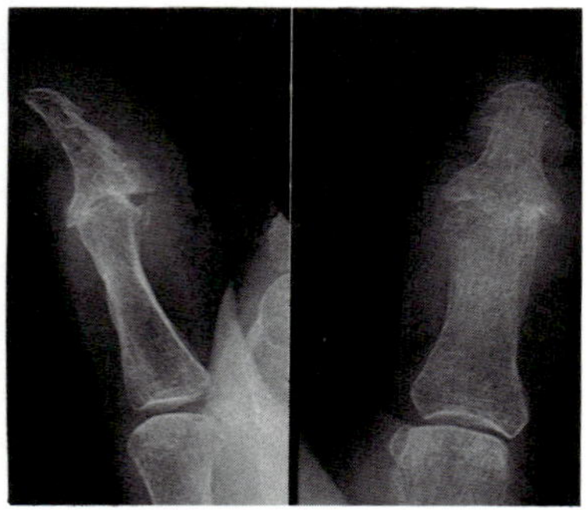

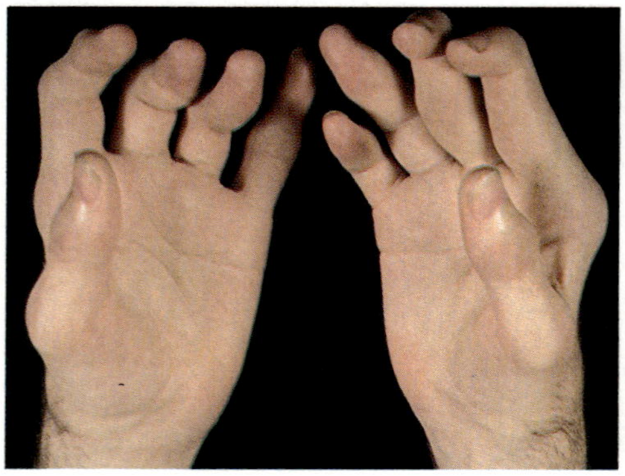

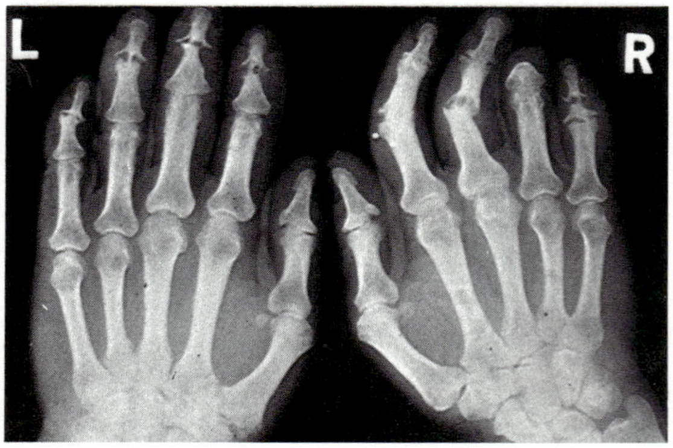

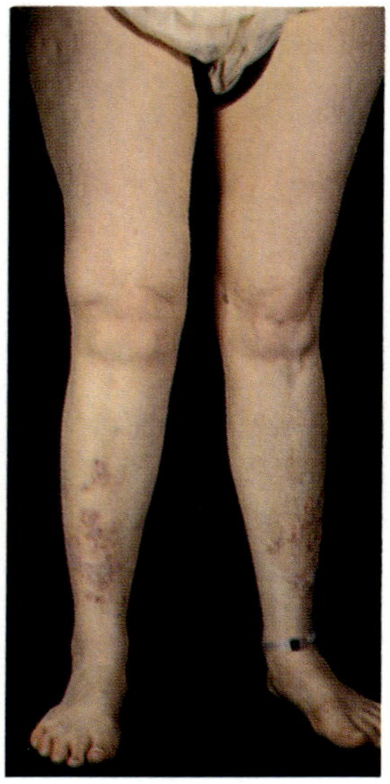

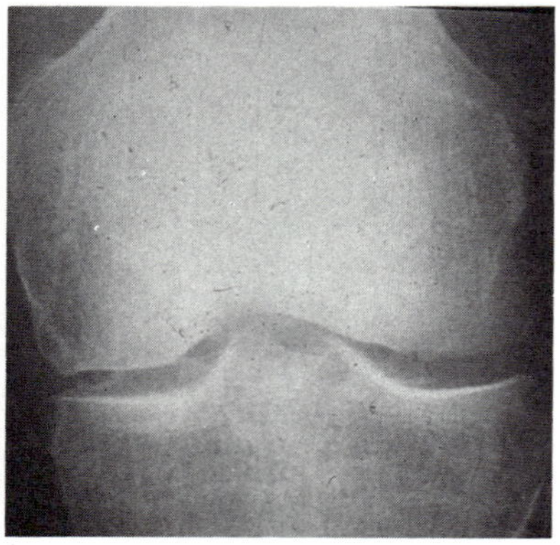

179–184 Psoriatic arthropathy.

Reiter's syndrome

This is a disease almost exclusively of males. There is a history of sexually transmitted non-specific urethritis or, less commonly, dysentery. The triad of urethritis, conjunctivitis and arthritis is classical.

The arthritis most commonly affects the weight-bearing joints of the lower limbs; toes, ankles and knees.

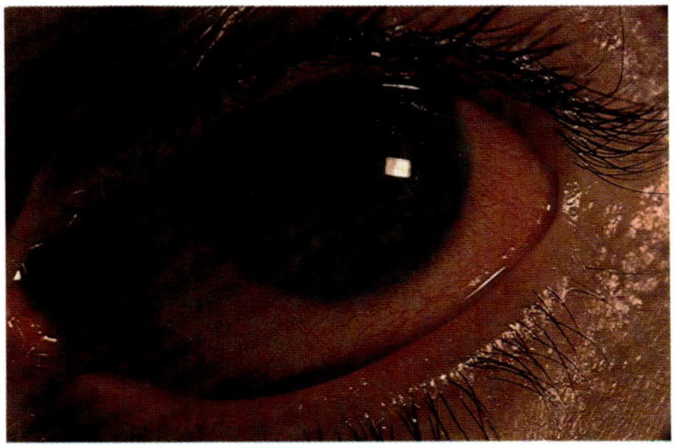

185 Subacute conjunctivitis in a case of Reiter's syndrome.

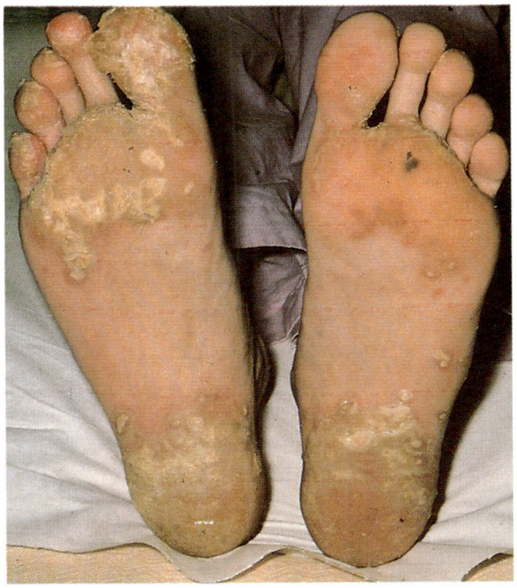

186 Skin lesions are a frequent accompaniment. Keratodermia blennorrhagia closely resembles pustular psoriasis.

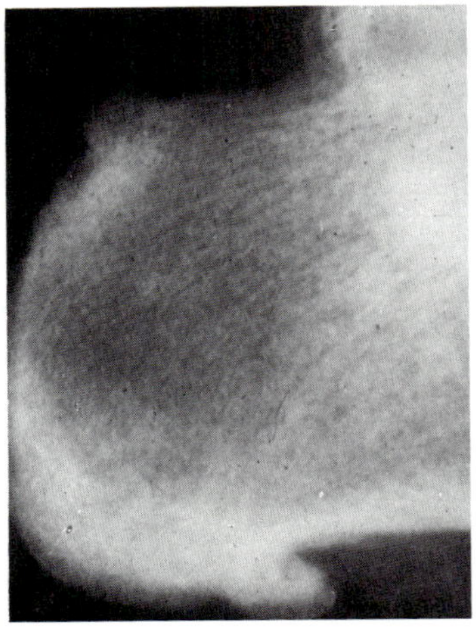

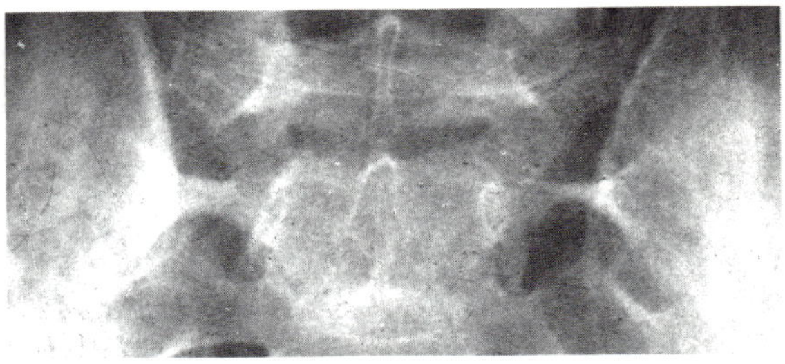

187, 188 As in ankylosing spondylitis heel pain caused by spur formations and a sacroileitis are common occurrences in Reiter's syndrome; indeed, HLA-B27 is positive in 75% of cases.

Infection of bone and joint

Acute pyogenic osteomyelitis and acute pyogenic arthritis, (which is almost always secondary to intra-articular osteomyelitis), was at one time very common, and even severe enough to be fatal.

The advent of antibiotics has completely altered the incidence, course and destructive potential of the disease. The beneficial effects of early antibiotic therapy prevents many of the ghastly consequences of the infection, but does carry with it the problem of masking the early diagnosis.

Infection may occur by direct innoculation, e.g. from an open fracture, or, more commonly, by haematogenous spread from a distant septic focus.

The causal organism is usually *Staphylococcus aureus*, although a wide range of infecting organisms may be implicated with particular predilections depending upon the age, site and predisposing conditions.

Osteomyelitis caused by salmonella infection is frequently multifocal, particularly in patients suffering from sickle cell disease.

Even viral osteomyeleitis, in particular the smallpox virus, has been found to cause acute and subsequently chronic infestation of bone and joint.

Although the pathological reaction to infection in bone does not differ in essence from that in other tissues, it is considerably modified by the loss of blood supply to bone owing to endosteal infection when, simultaneously, an abscess has stripped off the periosteum. Even when the focus of infection has been sterilised by antibiotic therapy, the mineralised structure of bone creates special problems of healing, which may lead to late development of sequestra in which an adequate concentration of antibiotics at the site of infection cannot be obtained. For this reason the early diagnosis, isolation of infecting organism and the relief of tension within any abscess which may lead to avascular necrosis of bone, is imperative.

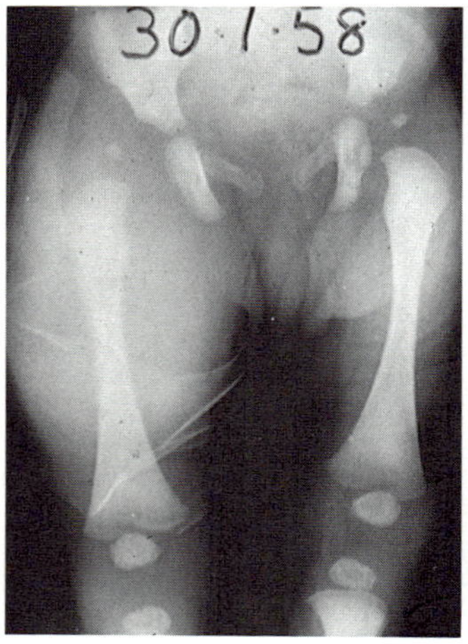

189 In the neonate and infant streptococci, pneumococci, haemophilus and meningococci may be responsible. In the case shown, osteomyelitis of the right upper femoral metaphysis has spread to the adjacent hip joint with consequent dislocation of the hip.

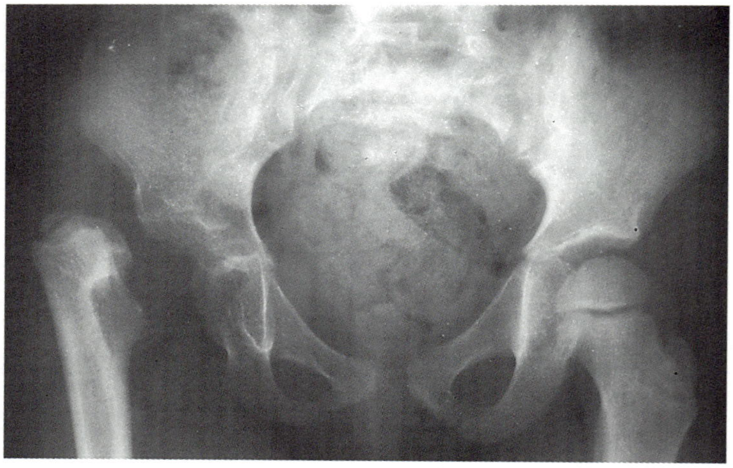

190 The consequences of inadequately treated infections such as that shown in **189** are a permanently destroyed and unstable hip (Tom Smith's arthritis).

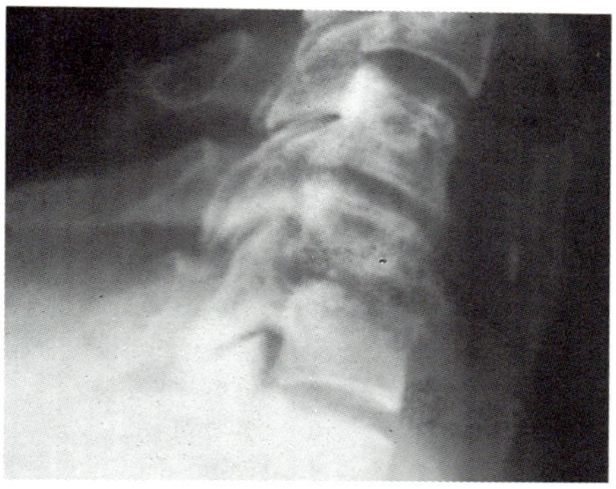

191 Brucellosis. Where brucellosis is endemic bone infections sometimes occur with particular prediliction for the spine.

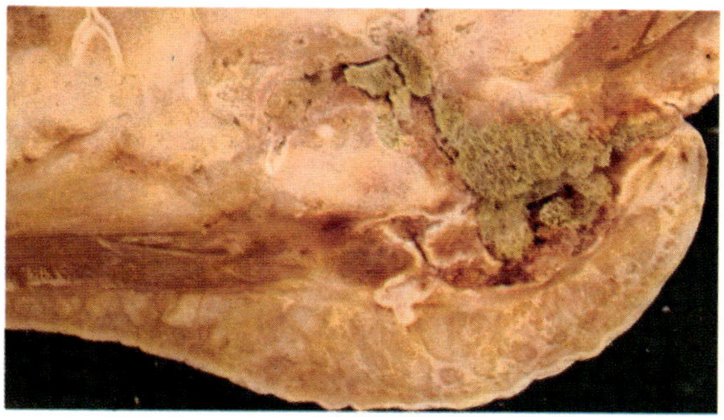

192 Infection of the os calcis frequently develops from penetrating injuries. *Pseudomonas* is a commonly isolated organism in this site resulting in an indolent infection.

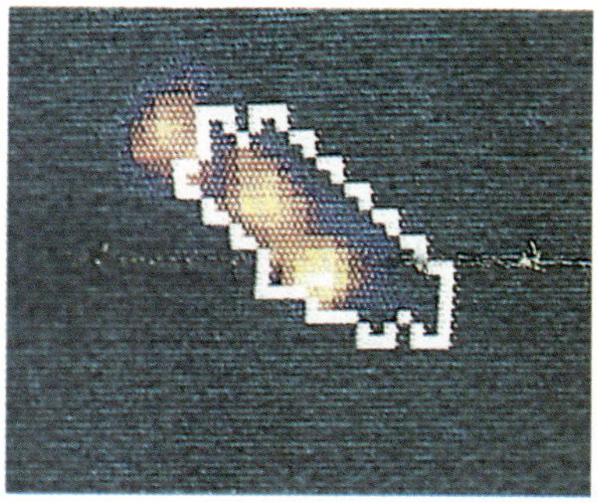

193 A labelled white cell scan of the os calcis (outlined white) showing increased isotope uptake within the os calcis and associated sinus representing persistent chronic infection.

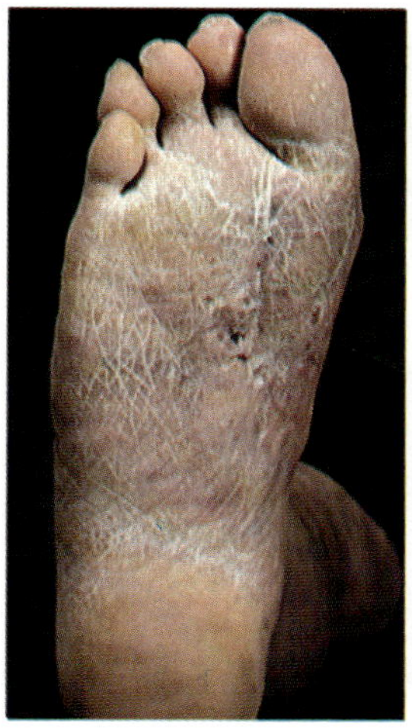

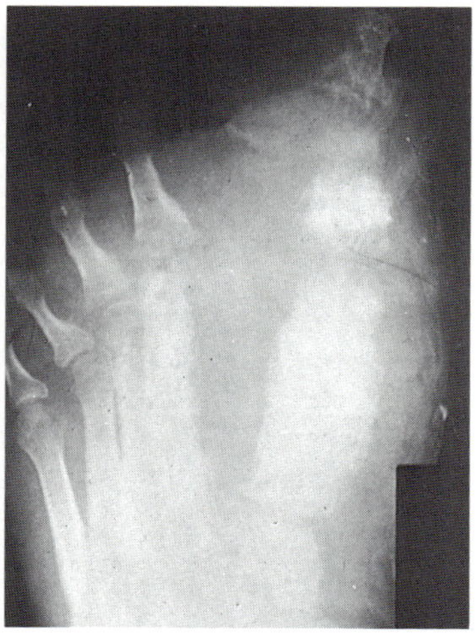

194 & **195** Madura Foot. In tropical regions the range of infecting agents is more extensive including fungi.

Diagnosis

Fever, malaise and pain over the affected bone or joint are typical features though in many instances the systemic disturbance may be misleadingly mild possibly owing to the institution of antibiotic therapy for some other condition. A high index of suspicion is therefore required.

Typically the ESR is elevated, with a polymorphonuclear leucocytosis. Blood cultures should be taken to isolate the organism before commencing antibiotics.

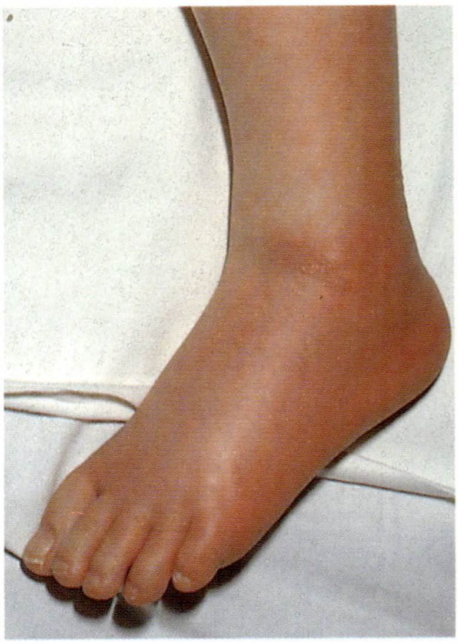

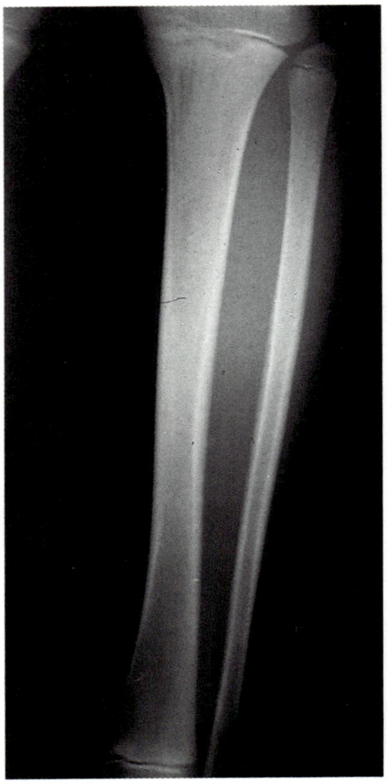

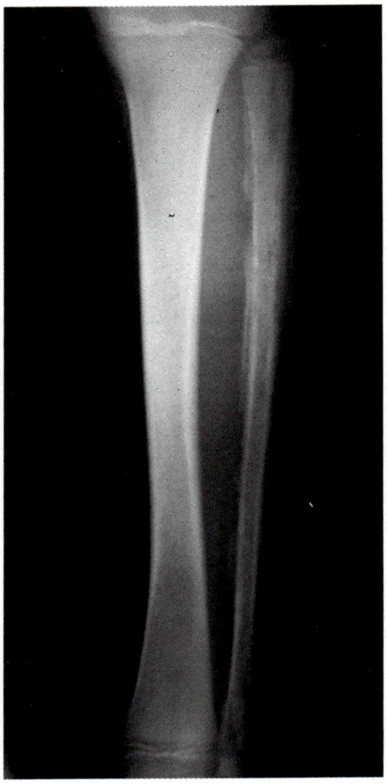

196–198 Local inflammation around the foot and ankle led to a clinical diagnosis of osteomyelitis. Radiographs soon after presentation were normal and unhelpful. A periosteal reaction was not seen until some days later.

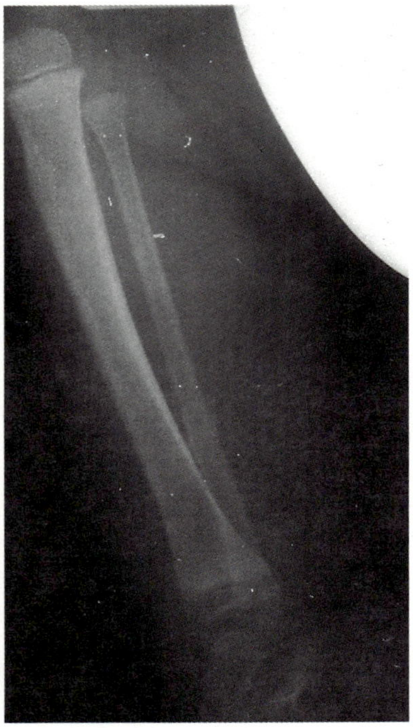

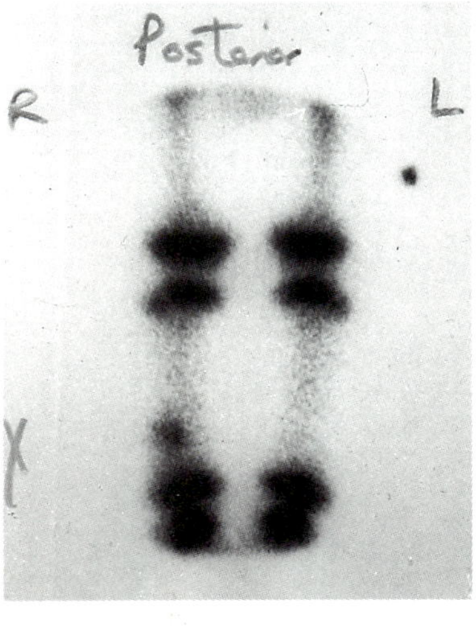

199 & 200 An isotope bone scan will be positive at an early stage and may warn of multifocal infection. In this case radiographs of the right leg were normal, the septic focus in the fibula being detected by radioactive Tc scan.

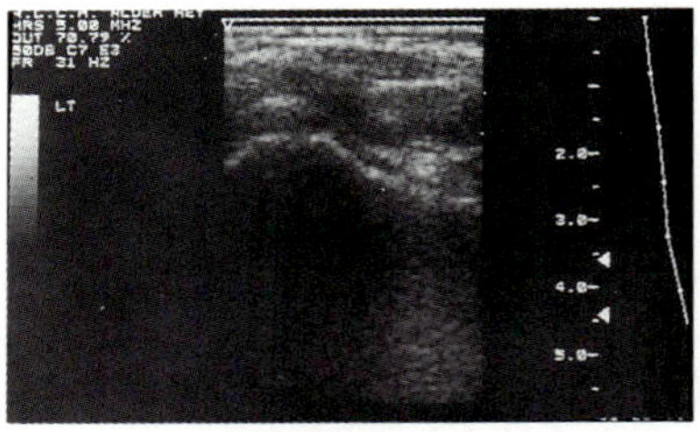

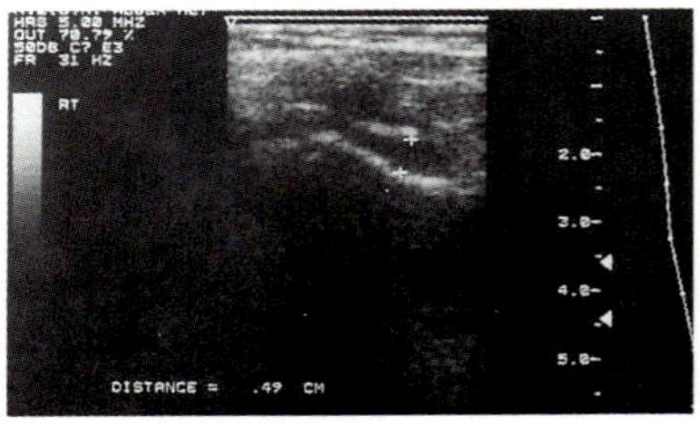

201 In the case of a suspected deep joint infection an ultrasound scan may help in confirming increased fluid in a joint.

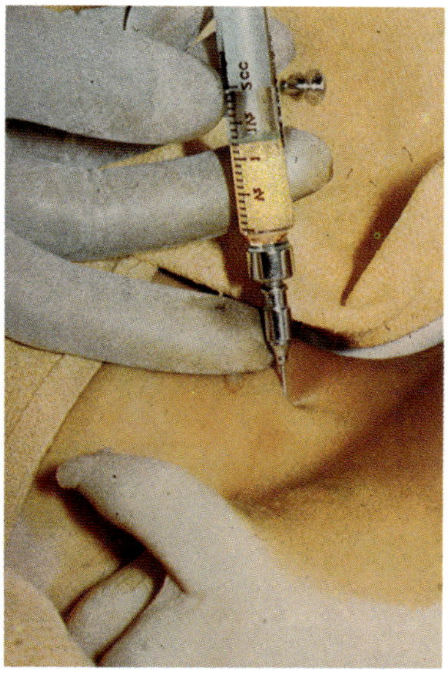

202 Aspiration of pus containing *Staphylococcus aureus* from the hip joint of an infant. This technique may be useful as an adjunct to investigation; the editors, however, do not attach any therapeutic value to the procedure. A positive tap confirms the diagnosis of infection; aspiration, however, does not satisfactorily decompress the joint, which should be completed by formal arthrotomy. A negative tap confirms nothing. If other clinical indicators suggest infection formal arthrotomy is again required.

Chronic osteomyelitis

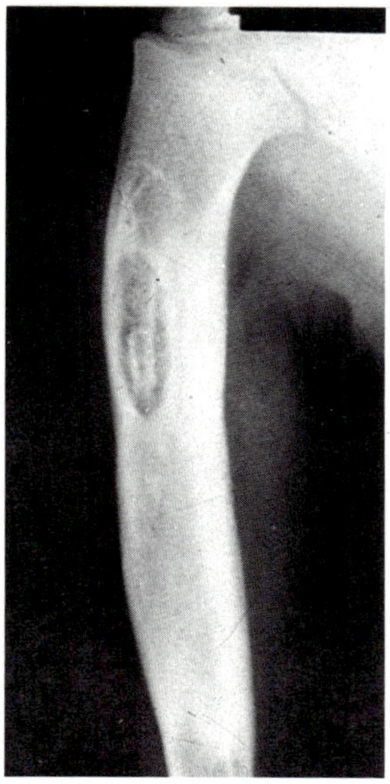

203 If treatment has been delayed or the initial treatment has not controlled the infection, a chronic bone abscess (a Brodie's abscess), may develop. The abscess contains necrotic debris and bacterial colonies that are walled off by fibrous tissue and surrounding dense woven bone. Such an abscess may persist for years before giving rise to symptoms. When symptoms do arise the flare-up is characterised by episodes of local swelling, erythema and pain. The abscess cavity may discharge to the surface through sinuses which themselves may chronically persist.

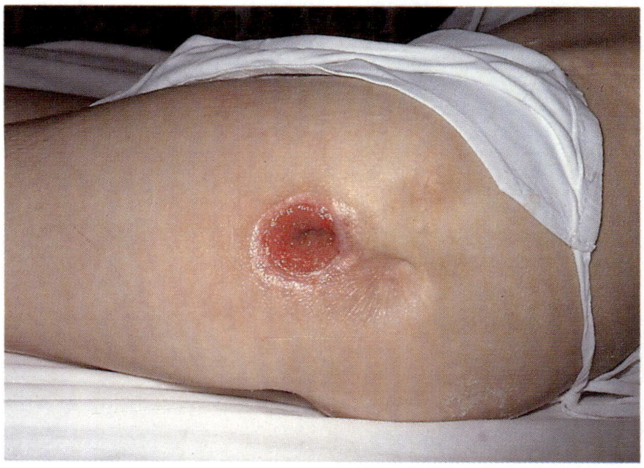

204 Marjolin's ulcer. Rarely, a chronically discharging sinus will give rise to a malignant ulcer, usually a squamous cell carcinoma. Another rare complication of the condition is the development of amyloidosis.

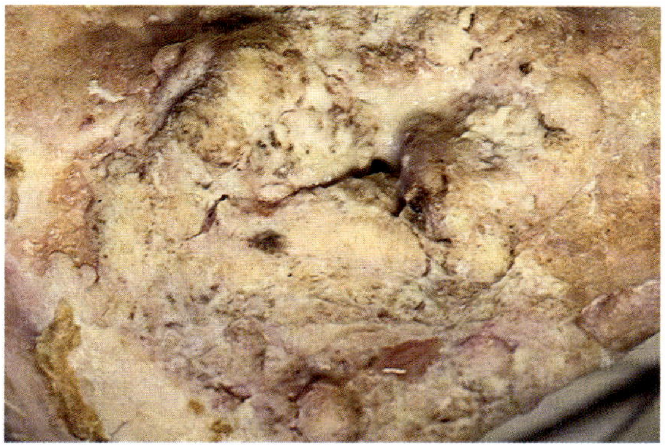

205 Squamous cell carcinoma complicating chronic osteomyelitis.

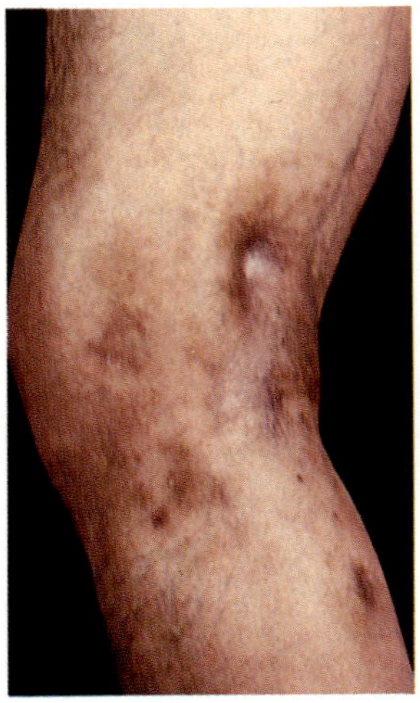

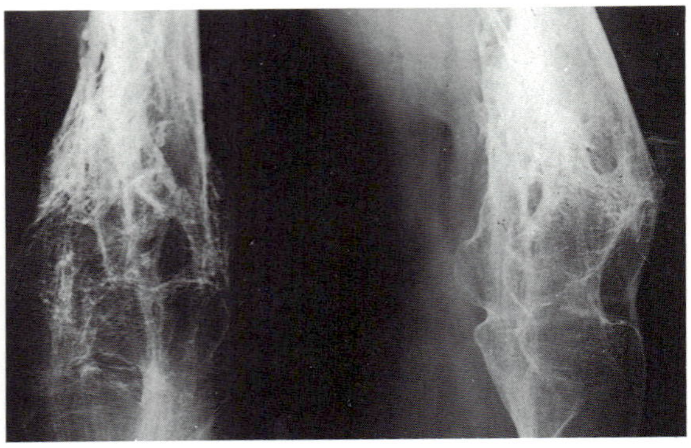

206 & **207** Bony ankylosis. The end result of a severe case of septic arthritis of the knee.

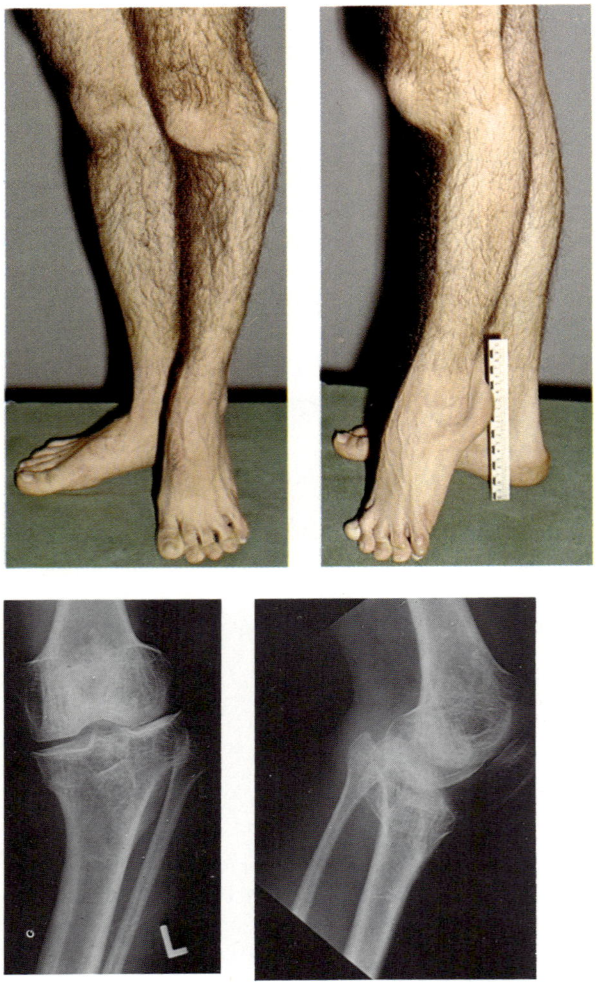

208–211 'Frame knee'. Premature epiphyseal arrest may arise from infection involving the growth plate or, as occurred in the past, from prolonged immobilisation on a frame with the knee extended.

Tuberculosis infection

Tuberculosis of bone or joint is the local manifestation of general disease, although it may be the most obvious and important presenting feature. The initial lesion is usually in lung or intestine, caused by the human or bovine tubercle bacillus. Formerly 85% were bovine in origin, but in the economically developed world where the disease is now very much less common, pasteurisation and TT testing (tuberculin) has reduced bovine cases to 25% of the total. Orthopaedic hospitals in the 19th century were built in the countryside with the main object of treating tuberculosis of bone and joint in young people. The disease is now far less common, but is still occasionally seen either as an acute episode, or as the result of past infection. In the economically developing countries orthopaedic tuberculosis still presents a very serious problem. A few examples are shown here.

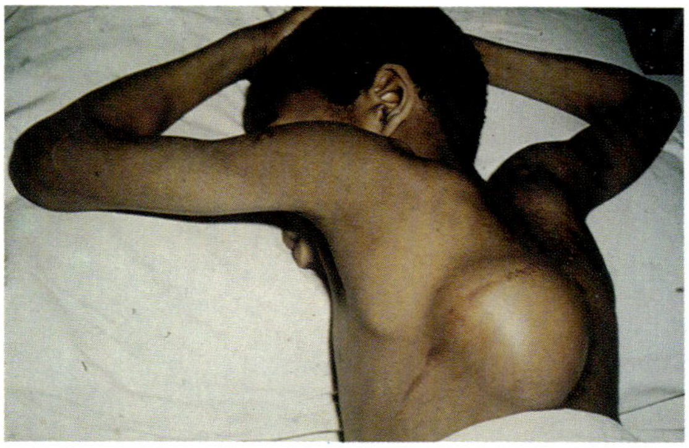

212 A 'cold' abscess in a child presenting in the loin as a painless swelling arises from infection of the spine.

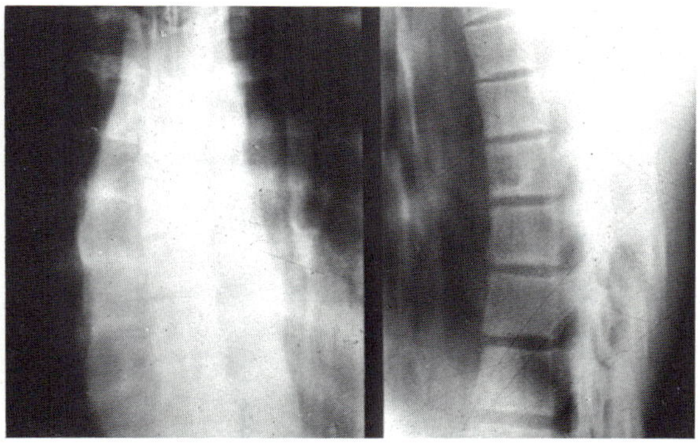

213 The tuberculous focus seen in the dorsal spine with its surrounding abscess formation.

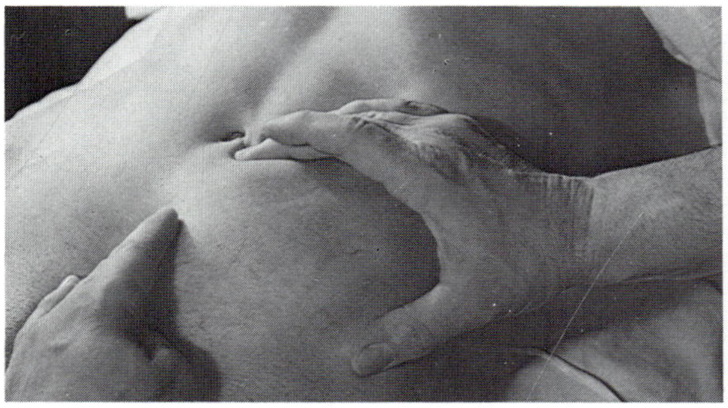

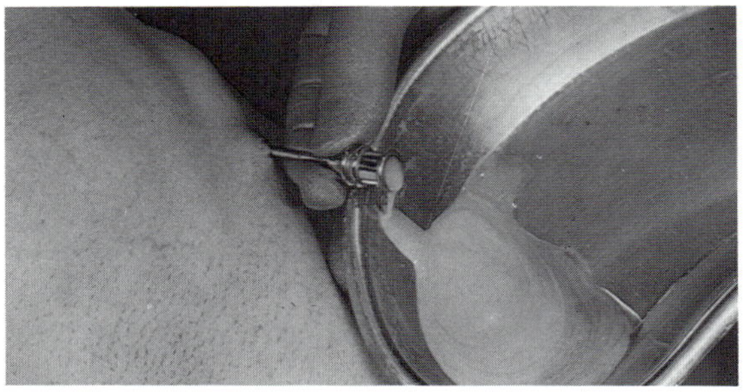

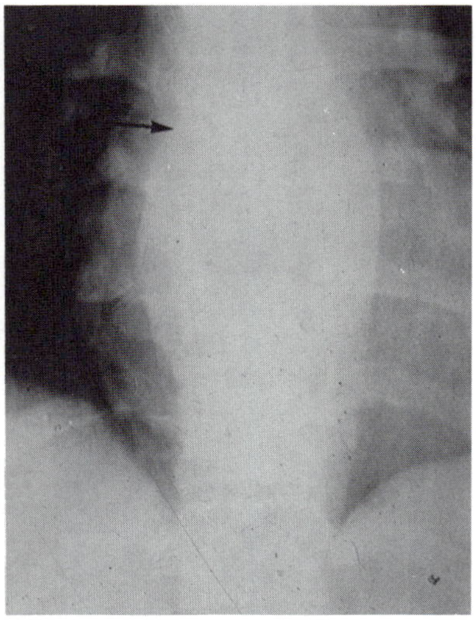

214–216 A cold abscess arising in the retroperitoneal tissues from the dorsal spine may present as an abdominal mass.

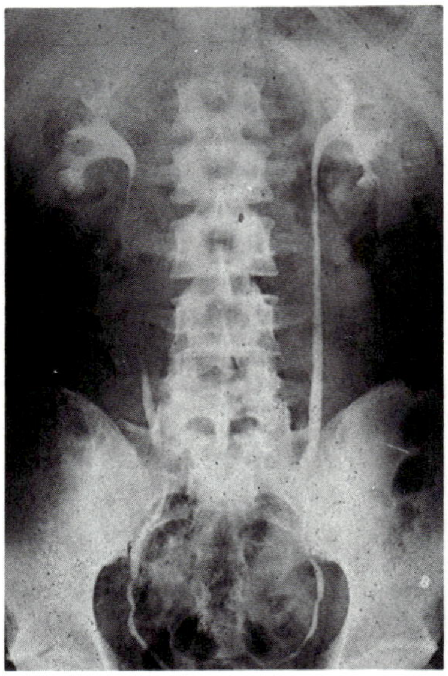

217 The cold abscess may lie within the sheath of the psoas muscle and may then present as a psoas abscess. An intravenous pyelogram shows the right ureter slightly obstructed and displaced by the psoas abscess.

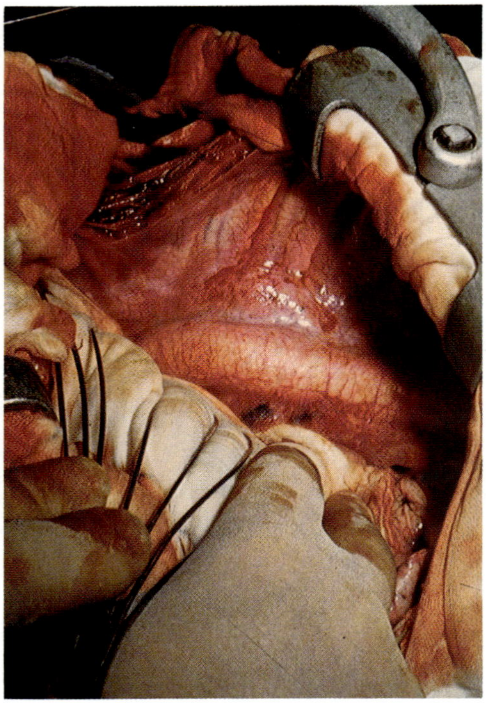

218 A tuberculous cold abscess of the dorsal spine seen above the thoracic aorta at operation.

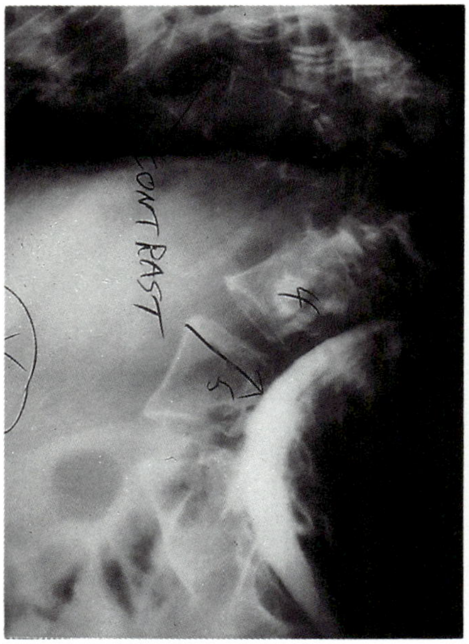

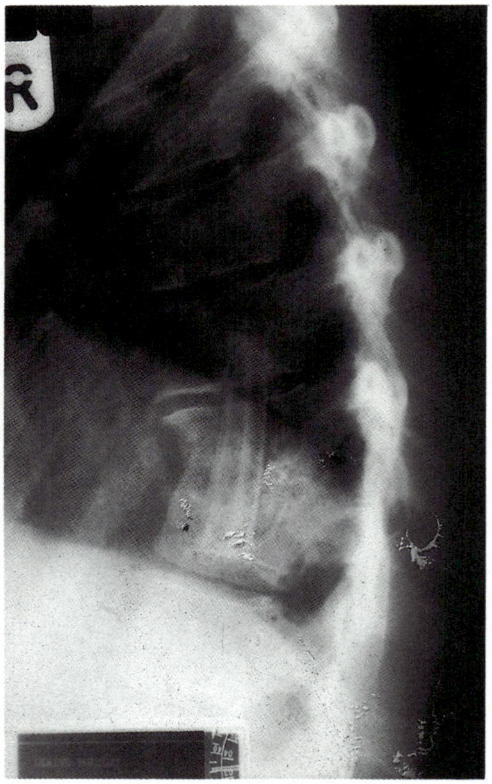

219 & **220** Spinal tuberculosis can lead to severe collapse and kyphos formation with paralysis. Early surgical debridement and bone grafting can prevent the deformities and sequelae seen in the past.

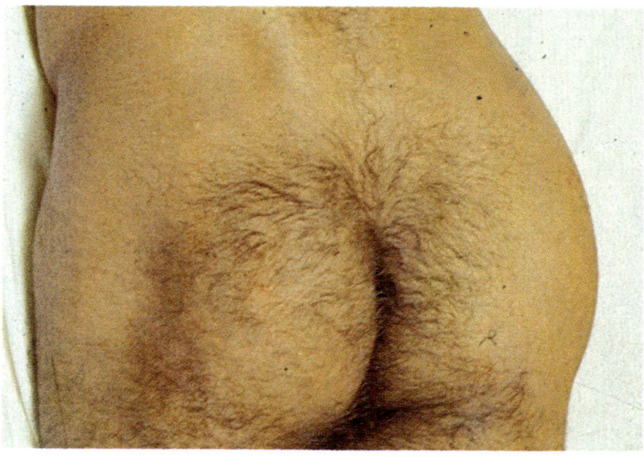

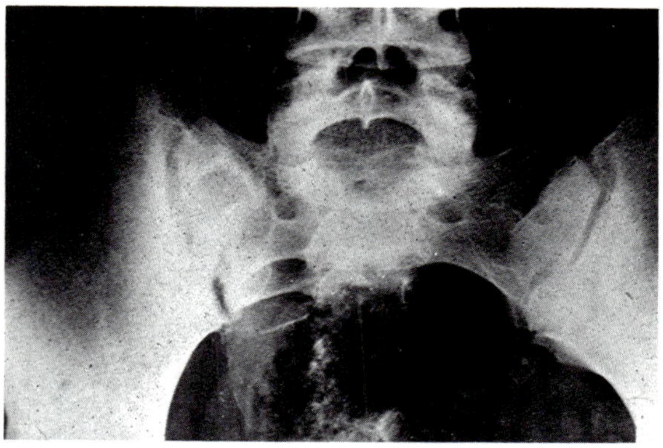

221 & **222** Tuberculosis of the right sacro-iliac joint presenting as a cold abscess in the buttock.

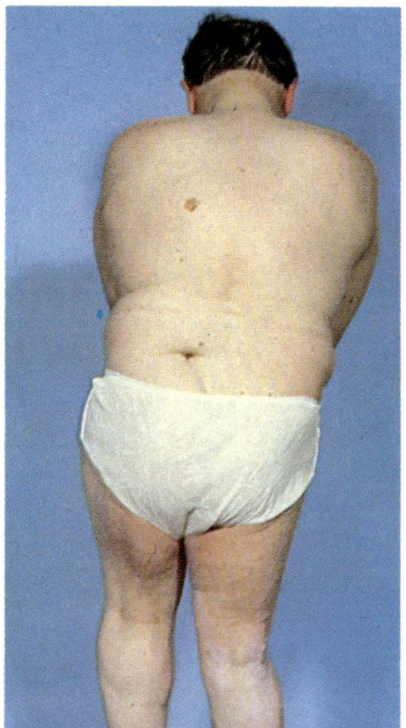

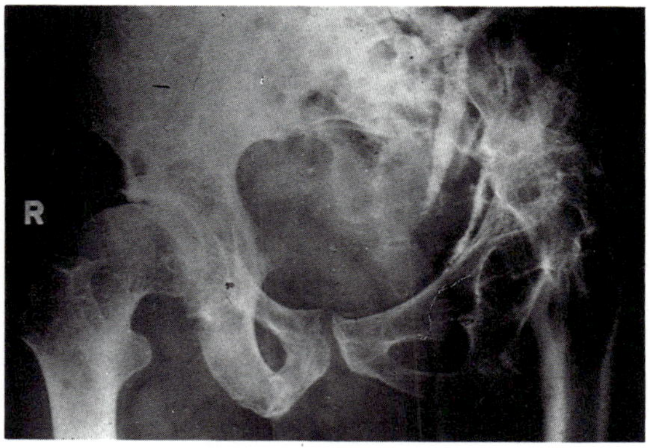

223 & **224** Old tuberculosis of the left hip joint causing destruction and a fibrous ankylosis with adduction deformity and shortening.

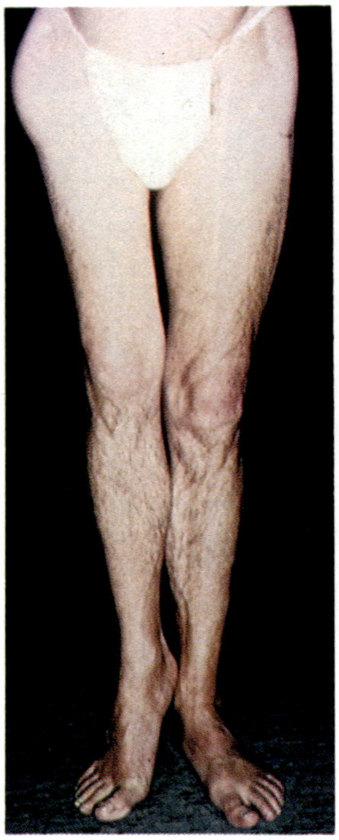

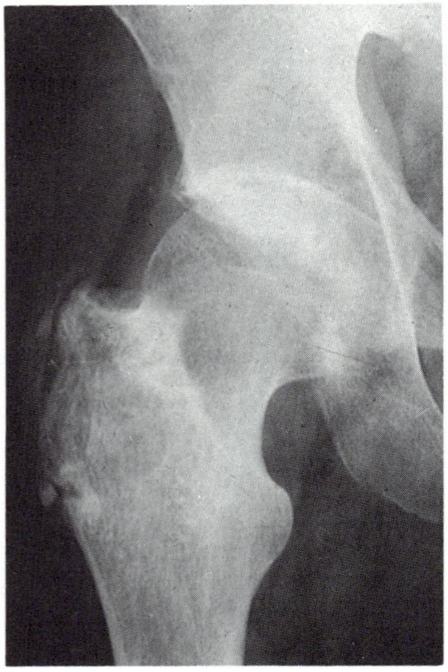

225 & **226** Tuberculosis of the trochanteric bursa. The cold abscess is visible and palpable over the greater trochanter, which is seen to be eroded.

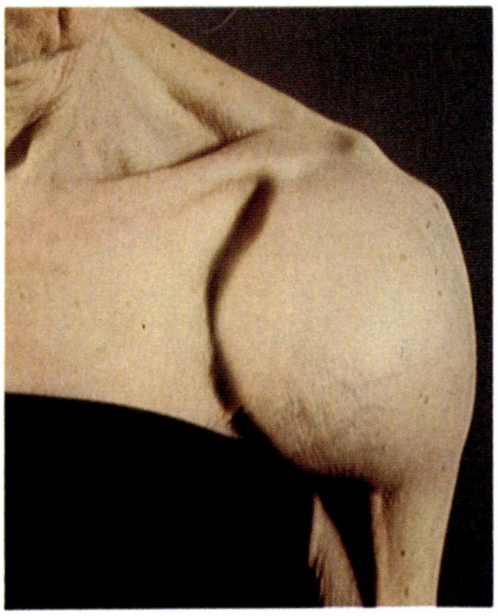

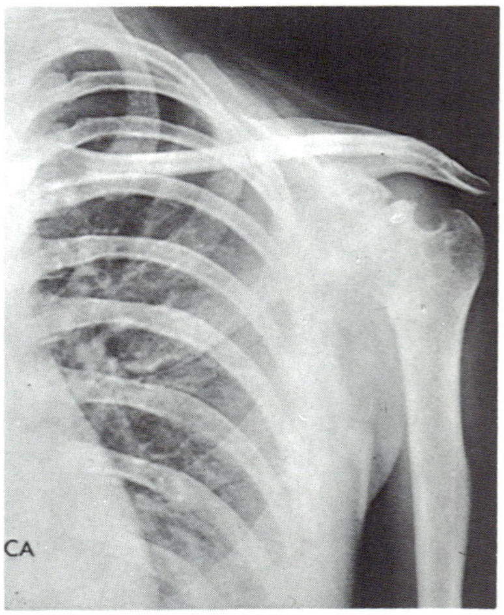

227 & **228** Tuberculosis of the shoulder joint with cold abscess formation. Sometimes tuberculosis occurs in the shoulder with little or no pus formation, and is called caries sicca.

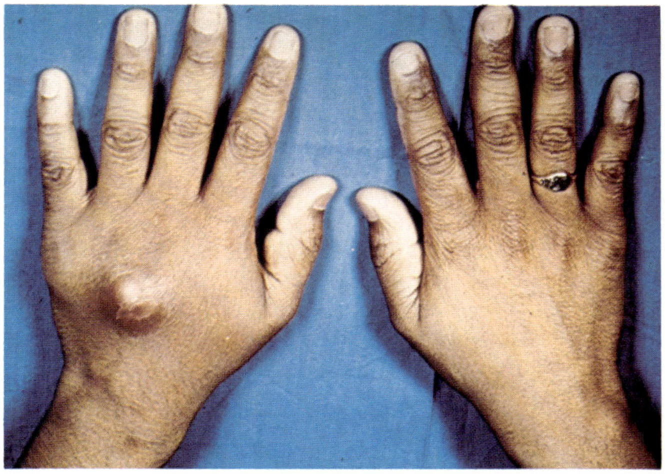

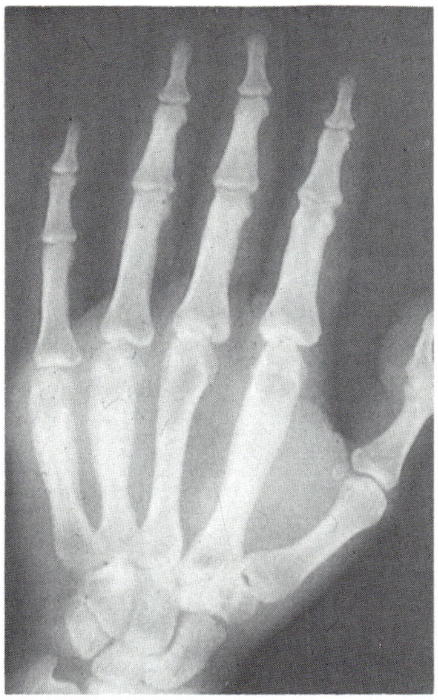

229 & **230** Tuberculous dactylitis. The focus is seen in the shaft of the fourth metacarpal bone of the left hand.

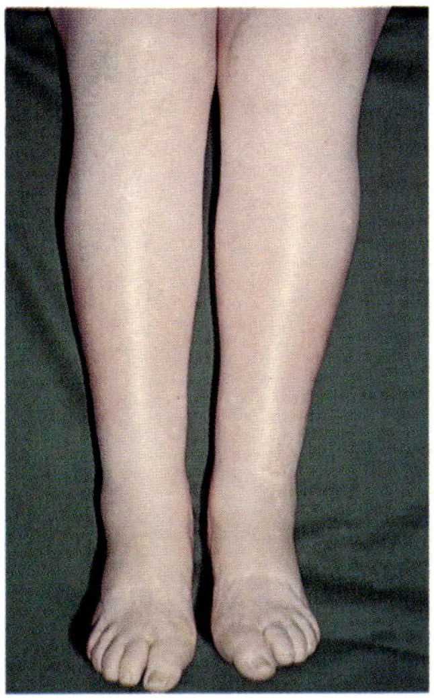

231 Scrofulous oedema. A case of longstanding tuberculous infection of the spine in which the lymphatic flow from the lower limbs is obstructed.

Disorders of joints and soft tissues: Connective tissue

Ehlers–Danlos syndrome

Excessive mobility of joints or being 'double-jointed' varies from comparatively mild ligamentous laxity, which may be a familial trait, expressed in an ability to hyperextend knees, elbows, wrists and fingers, to a more severe disorder.

Ehlers–Danlos syndrome is an inherited disorder of autosomal dominance in which there is a disorder of connective tissue affecting skin, ligaments and blood vessel walls.

Although the disease is rare, its importance lies in the associated vascular fragility resulting in a tendency to bruising, aneurysm formation and spontaneous vessel rupture.

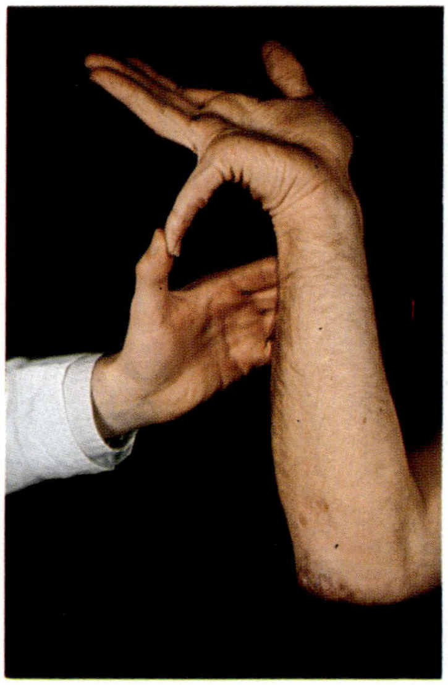

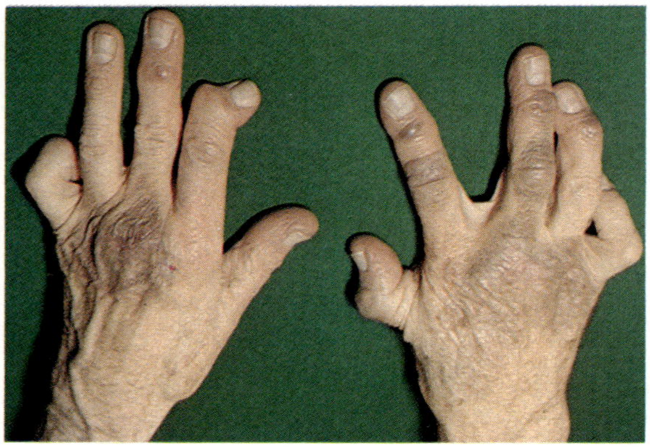

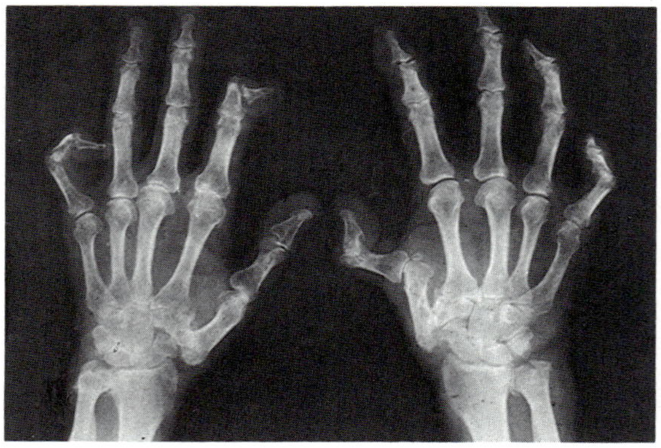

232–234 Excessive mobility of joints is a feature often resulting in recurrent dislocations and effusions of joints. A destructive arthropathy in which the basal joint of the thumb is particularly affected, may eventually develop.

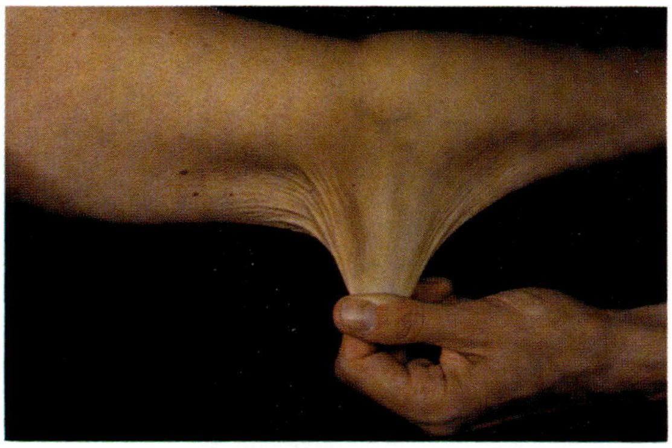

235 In Ehlers–Danlos syndrome the excessive ligamentous laxity is only one aspect of a widespread connective tissue disorder expressed, for example, in hyperelasticity of the skin which frequently has a characteristically velvety feel.

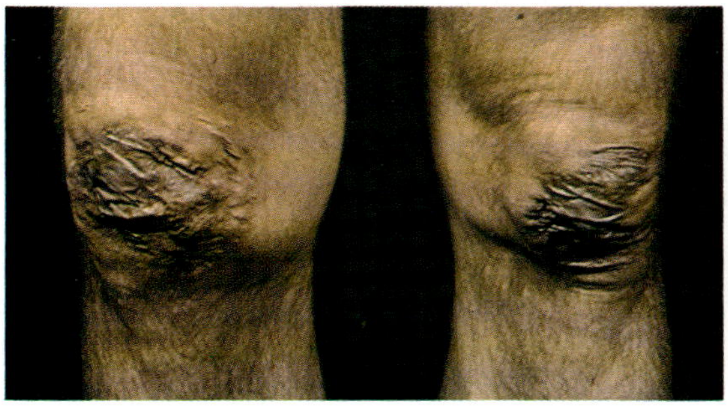

236 The skin has a tendency to split easily and leave pigmented tissue paper scars.

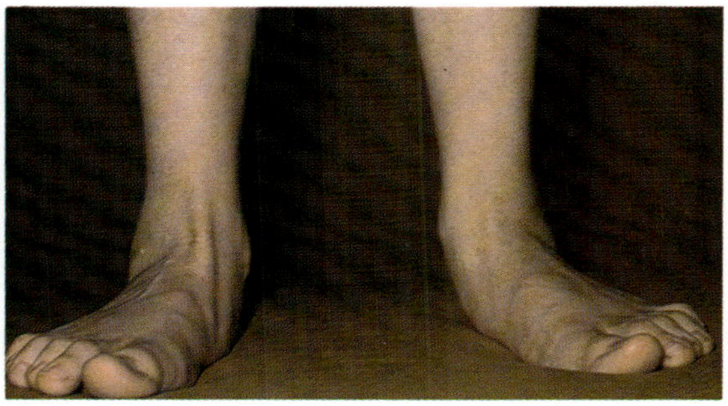

237 Ehlers–Danlos syndrome is a rare cause of flat foot.

Marfan's syndrome

Marfan's syndrome is of autosomal dominant inheritance and is characterised by a generalised disorder of connective tissue owing to a defect in elastin and collagen. Generalised joint laxity, ocular lens dislocation and aortic aneurysms are common features.

Patients are tall with disproportionately long limbs, particularly in distal segment bone, e.g. metacarpals, resulting in arachnodactyly.

Other features include a high-arched palate, scoliosis and herniae.

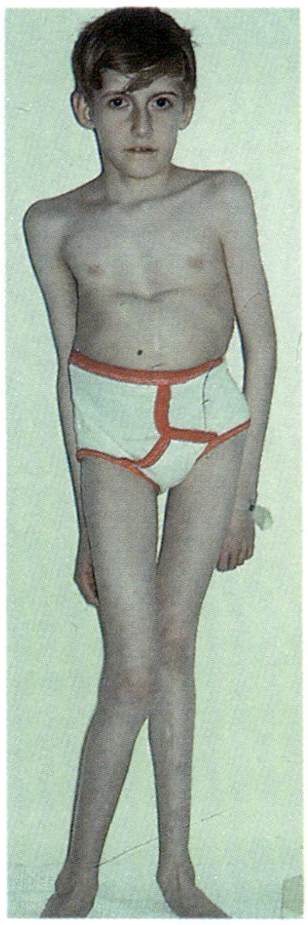

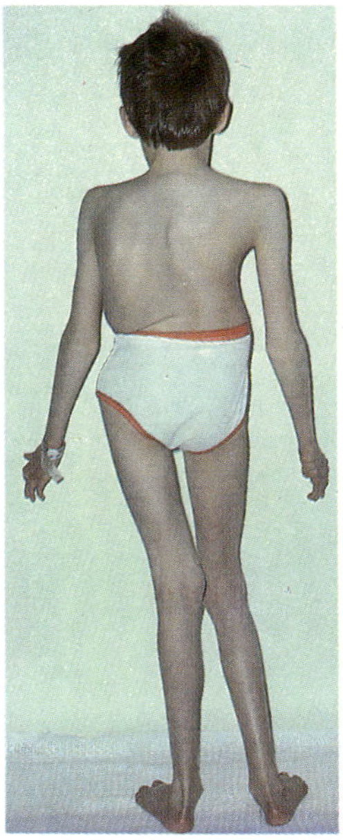

238 & **239** General appearance. The disproportionately long limbs are well shown. Other deformities include a scoliosis, genu valgum and plano-valgus feet.

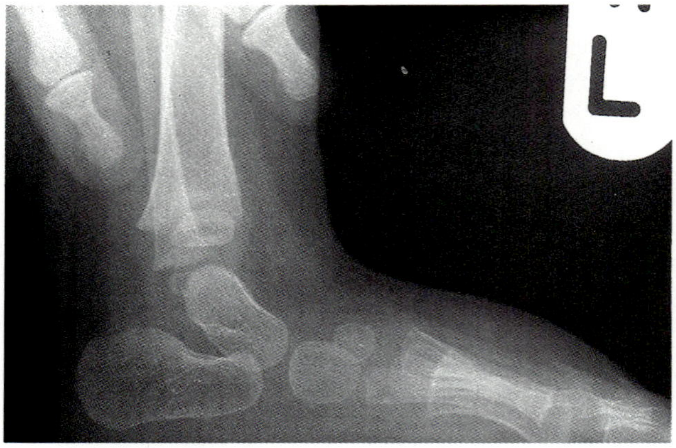

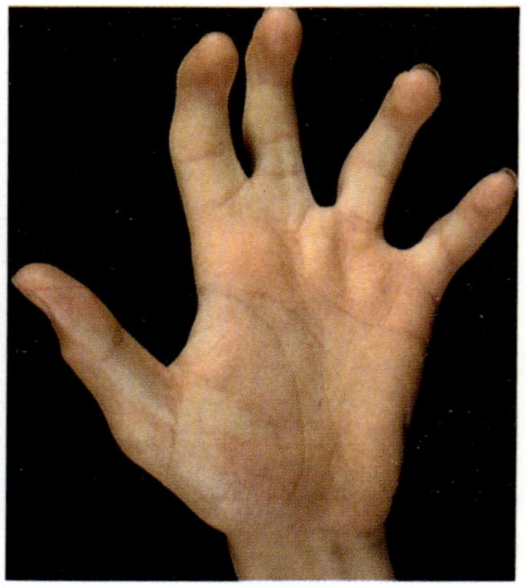

240 Congenital vertical talus. The flat foot in this case was due to a congenital vertical talus.

241 Arachnodactyly.

Disorders of joints and soft tissues: muscle and fascia

Arthrogryposis multiplex congenita

This condition is characterised by stiffness and contracture of joints from birth due to the absence of muscle development around joints. It occurs sporadically and the condition undoubtedly represents a heterogeneous group of arrested intrauterine myopathies and neuropathies.

The condition affects the lower limbs only in 40%, the upper limbs only in 10% and upper and lower limbs in 50%. The condition does not progress after birth and mentality is usually normal.

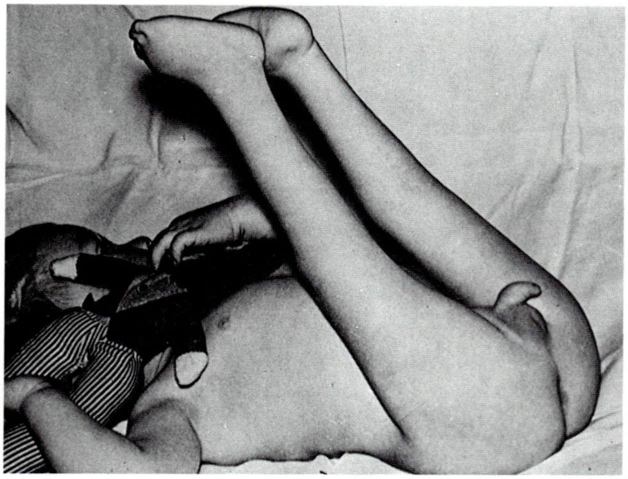

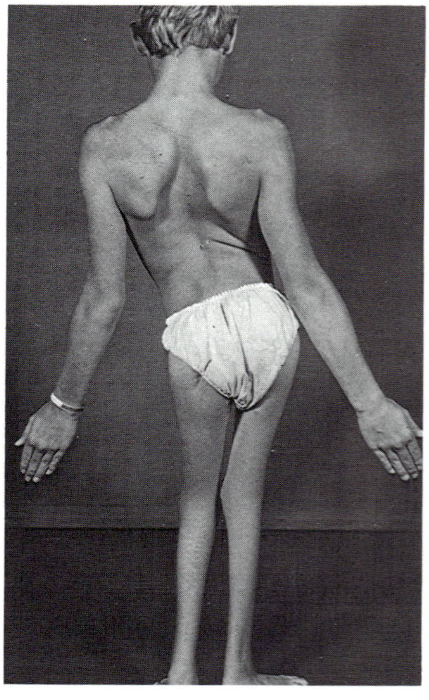

242 & **243** The normal contours of affected joints are lost and skin creases around the joints are absent. The limbs have a cylindrical, pipe-stem appearance.

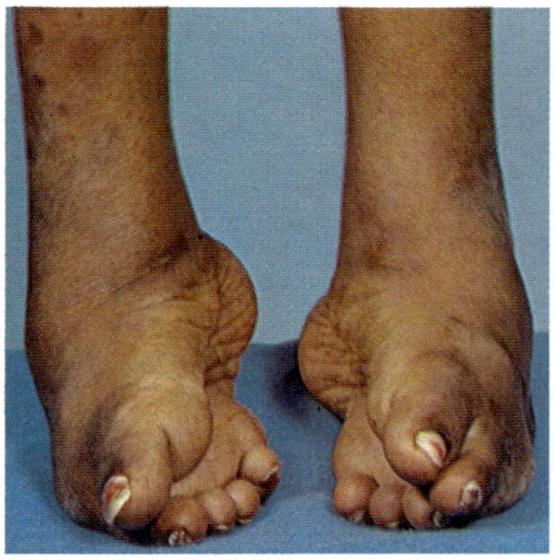

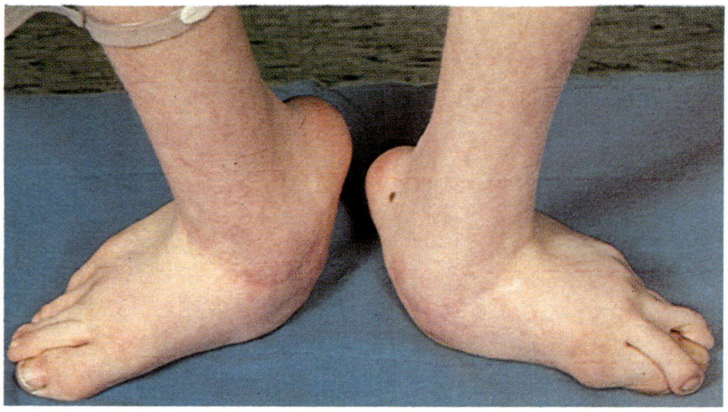

244 & **245** Deformities such as talipes, vertical talus, scoliosis and hip dislocations are frequently present.

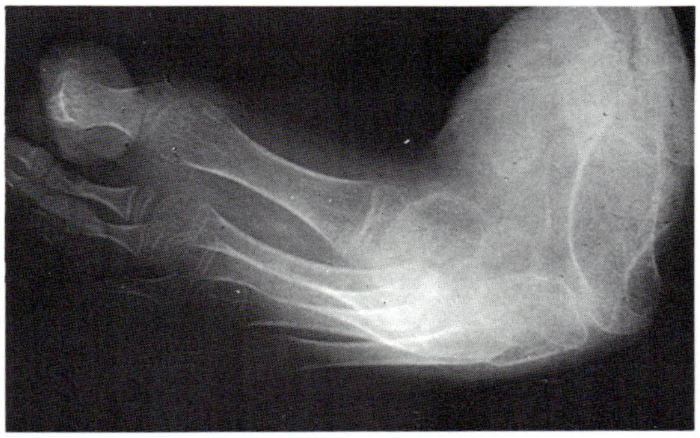

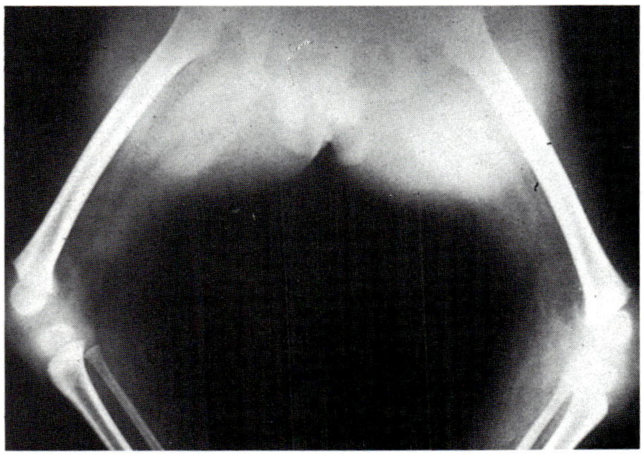

246 & **247** Radiographs show normal bone pattern but gross deformity of joints, which often includes dislocation. Radiographs of long bones show the diminished muscle mass and muscle pattern in the limb.

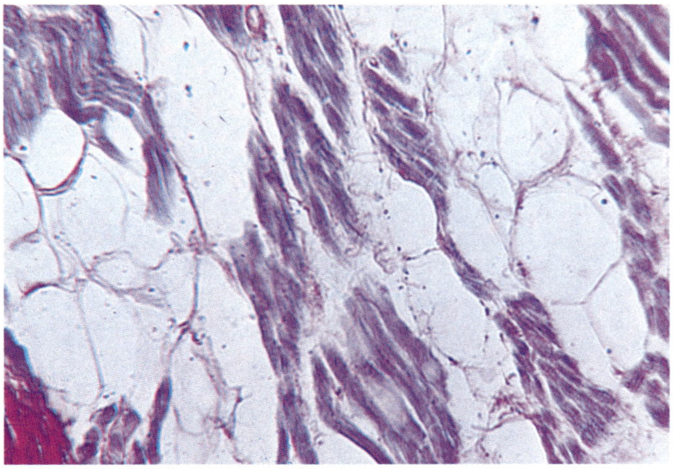

248 Histopathology shows fatty infiltration of muscle. (*x 75*)

The muscular dystrophies

This group of inherited conditions have a variable clinical presentation, some being manifest in early childhood and others not being apparent until adolescence or early adulthood. They also demonstrate variable patterns of inheritance.

Duchenne's muscular dystrophy (X-linked recessive)

This is the commonest (80% of all cases) and the severest of the muscular dystrophies. It is of X-linked recessive inheritance, affecting only males and becomes clinically apparent within the first 3 years of life. Affected children show a characteristic technique of rising to the feet by pushing themselves upright with their hands progressively working up their legs (Gower's Sign) (**249**). There is progressive muscular weakness, in the early stages the muscles are enlarged, particularly the calves (pseudohypertrophy) (**250**). Scoliosis may occur due to progressive weakness of trunk muscles. The patient usually becomes unable to walk in early adolescence and death by the age of 20 years is usual (**251**). The serum creatinine phosphokinase (CPK) level is elevated in affected individuals and in the female carrier.

There are other, less severe varieties of X-linked recessive muscular dystrophies characterised by the later onset of weakness in adolescence or even adulthood. Frequently weakness is localised to the pelvic or shoulder girdle musculature in the early stages, though progressive weakness does slowly occur.

249

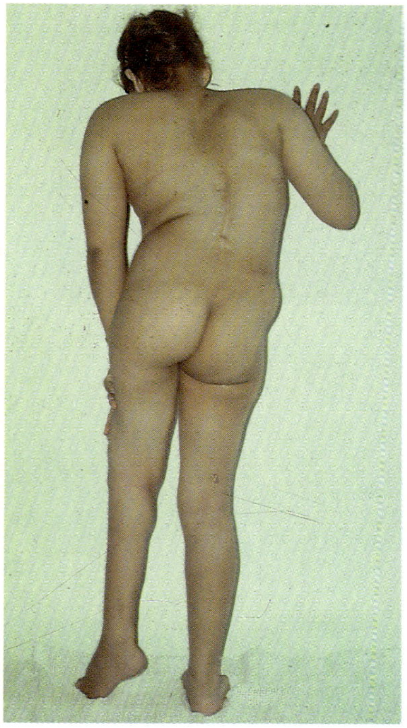

250

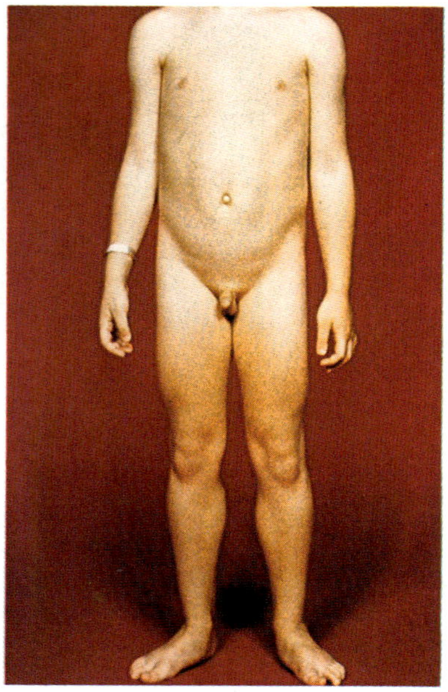

249–251 Duchenne's muscular dystrophy

251

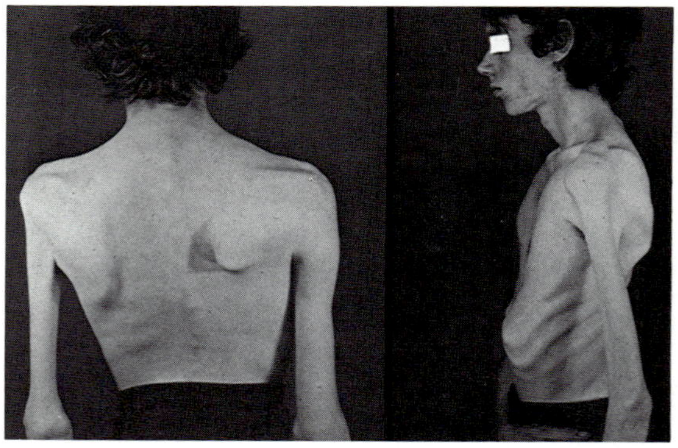

Muscular dystrophies of autosomal recessive inheritance

A Duchenne type of muscular dystrophy affecting both males and females does occur, the clinical course, however, is milder than the classical disease.

Limb girdle muscular dystrophy has its onset in the twenties or thirties age group. Proximal limb muscles are most severely affected resulting in contractures. Death occurs in middle age.

Muscular dystrophies of autosomal dominant inheritance

Facioscapulohumeral dystrophy becomes apparent during the second decade of life. Progress of the disease is slow and relatively benign. The expectation of life is good.

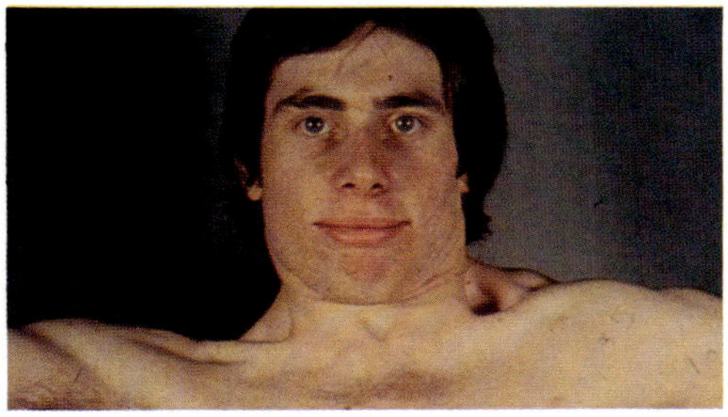

252 Tapir mouth. The characteristic facies with pouting lips owing to weakness of the orbicularis oris muscle.

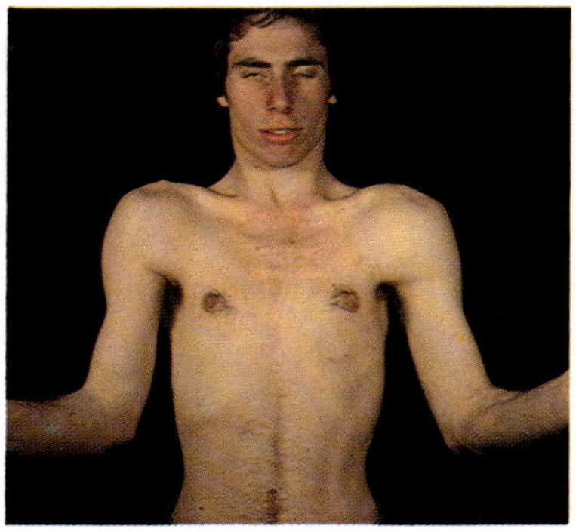

253 Note the discrepancy between the powerful arms and loss of muscle bulk of the chest.

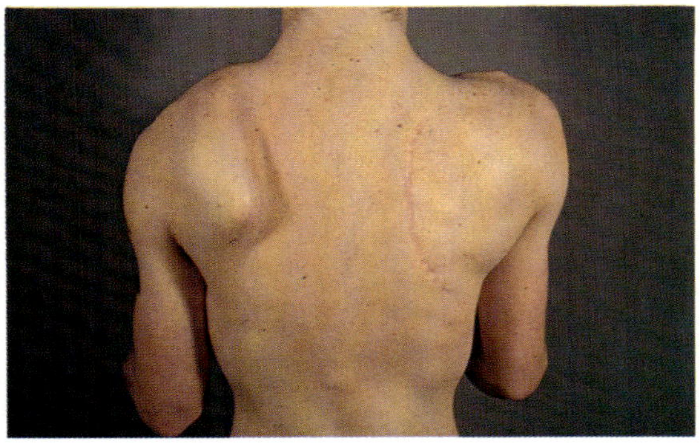

254 The right scapula has been fused to the chest wall at operation, and its stabilisation has improved shoulder girdle function on the right side. Characteristic winging of the scapula can be seen on the unoperated side.

Metabolic and endocrine disease

Bone is a dynamic structure continually being remodelled with bone resorption and mineralisation occurring simultaneously at various sites.

This remodelling process is dependent upon adequate dietary calcium and Vitamin D and a normally functioning endocrine system. Disturbances in either can lead to bone disease.

Rickets and osteomalacia

Rickets and its adult equivalent osteomalacia have a variety of causes behind the common finding, at cellular level, of a failure of bone mineralisation.

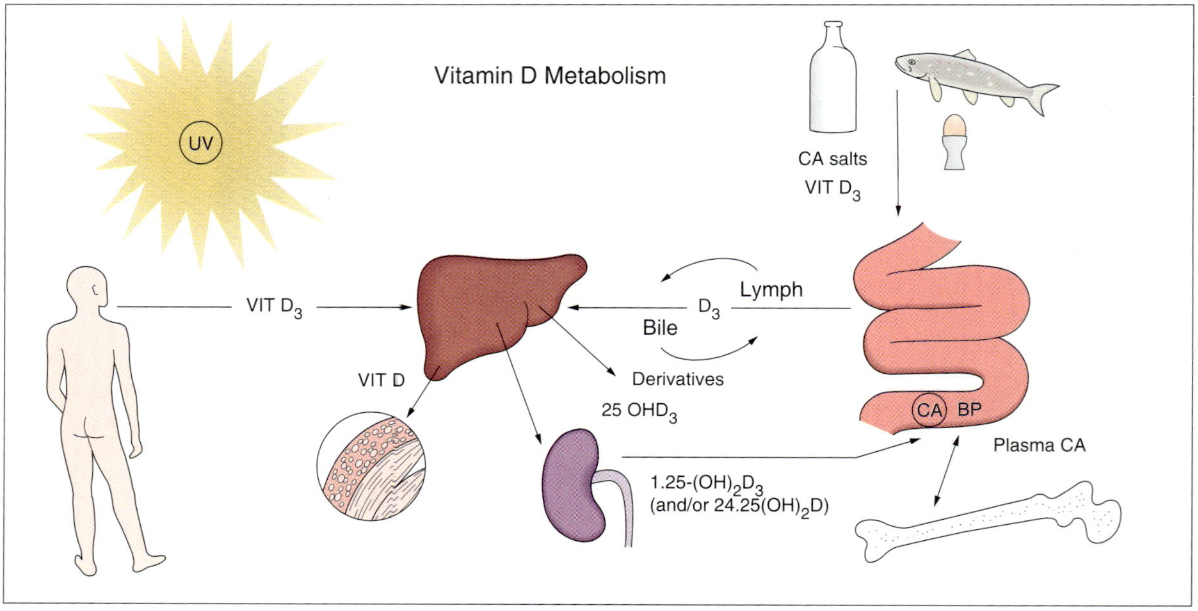

255 Vitamin D metabolism. Dietary vitamin D deficiency and poor solar irradiation with failure of the synthesis of skin cholecalciferol are among the commonest causes of rickets and osteomalacia. Failure of intestinal absorption, pancreatic and liver disease are often compounded with calcium and magnesium deficiencies. Phosphate or bicarbonate loss from the kidneys or the failure of the kidneys to elaborate vitamin D are the mechanisms behind most cases of renal rickets. Other causes include anticonvulsant drugs and excessive use of diphosphonates or aluminium hydroxide.

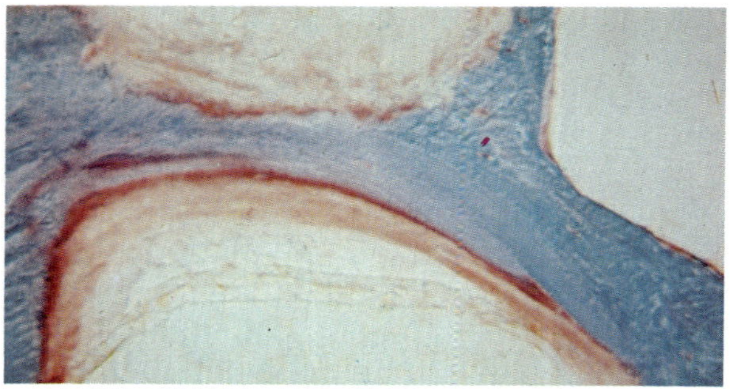

256 Normal bone. The bone salts are dyed blue; the osteoid tissue is stained pink. The relation between mature calcified bone (blue) and immature unmineralised osteoid (pink) is noted. On the right-hand side of the section a resorption cavity can be seen. (*Solochrome–cyanin x 100*)

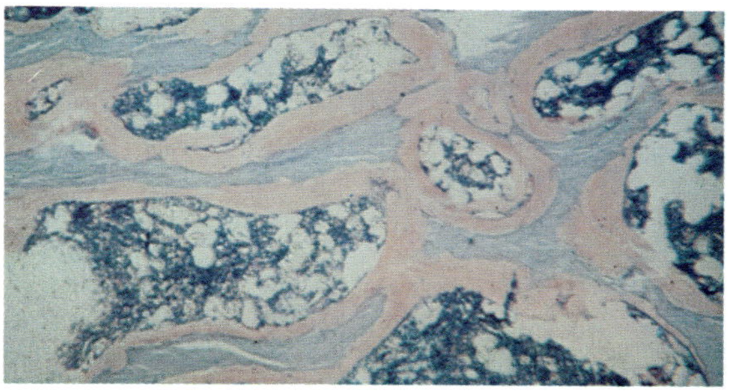

257 Osteomalacia. There is inadequate mineralisation. A decrease of mature bone (blue) compared with osteoid tissue (pink). (*× 50*)

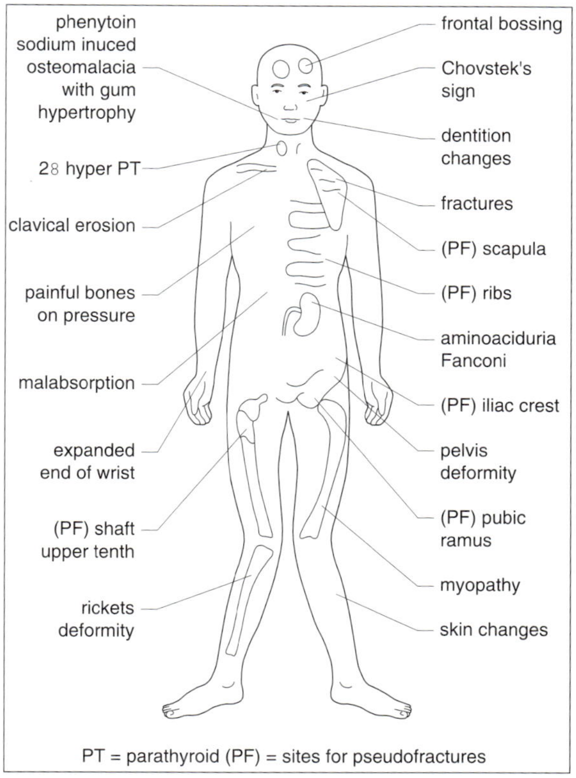

258 Rickets and osteomalacia – clinical features.

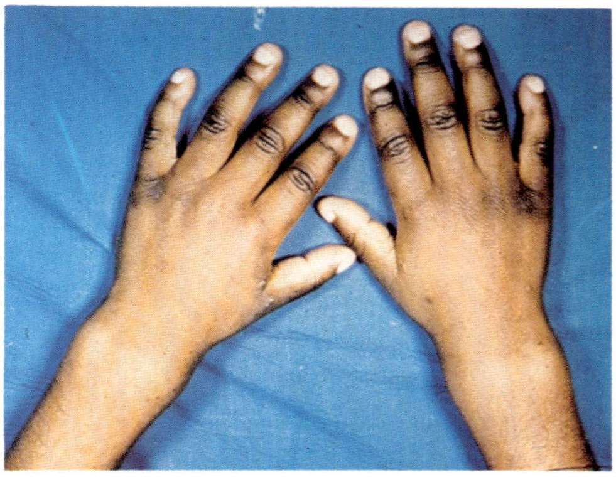

259 Nutritional rickets. The swollen wrists of a child suffering from inadequate vitamin D intake. The swelling is caused by enlargement of the radius and ulna at their lower end where most growth occurs.

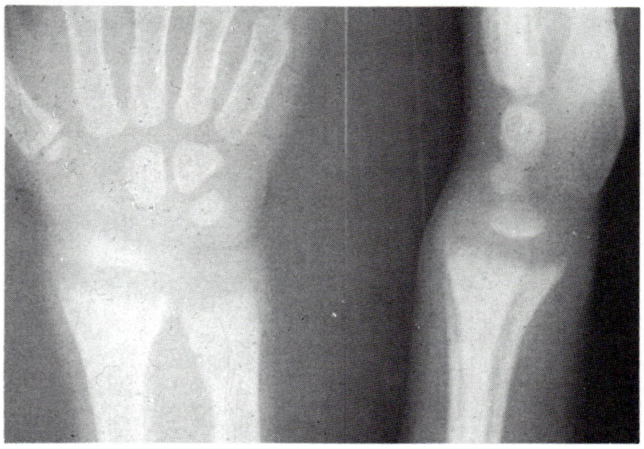

260 Radiograph to show the abnormal and enlarged growth-plates of radius and ulna due to the impairment of normal ossification of growth cartilage.

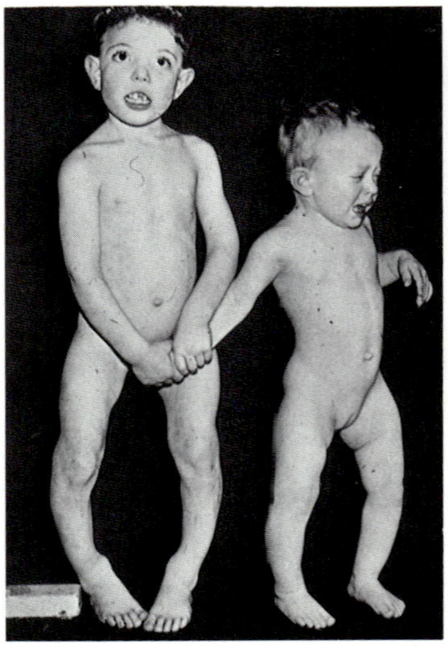

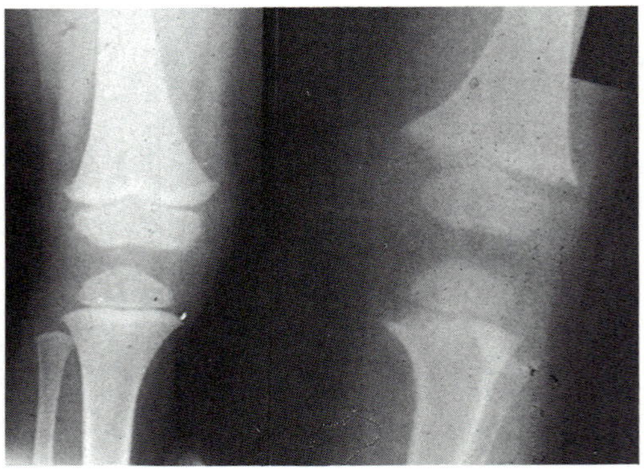

262 Rickets. Radiographs of the knee joints of a normal and rachitic child for comparison. The enlarged and irregular growth-plates and the relative loss of bone density are obvious.

261 Hereditary hypophosphataemic rickets. In this condition the renal tubules fail to re-absorb phosphorus, thereby interfering with the normal metabolism of bone salt. Only one type of renal tubular deficiency rickets occurs.

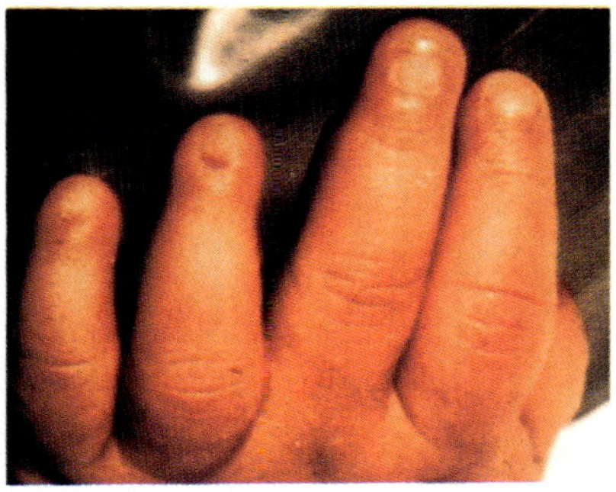

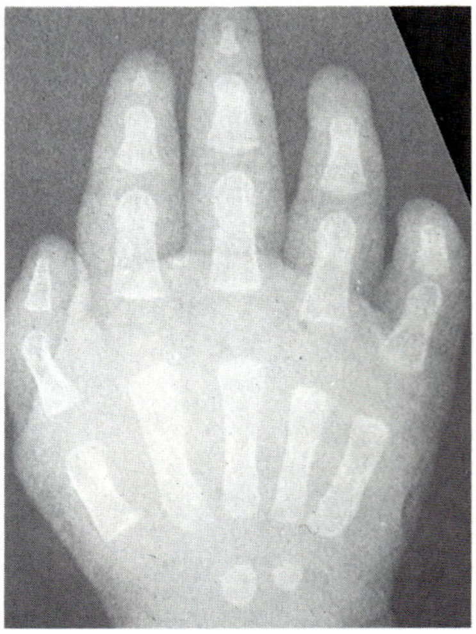

263 & **264** Phenytoin rickets. This is an example of the interruption of vitamin D metabolism in the liver. Prolonged anticonvulsant therapy with phenytoin may impair vitamin D metabolism, probably by an enzyme failure in the liver. Radiographs show the severe atrophy of the distal phalanges.

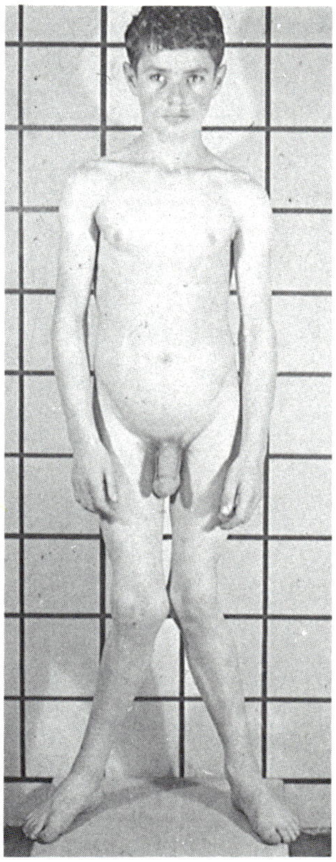

265 Rickets in a child due to renal damage. Because of impairment of renal function by kidney disease in childhood, the normal calciumphosphorus metabolism has been altered.

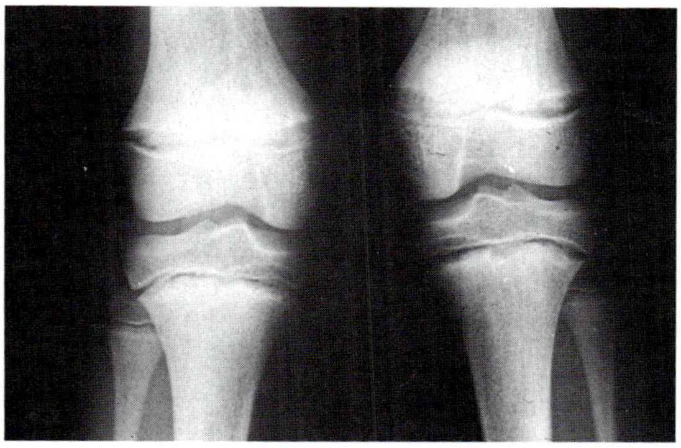

266 Radiographs of the knees in the same patient.

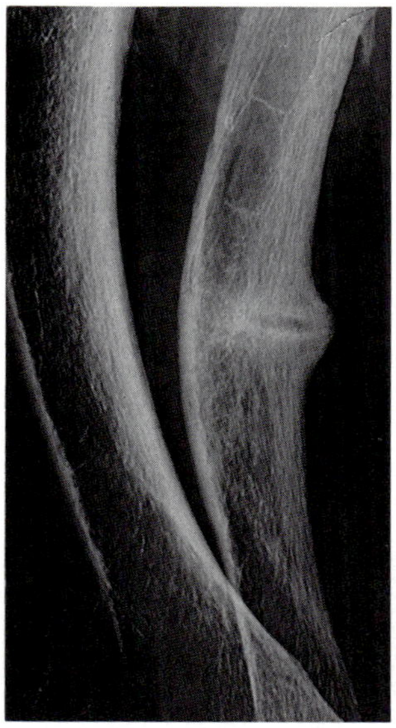

267 A typical osteoid seam (Looser's zone) in a rib; a form of pathological fracture in osteoporosis and osteomalacia.

Osteoporosis

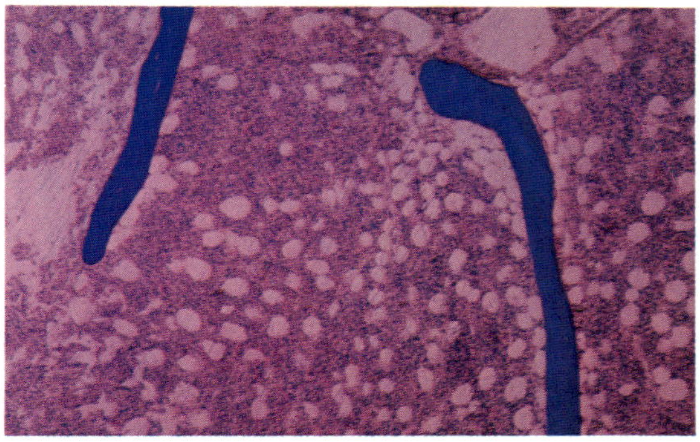

268 The bone that has been formed is of normal composition, but there is an insufficient total amount. An undecalcified section shows that the mature bone (deep blue) is of normal structure, but considerably diminished. It lies in haemopoietic marrow.

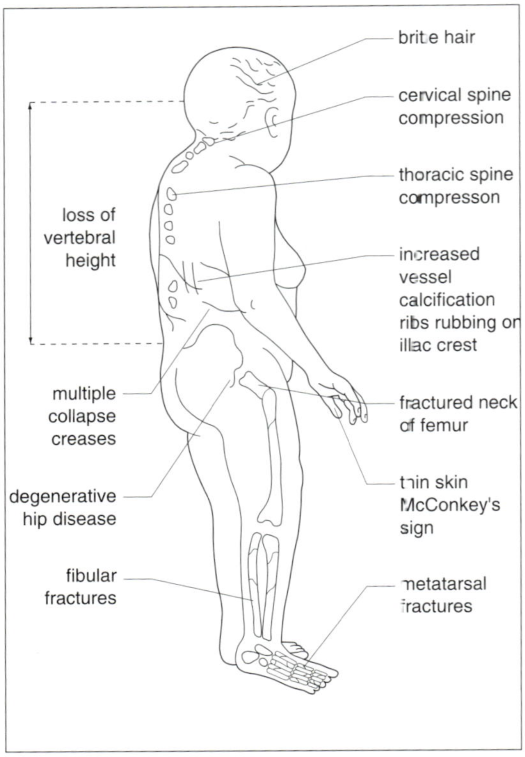

269 Osteoporosis – clinical features.
Causes of osteoporosis:

- Senile or post-menopausal
- Endocrine: Cushing's disease Thyrotoxicosis.
- Idiopathic juvenile osteoporosis
- Disuse osteoporosis

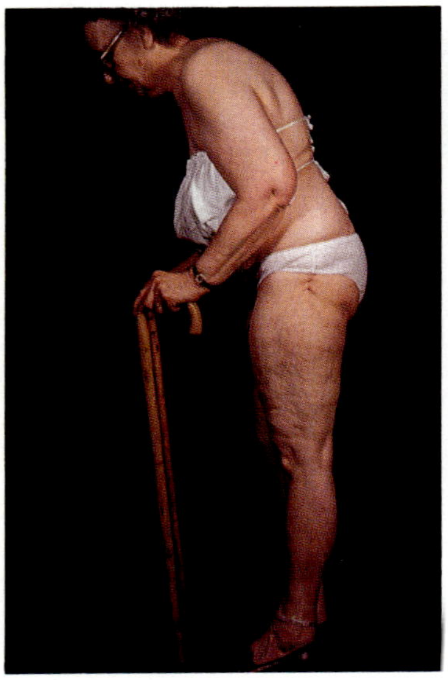

270 Senile osteoporosis. A common disorder probably related to hormonal disturbance of bone metabolism. The first clinical evidence is often the development of a simple forward spinal curvature.

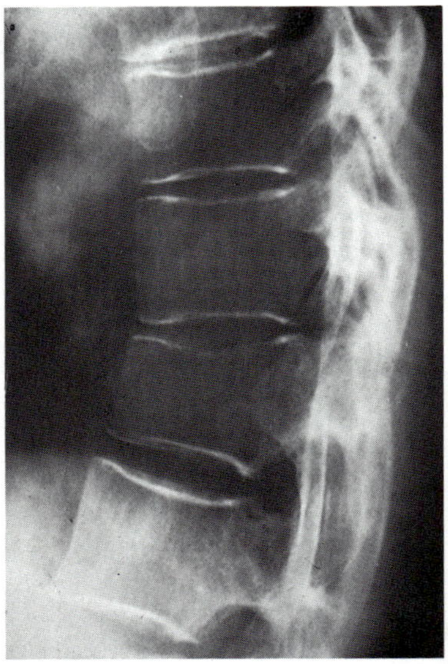

271 Senile osteoporosis. Lateral radiograph of an early case.

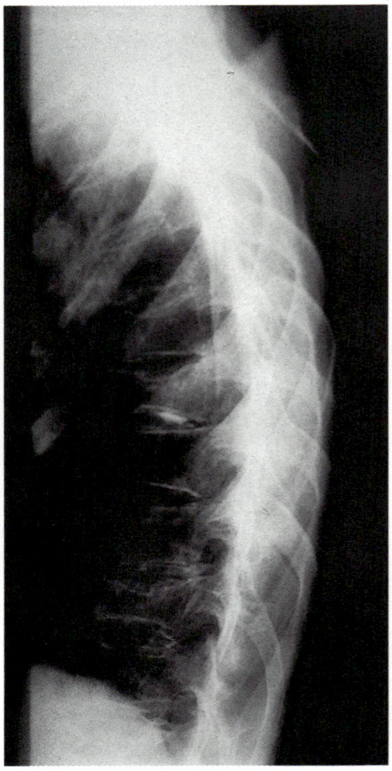

272 In late cases spontaneous vertebral collapse occurs.

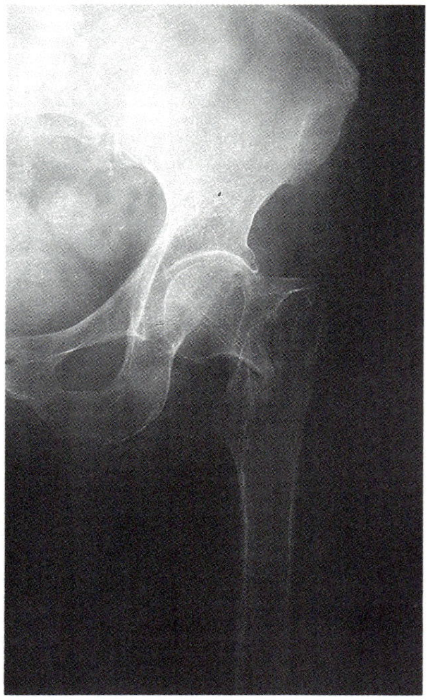

273 Pathological fractured neck of femur. Osteoporosis is the commonest cause of pathological fracture. The subcapital portion of the femoral neck being one of the commonest sites. In many cases this proves to be a terminal event with the later development of deep venous thrombosis and pulmonary embolus.

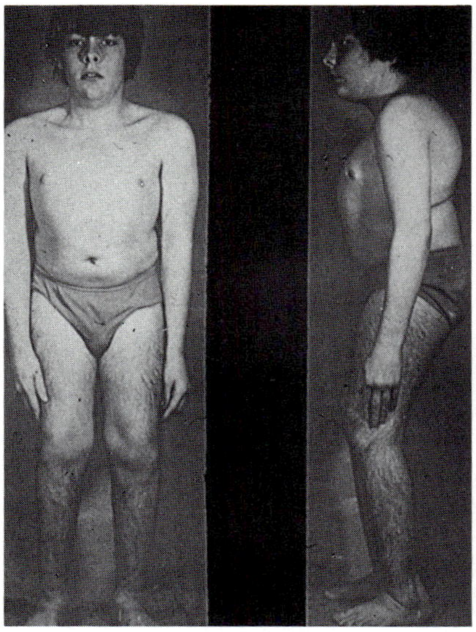

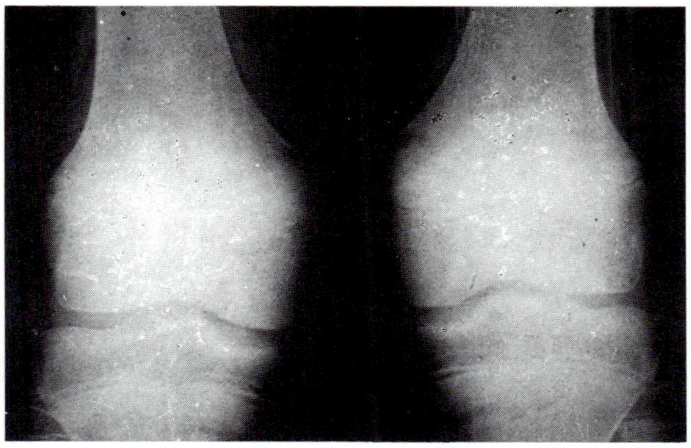

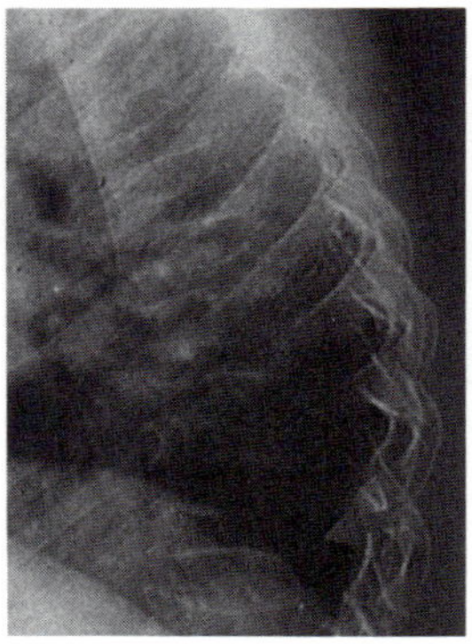

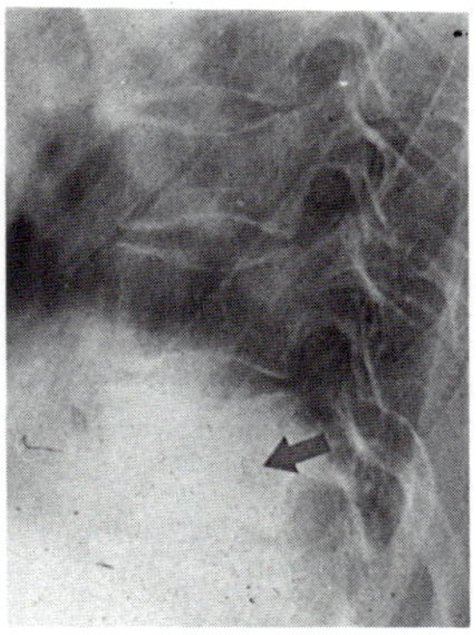

274–277 Idiopathic juvenile osteoporosis. No disturbance of vitamin D metabolism can be established and the bone that is formed is of normal density and structure, but there is too little of it. The dorsal vertebrae in this case show early collapse and a tendency to a biconcave shape.

Paget's disease of bone

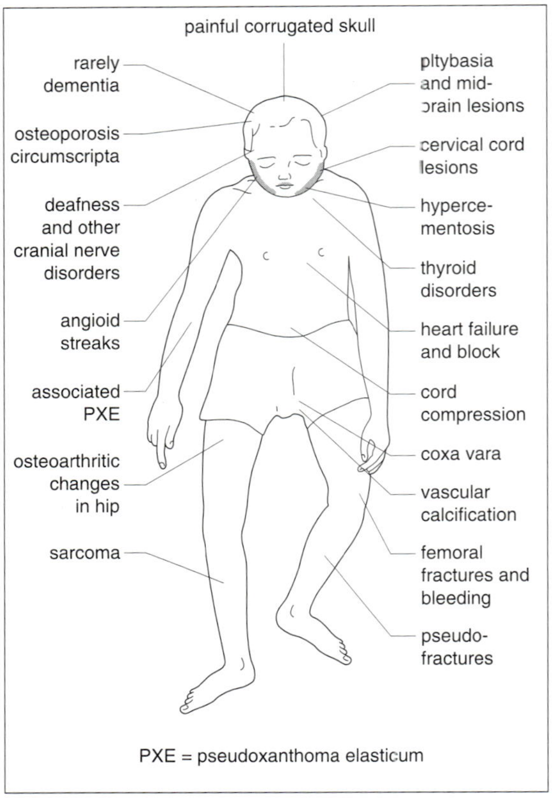

278 This is a disease of unknown origin which mainly affects the skeletal system of middle-aged and elderly people; it is most common in Great Britain, United States and Australasia. Night pain, deformity, progressive enlargement of the head, bone deafness and other complications may occur. There are three phases: destructive, bone forming, and combined.

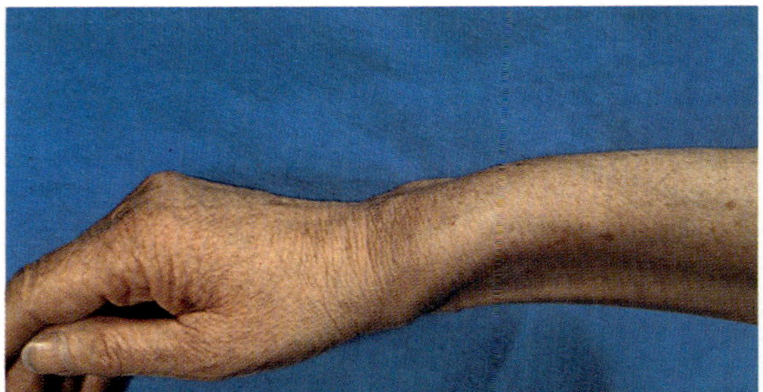

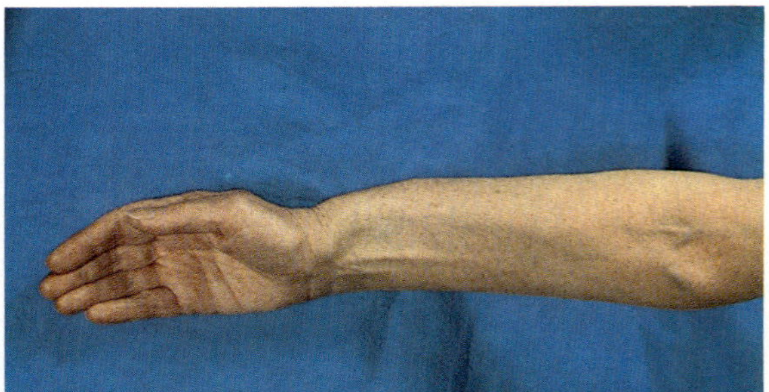

279, 280 Deformity of the forearm due to enlargement and elongation of the radius.

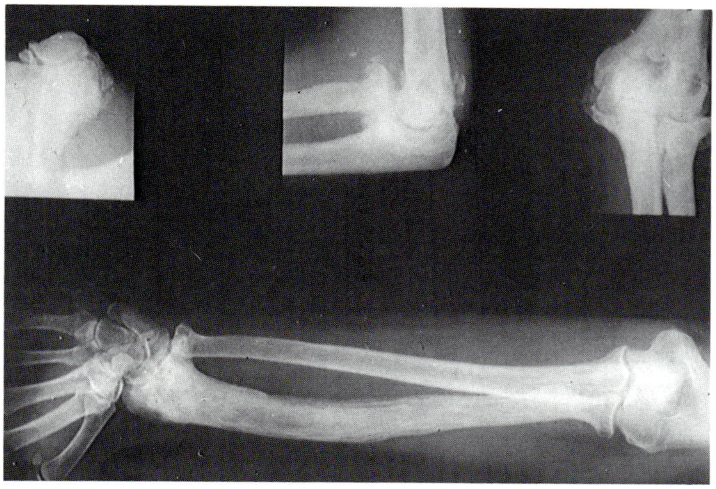

281 A skeletal survey showed that the opposite elbow joint was also affected.

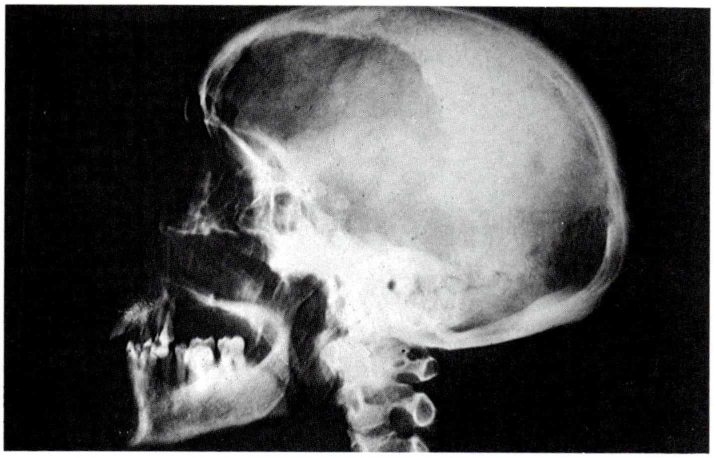

282 The skull showed typical changes of the acute phase of Paget's disease, known as osteoporosis circumscripta.

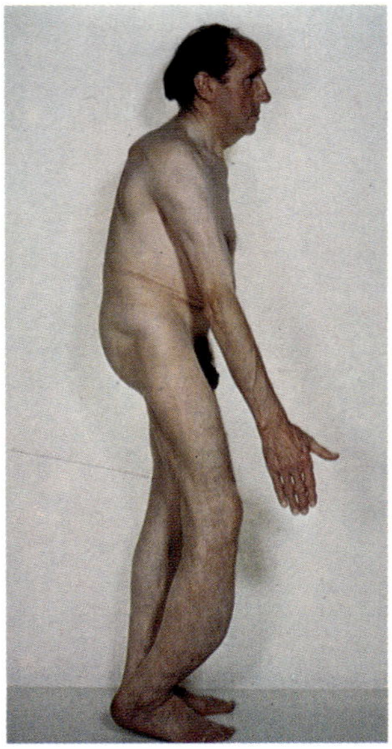

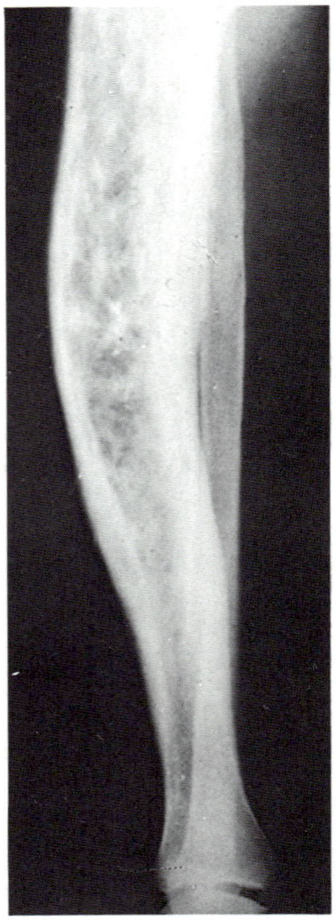

283–286 Paget's disease of bone in its more advanced stage. The patient has a 'sabre' tibia due to actual enlargement of length and bulk of the tibia with anterior bowing. Almost the entire skeleton was involved. The skull shows a more advanced stage of the disease with new bone accretion on the cortex.

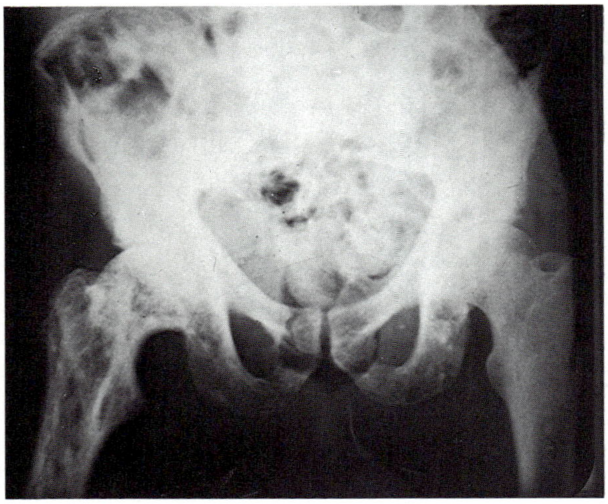

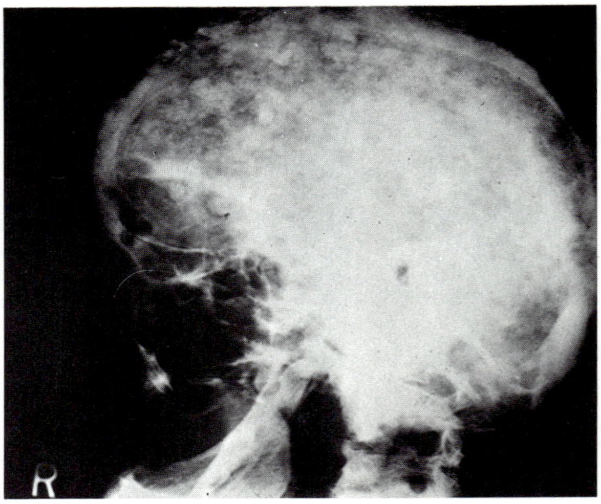

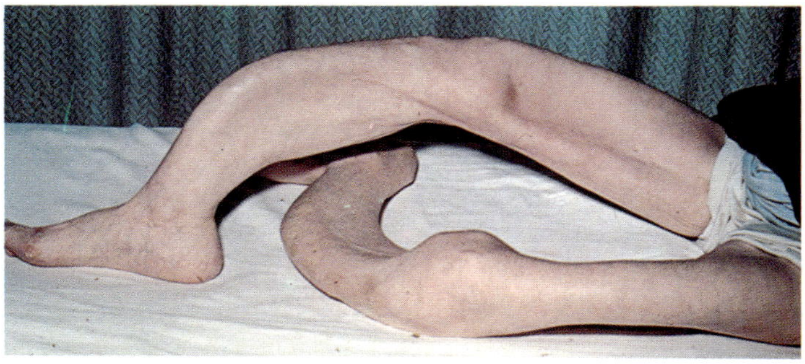

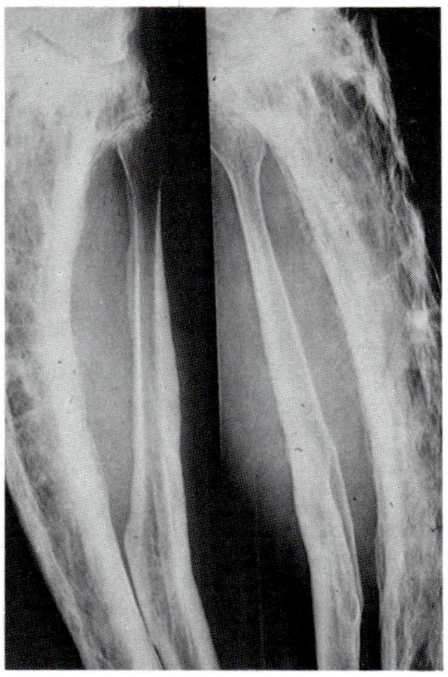

287 & **288** Advanced form of Paget's disease with gross bowing of the tibia and alteration of architectural pattern. The alkaline phosphatase level of this patient was raised to between 65 and 100 *Ka* units (about 10 units is normal).

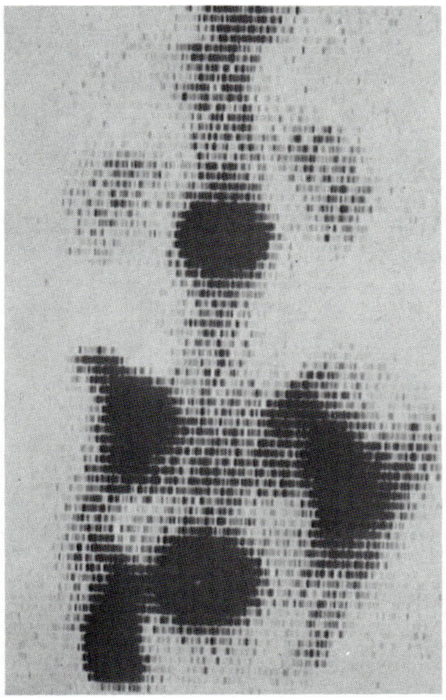

289 Radio-isotope scanning shows considerable increase of uptake of the bone-seeking isotope technetium by the most affected parts of the skeleton.

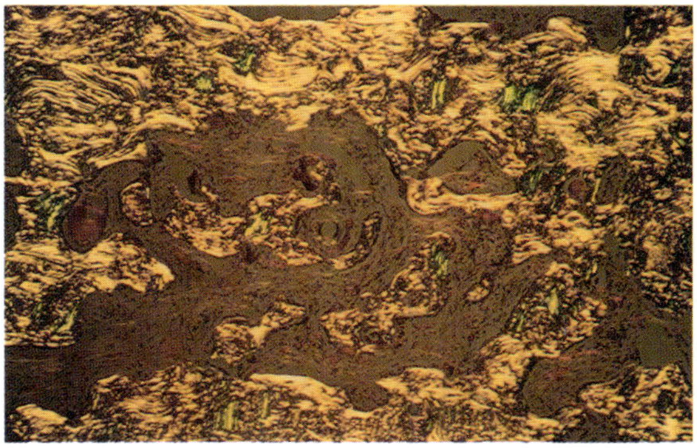

290 Non-lamellar arrangement (woven) bone in Paget's disease viewed in polarised light. (*x 75*)

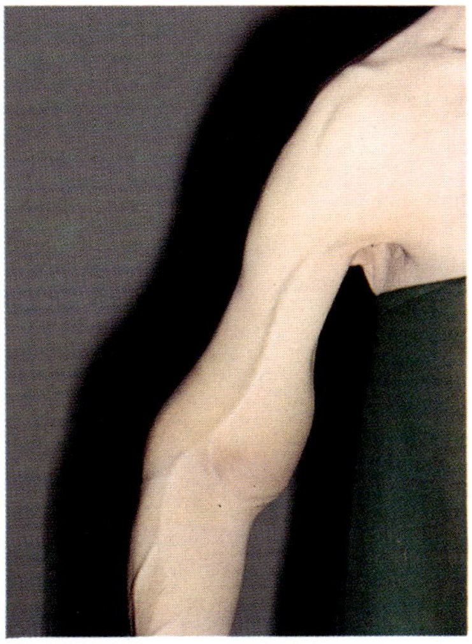

291 Paget's sarcoma of the humerus. Approximately 1% of cases of Paget's disease may advance to develop a sarcoma of variable cell type.

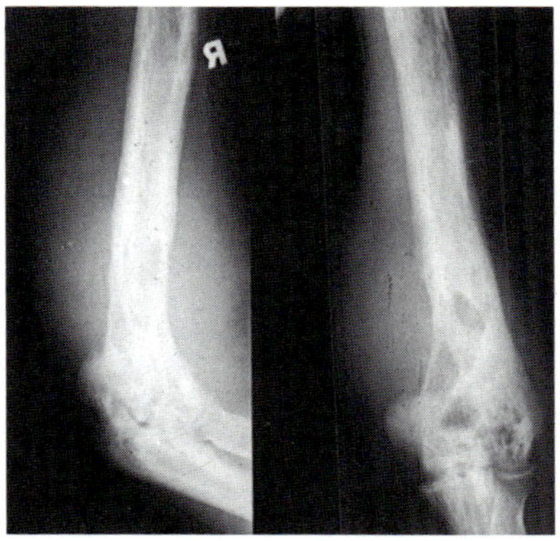

292 Radiograph of the same patient. Note the soft tissue swelling, as well as destruction of the medial cortex.

Parathyroid osteodystrophy and renal osteodystrophy

The parathyroid glands play a vital role in calcium–phosphorus metabolism and disturbance of their function is consequently noted in the skeleton. Primary hyperparathyroidism is caused by a tumour in the gland. Secondary hyperparathyroidism (the more common) is caused by hyperplasia of the gland, and is usually associated with chronic renal failure.

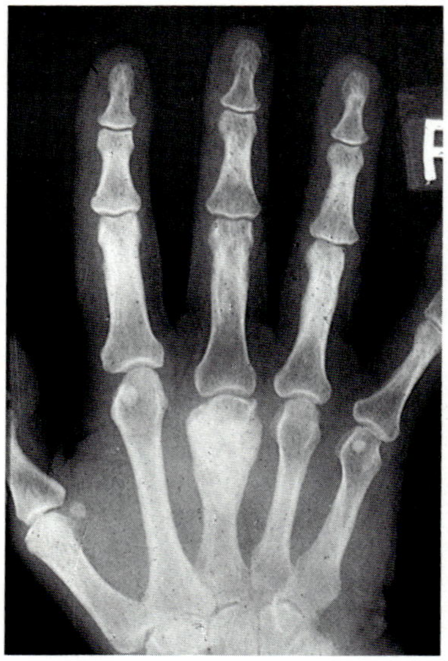

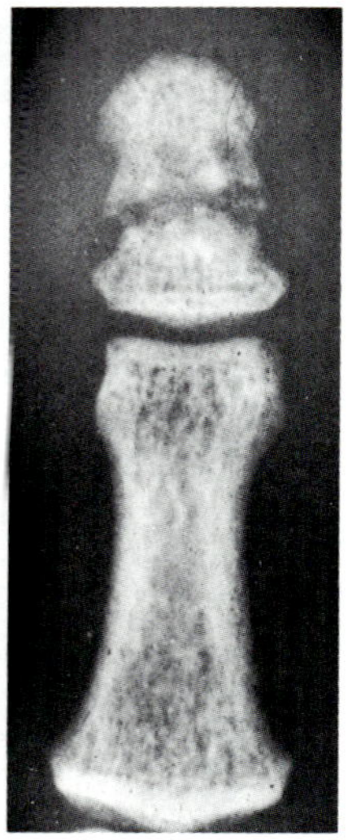

293 & **294** Primary hyperparathyroidism. Approximately 20% of patients have a skeletal lesion, most commonly in the hands. Sub-periosteal resorption of the phalanges in the middle and ring fingers is noted. A 'brown tumour' expands the middle metacarpal bone.

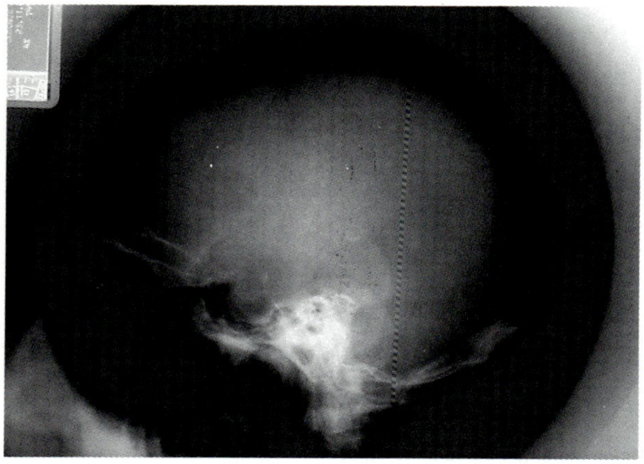

295 The skull shows a characteristic punctate loss of bone density resulting in the 'pepper-pot skull' appearance.

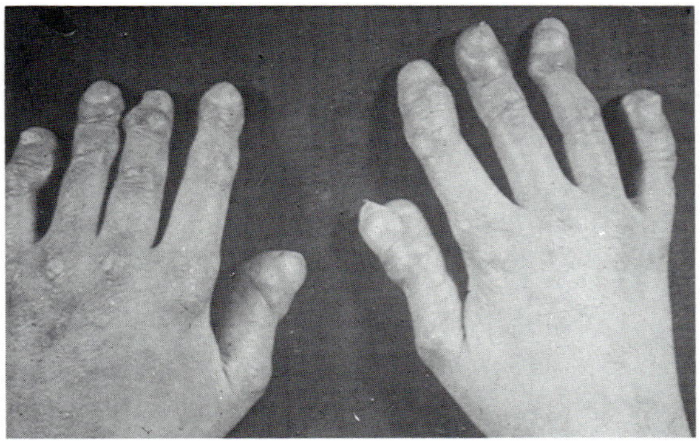

296 Secondary hyperparathyroidism to show pseudoclubbing.

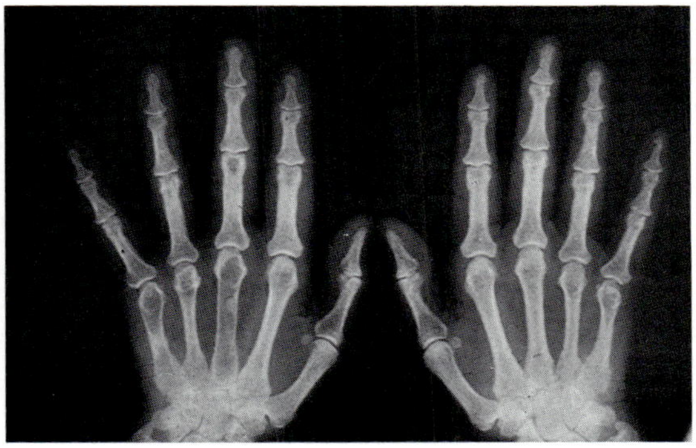

297 Radiographs show resorption of the terminal phalanges.

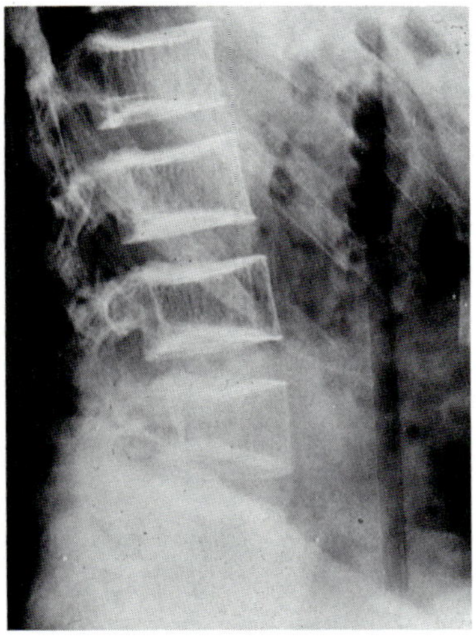

298 Typical 'rugger-jersey' effect in the spine in secondary hyperparathyroidism caused by demineralisation of the vertebral bodies, with simultaneous new bone formation at the subchondral plates.

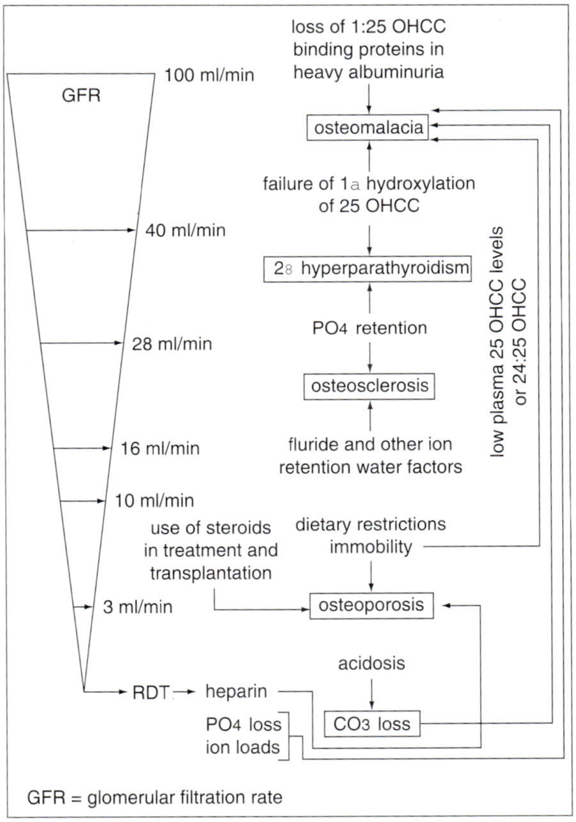

299 Renal Osteodystrophy. The bone lesions in chronic renal disease include osteomalacia, osteitis fibrosa cystica caused by secondary hyperparathyroidism, osteosclerosis and osteoporosis. The mechanisms by which these bone lesions are brought about are shown.

Soft tissue 'calcification' syndromes

These are a heterogeneous group of conditions, and in many, the aetiology and mechanism of calcium or in some cases osseous deposition remains obscure. The deposition of calcium or heterotopic calcification may usefully be divided into two groups:

- **Metastatic calcification:** the precipitation of calcium salts in apparently normal tissues and as a general rule has a metabolic cause, resulting in a disturbance of calcium and phosphate metabolism. There is frequently, but not always, hypercalcaemia.
- **Dystrophic calcification:** the deposition of calcium salts in dead or degenerate tissue and is the more frequently encountered type in orthopaedic practice. Dead or degenerate tissue includes post-traumatic haematomas, thrombi, or degenerate tendons. In many of the circumstances encountered in orthopaedic practice there has been an episode of trauma.

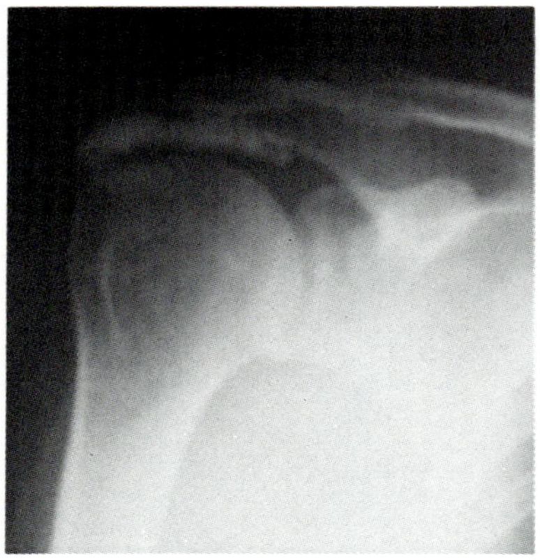

300 Acute calcific supraspinatus tendinitis. Although degenerative changes in the supraspinatus tendon may play a part, the condition frequently presents in the younger age groups and trauma to the tendon is very likely a major cause.

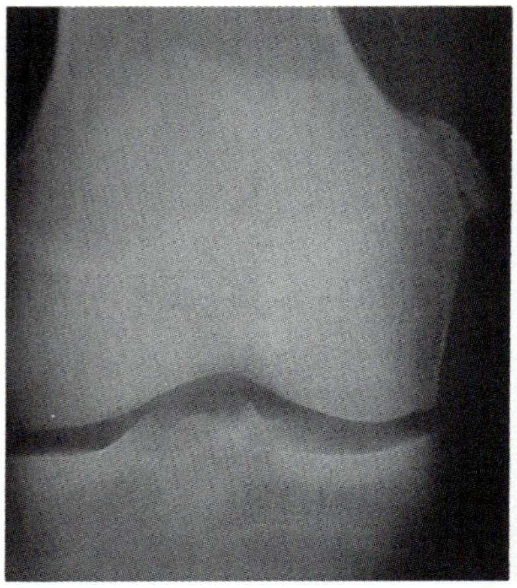

301 Pelligrini Stieda Lesion. Calcification at the femoral attachment of the medial collateral ligament of the knee at the site of a previous sprain.

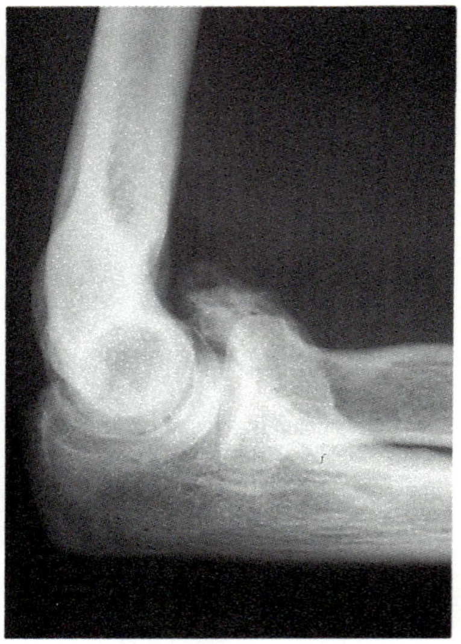

302 Following trauma around the elbow calcification in muscles and tendons is not unusual resulting in marked stiffness.

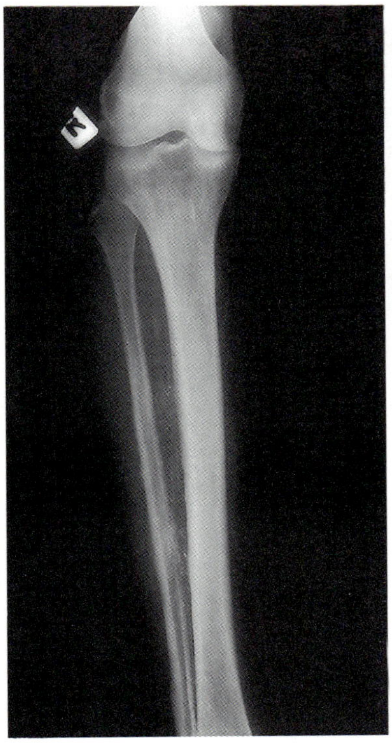

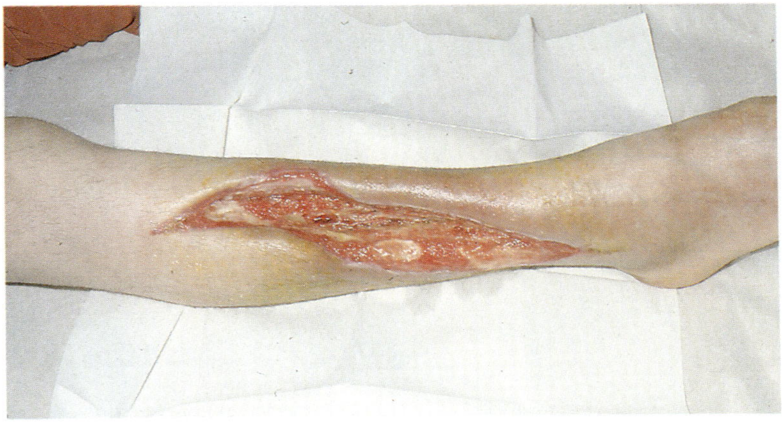

303 & **304** Following a dislocation of the knee this patient developed ischaemic necrosis of the anterior tibial compartment muscles. Years later, after dystrophic calcification had occurred, the calcium salts discharged through sinuses and debridement of the muscle compartment was required.

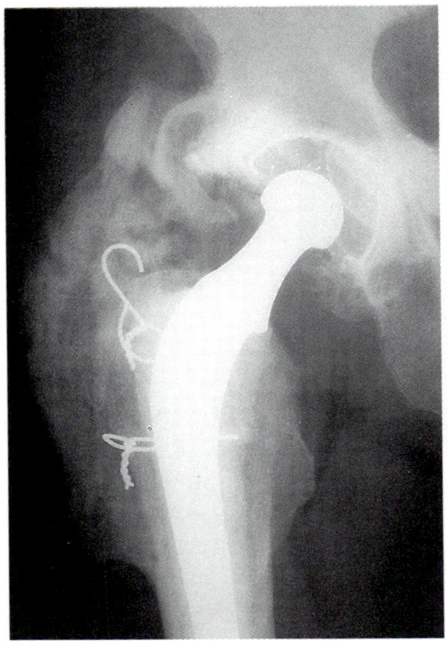

305 Heterotopic bone formation following total hip replacement.

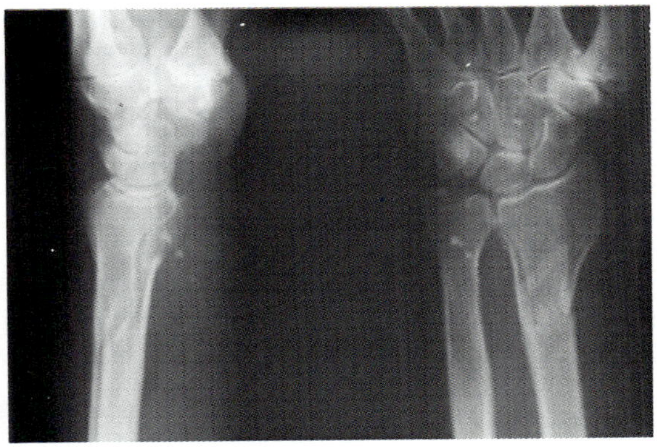

306 Phlebolithic calcification in a haemangioma of the wrist.

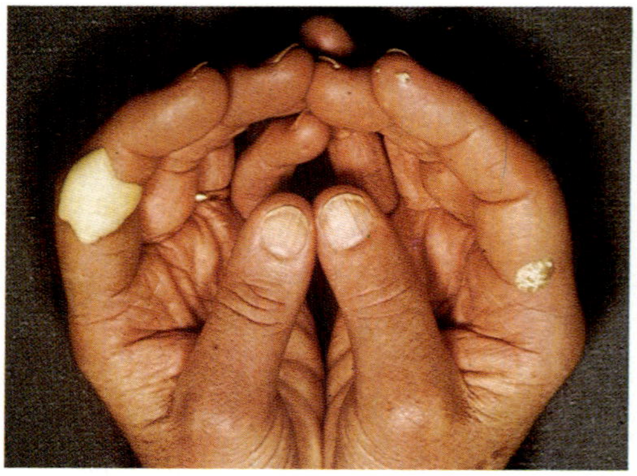

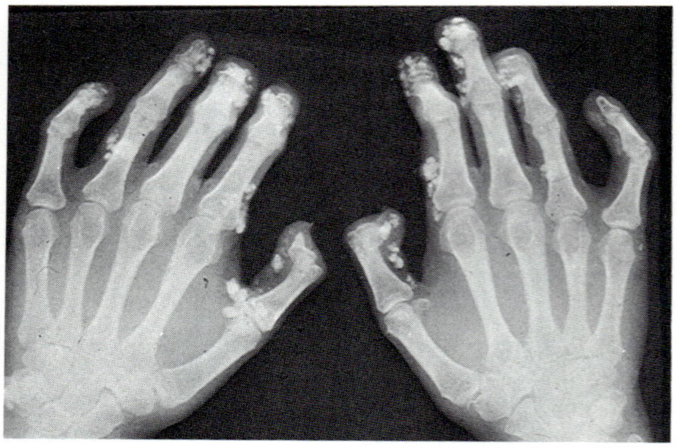

307 & **308** Calcinosis circumscripta. Diffuse calcinosis of the skin and subcutaneous tissues of the hands occurs in a number of the collagen diseases including rheumatoid arthritis. SLE and dermatomyositis but is most commonly seen in systemic sclerosis where it may be associated with scleroderma, Raynaud's phenomenon and cutaneous telangiectasia.

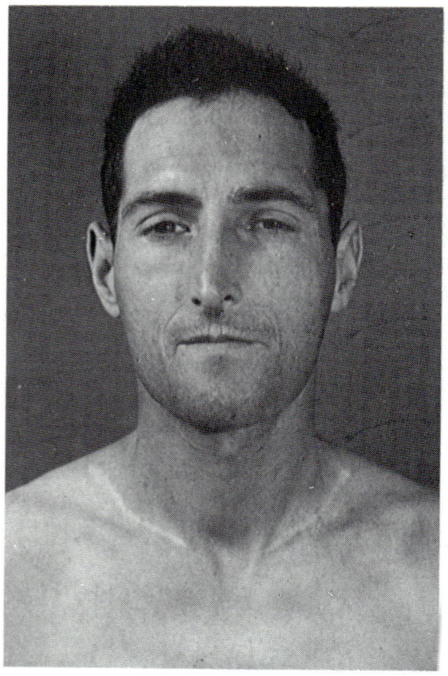

309 Scleroderma may affect the mouth at an early stage. Patients develop pinched, mask-like facies.

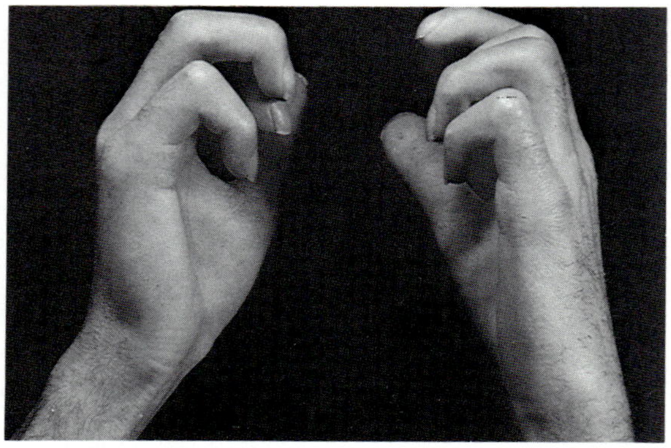

310 Scleroderma. The hands of a patient showing taut, shiny skin extending to involve all the joints with some atrophy of the distal segments of the fingers.

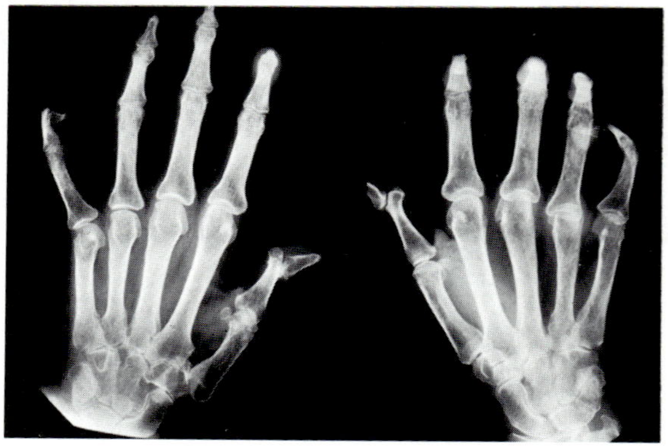

311 Radiographs show the conical pointing and resorption of the terminal phalanges.

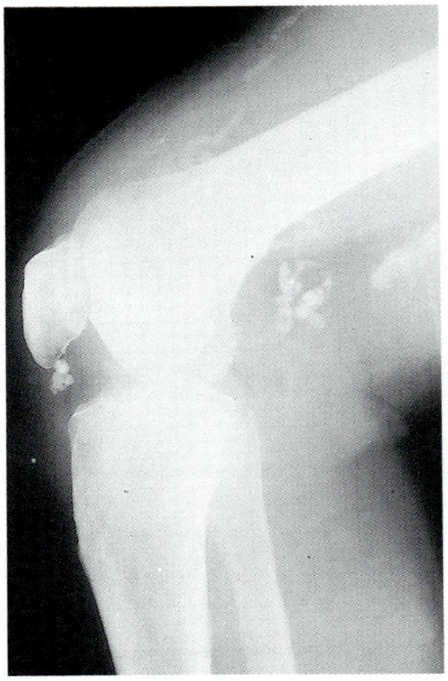

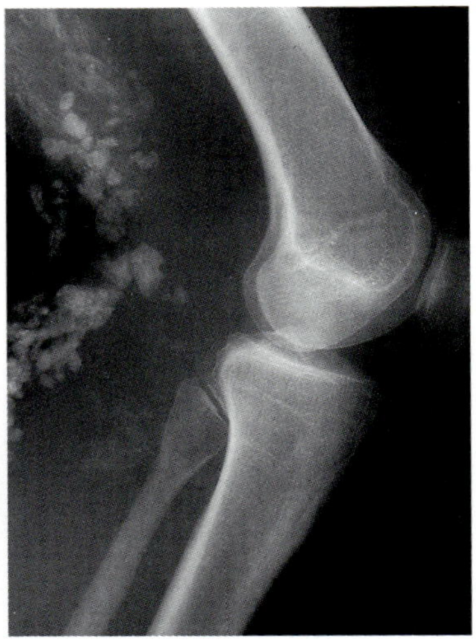

312 & **313** Calcinosis universalis. This is a rare more generalised calcinosis most commonly affecting the limbs. Lesions begin in the subcutaneous tissues, later extending to involve ligaments, tendons and the connective tissue of muscles.

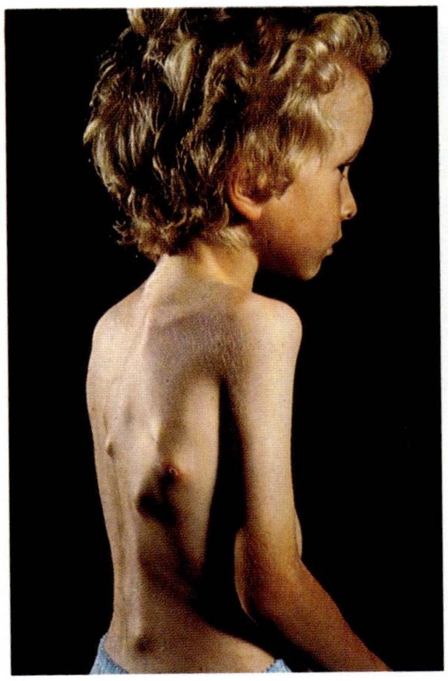

314 Myositis ossificans progressiva is a rare disease in which initially painful masses appear, usually first in the cervical and shoulder girdle regions.

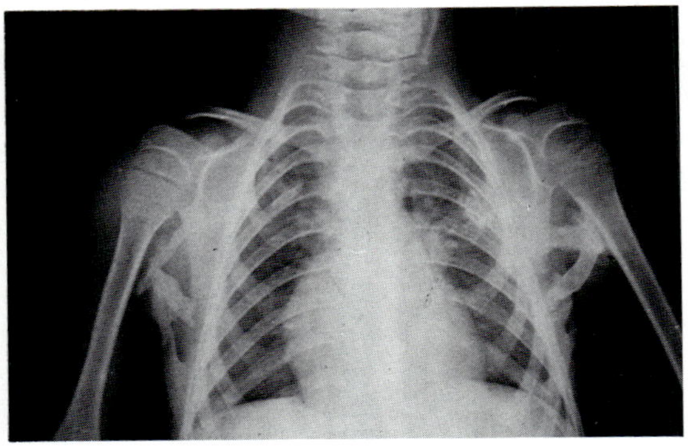

315 The masses of new bone formed in the soft tissues may restrict spine and shoulder movement as well as respiration. The condition should be distinguished from calcinosis universalis.

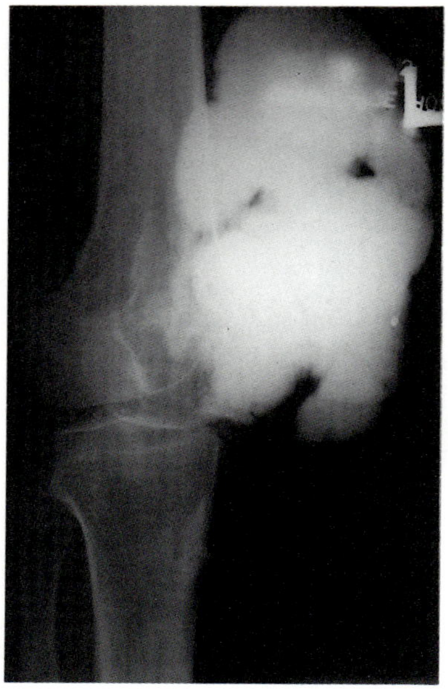

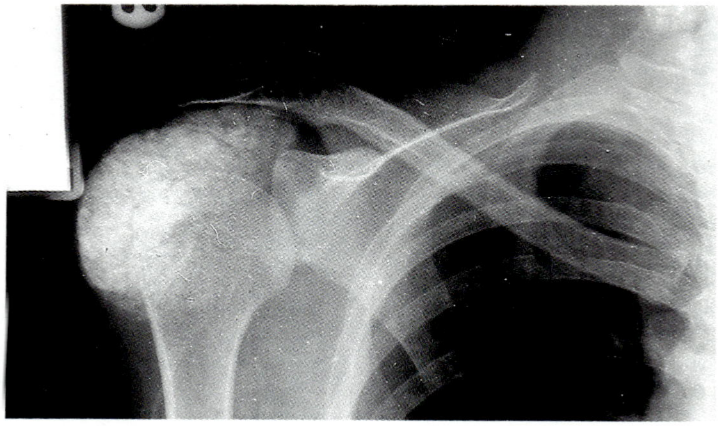

316 & **317** Tumoral calcinosis. Occasionally, heterotopic calcification can take on 'tumour-like' proportions.

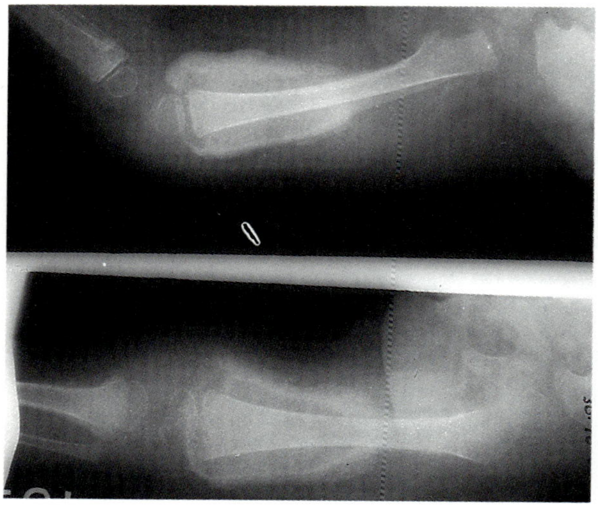

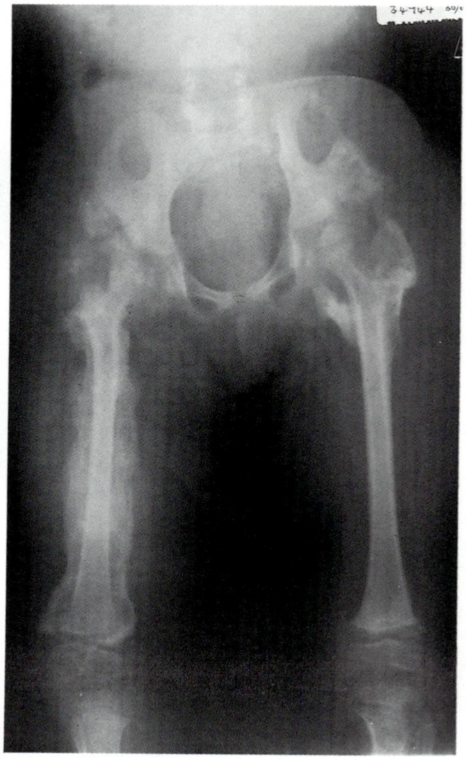

318 & **319** Minor trauma in patients with spina bifida can lead to excessive sub-periosteal new-bone formation and beyond.

Neurology in orthopaedics

There is an intimate clinical relation between orthopaedics and neurology. Since neurology pervades almost the whole of orthopaedic surgery, only a few examples of the more immediate and obvious relation can be shown here.

The effects following poliomyelitis (APM) are extremely variable. Deformities are occasionally due to gravity, but principally depend on the imbalance of muscles. The stronger surviving muscles produce the deformity: a limb that is totally paralysed usually has no fixed deformity. Occasional limb-length inequality develops, particularly if the disease occurred in early childhood.

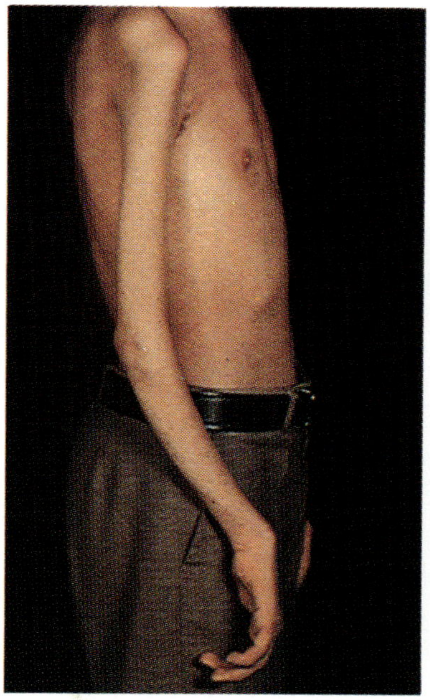

320 Flail arm following poliomyelitis in infancy.

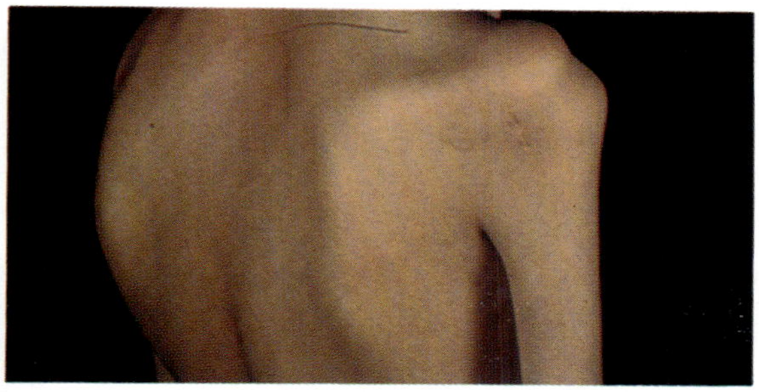

321 Paralytic subluxation of the shoulder. There is obvious wasting of the deltoid.

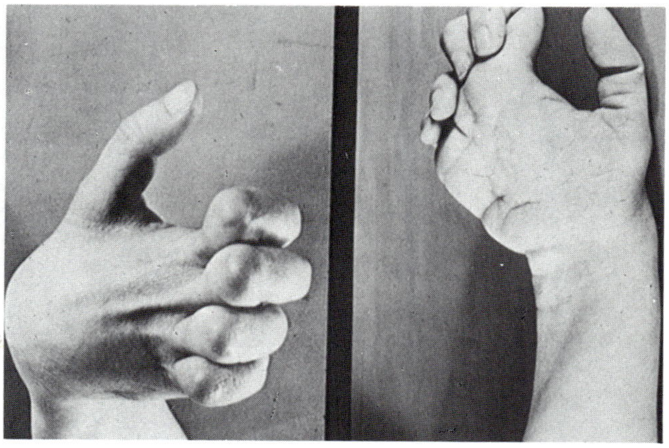

322 Severe claw-hand. Paralysis of the intrinsic muscles of the hand following poliomyelitis. The deformity is due to the fact that the long flexors and extensors of the fingers have not been affected. The claw-hand develops as a result of paralysis of their antagonists – the short intrinsic muscles.

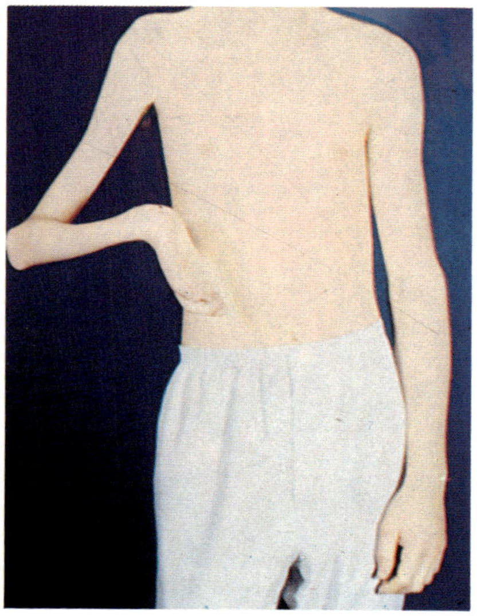

323 Poliomyelitis in infancy affected only the right upper limb in this young man. Weak active abduction of the shoulder and flexion of the elbow are all that remain in this withered and almost flail arm.

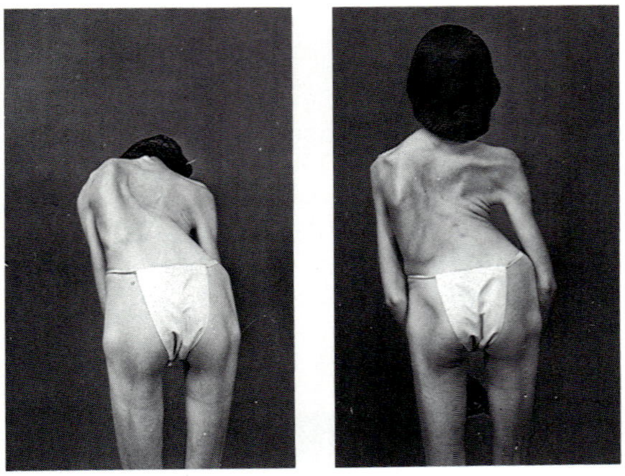

324 Paralytic scoliosis may follow pol omyelitis affecting the trunk muscles.

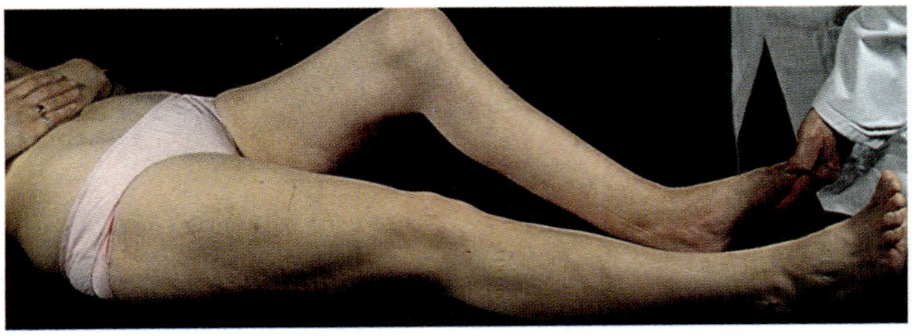

325 Contracture of tensor fascia latae muscle. Because the muscle traverses both hip and knee it can produce flexion deformities at both joints.

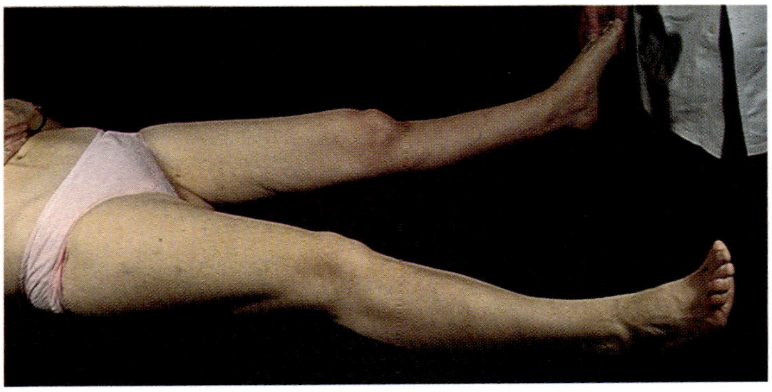

326 Yount's test. Both deformities of the hip and knee are corrected by simple abduction of the hip.

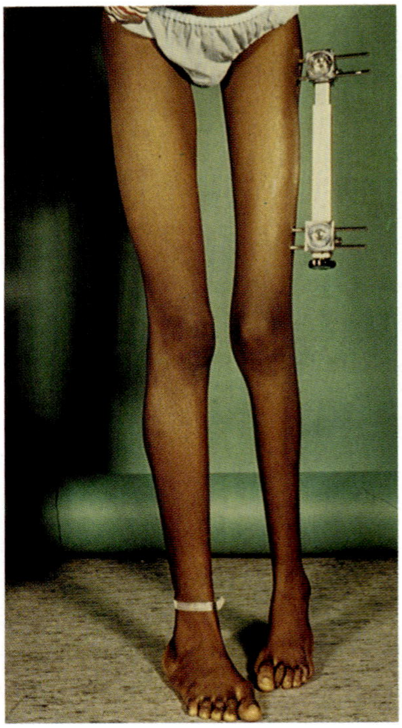

327 Dropped foot (paralytic equinus). Shortening of the left lower limb with equinus deformity of the ankle and foot.
The equinus may be beneficial to compensate for the shortened leg (the patient has a Wagner-type leg-lengthening apparatus *in situ*).

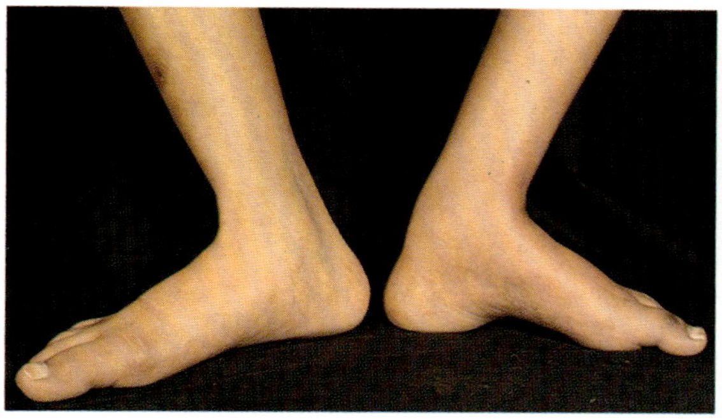

328 Pes calcaneo-cavus: the deformity is caused by paralysis of the calf muscles.

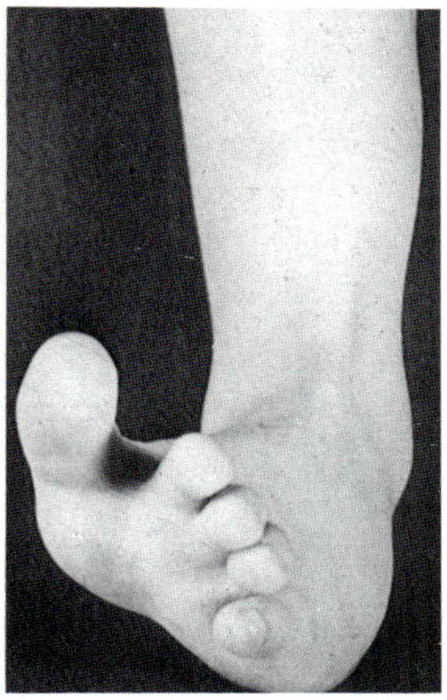

329 Weakness of tibialis anterior and the peroneal muscles. When the subject attempts to dorsiflex the ankle, the toes extend strongly in an attempt to compensate for the loss of ankle dorsiflexors. The deformity is a result of the unbalanced action of normal extensor toe muscles acting in the presence of paralysed tibialis anterior and peroneal muscles.

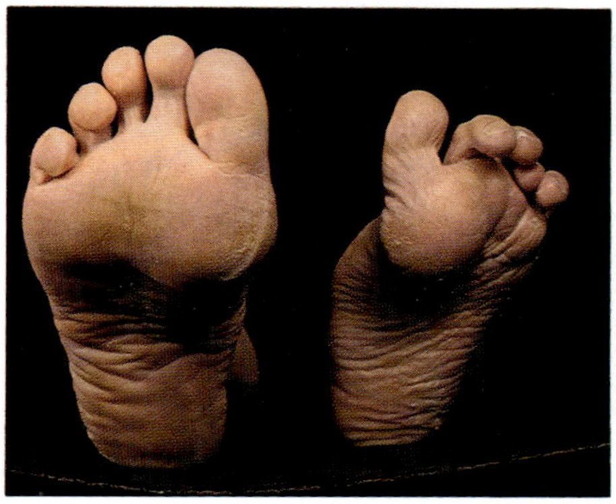

330 The opposite deformity is demonstrated here: the peroneal muscles are the stronger surviving group. The foot therefore moves into forcible eversion with depression of the head of the first metatarsal by the unopposed action of a strongly contracting peroneus longus muscle.

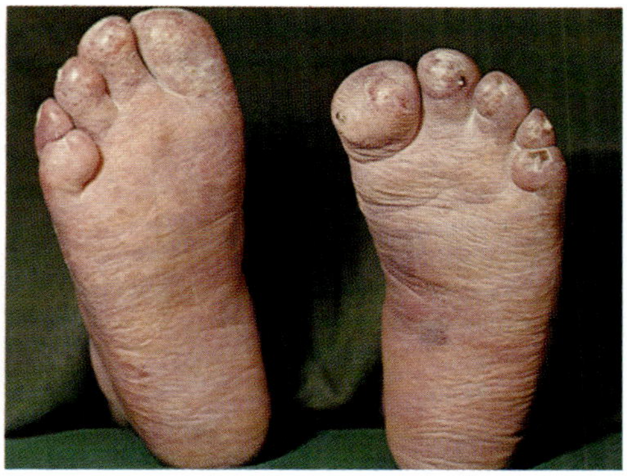

331 Polio-paraplegia in a middle-aged woman, who suffered an attack of poliomyelitis in infancy. There is no active muscle in the lower limbs and therefore no significant deformity. The patient has been living in a wheelchair and trophic changes are seen in the dependent feet.

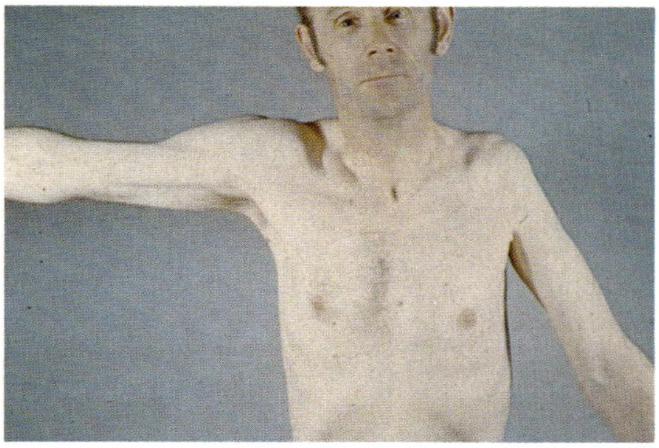

332 Neuralgic amyotrophy (shoulder girdle paralysis). The cause of this condition is uncertain but it is probably of viral origin, or follows immunisation serum. Following an episode of intense pain the patient has lost the ability to abduct his shoulder and there is gross wasting of the shoulder girdle musculature.

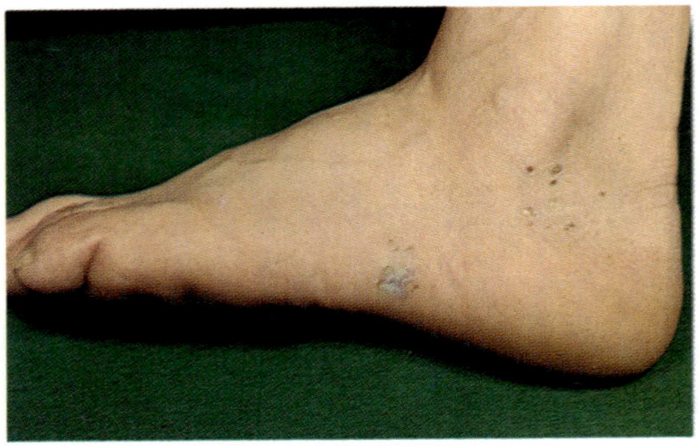

333 Simple herpes zoster skin lesion on the outer border of the foot. Prodromal or post-herpetic neuralgia may simulate 'sciatica'.

Pes cavus and progressive pes cavus

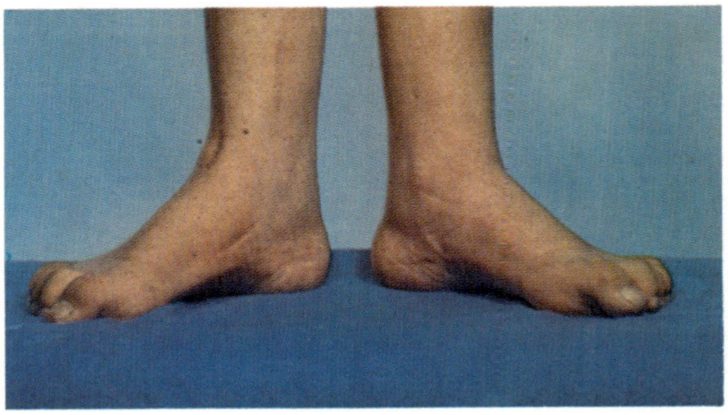

334 Pes cavus. Exaggeration of the arch of the foot is a common orthopaedic presentation of a neurological problem. A family history of high-arched foot is present in nearly half the cases of idiopathic pes cavus. It may be the only manifestation of peroneal muscular atrophy (HMSN Type I). The more carefully that any particular case of pes cavus is studied – particularly bilateral pes cavus – the more apparent becomes a neurological aetiology such as, e.g. Friedreich's disease (see **970**).

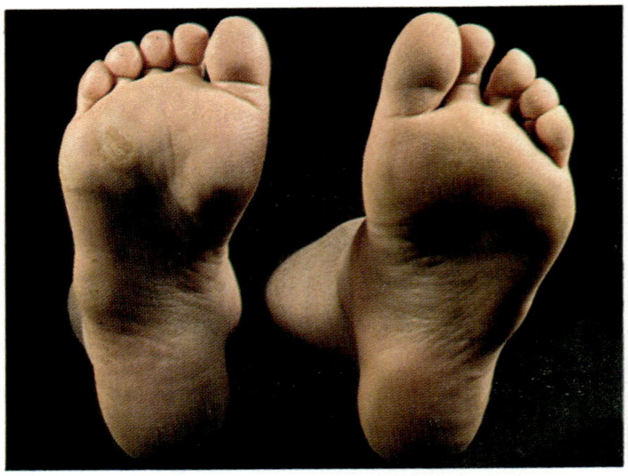

335 Progressive pes cavus: pressure points eventually develop under the heads of the metatarsals.

Peroneal muscular atrophy

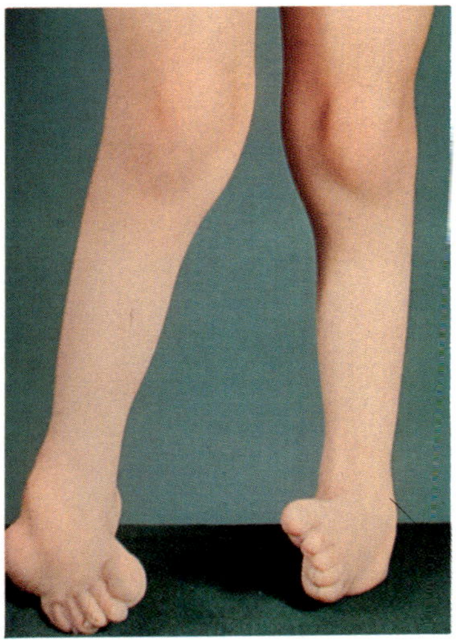

336 Peroneal muscular atrophy (Charcot–Marie–Tooth disease, HMSN Type I). Pes cavus is often the presenting symptom; shortening and distortion of the foot may, however, occur later. Wasting of the leg below the knee may be seen early in the disease. Severe talipes equino varus may develop. The gross deformity of a so-called 'Rooster's leg' is depicted here.

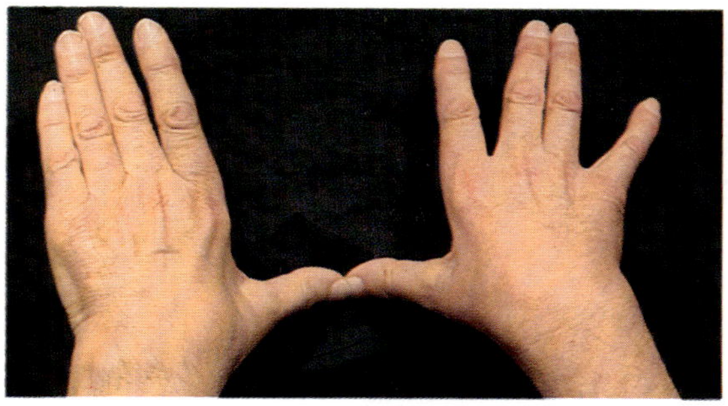

337 Wasting of the intrinsic muscles of the hands may develop late in the disease.

Spastic paralysis

Spastic paralysis may present as an orthopaedic problem, either as a consequence of cerebral palsy in infancy, or following a head injury or cerebrovascular disease.

Cerebral palsy embraces a group of disorders due to non-progressive brain damage occurring in the perinatal period from a variety of causes. Spastic, athetoid, ataxic, rigid and atonic varieties are described but the spastic variety demands most orthopaedic attention.

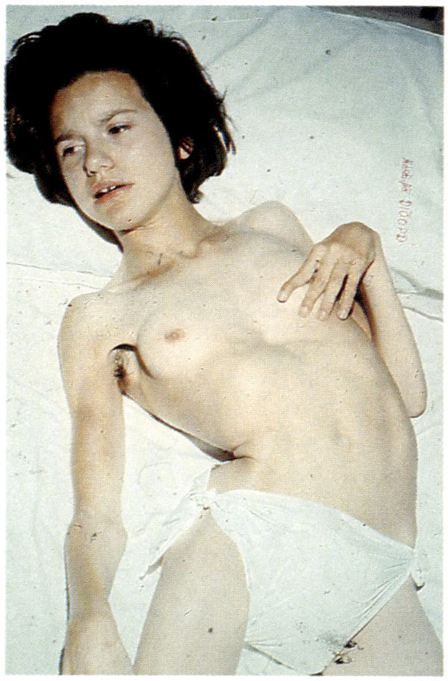

338 Spastic cerebral palsy. Characteristic posture of the left upper limb, adducted at the shoulder, flexed at elbow and wrist with a pronated forearm. A scoliosis is also present.

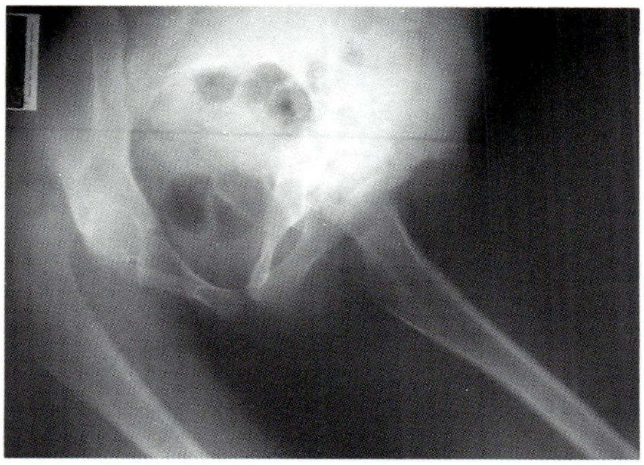

339 Muscle imbalance can lead to 'wind-swept' deformities of the lower limbs. On the adducted side the stability of the hip is compromised. In this case the hip has dislocated.

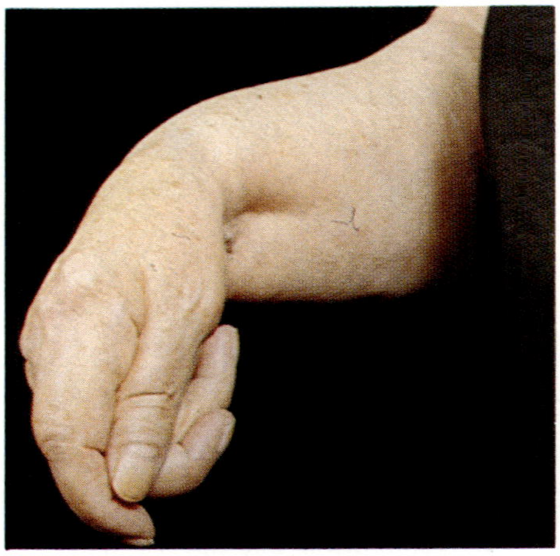

340 Spastic contracture of the wrist and forearm, characteristically held in full flexion and pronation.

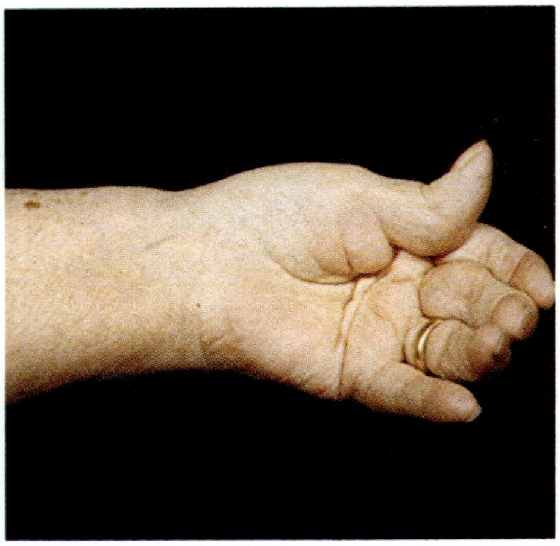

341 Adduction of the thumb in the same patient produces the 'thumb in palm' deformity.

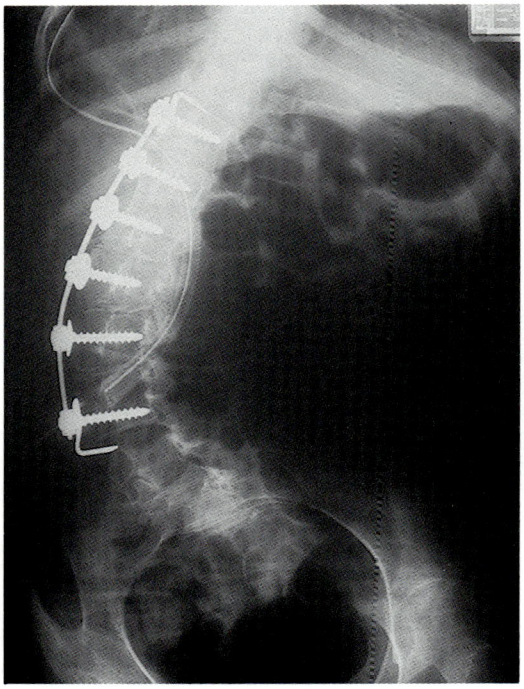

342 Scoliosis in spastic cerebral palsy can require extensive fusions to control the deformity.

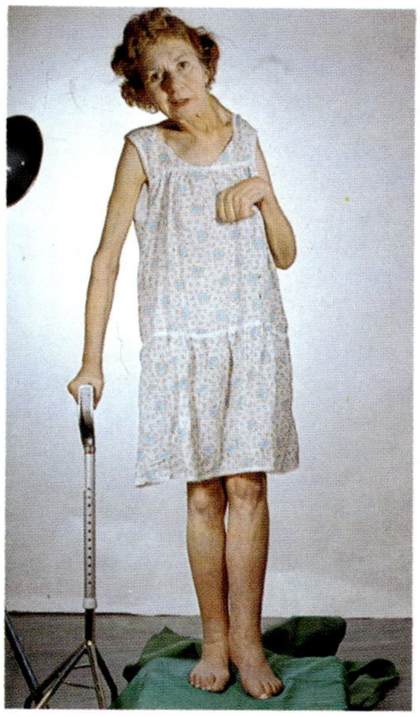

343 Hemiplegia following a cerebrovascular accident.

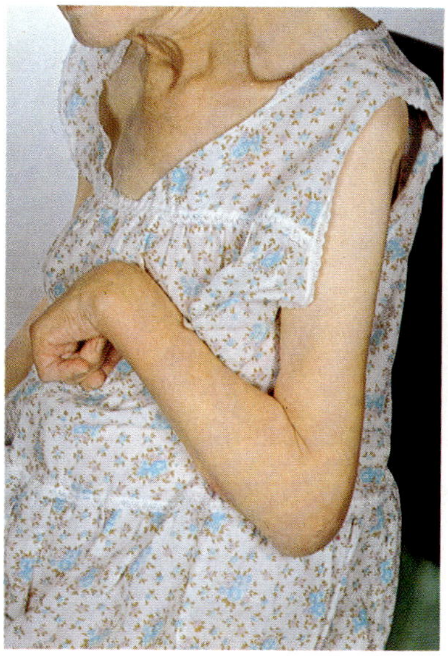

344 The upper limb is held in characteristic adduction at the shoulder, flexion at the elbow and wrist. The fingers are flexed, with thumb-in-palm position.

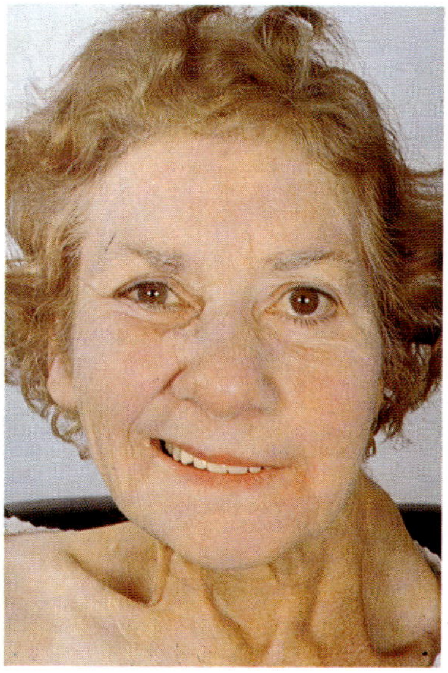

345 Facial paralysis may occur depending on the precise site of the vascular lesion.

Neuropathic arthropathy

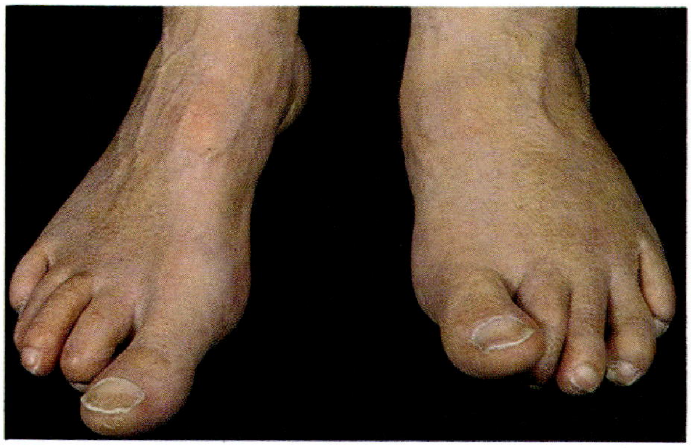

346 Diabetes. The feet of a diabetic patient with a combination of anaesthesia and peripheral vascular disease.

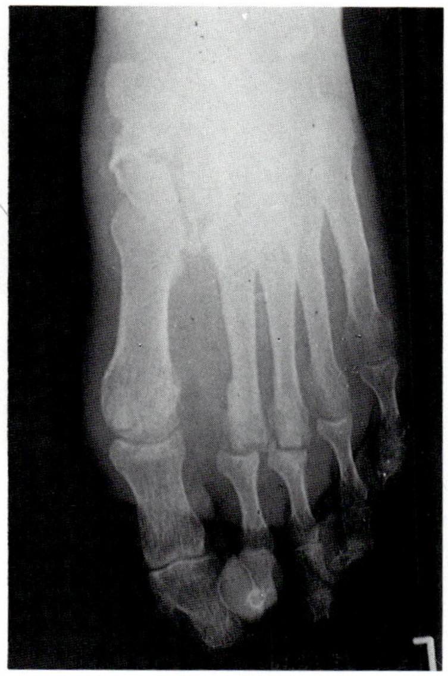

347 Radiographs show the disorganisation of the distal joints of the patient's foot.

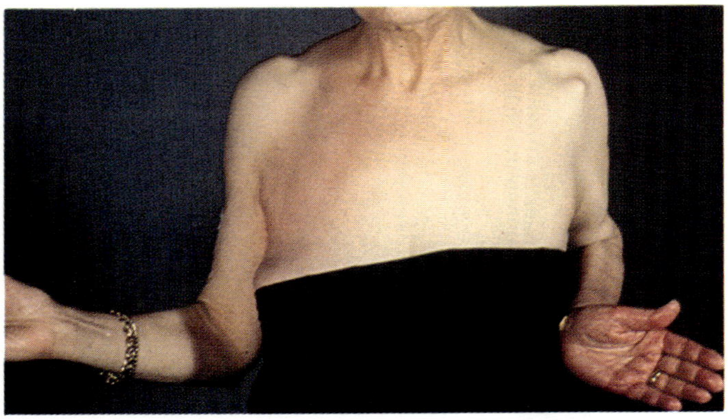

348 Syringomyelia resulting in a destructive arthropathy of the shoulder joint.

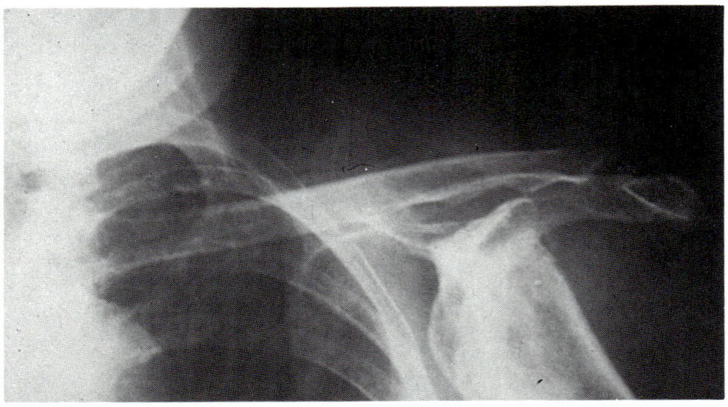

349 Radiograph of the same patient.

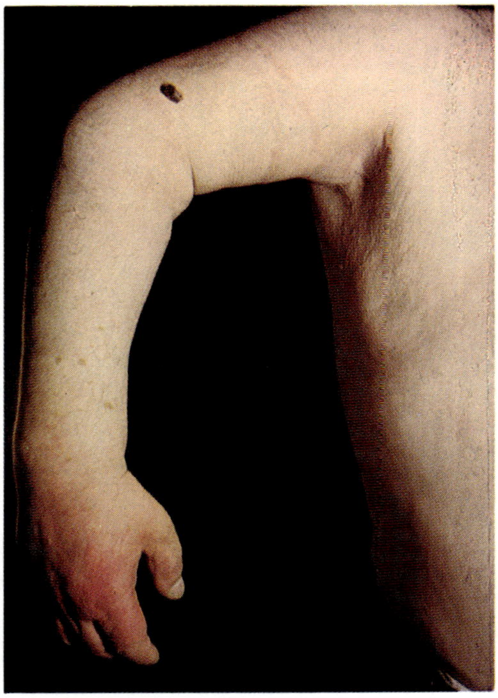

350 Syringomyelia. Flail painless elbow joint.

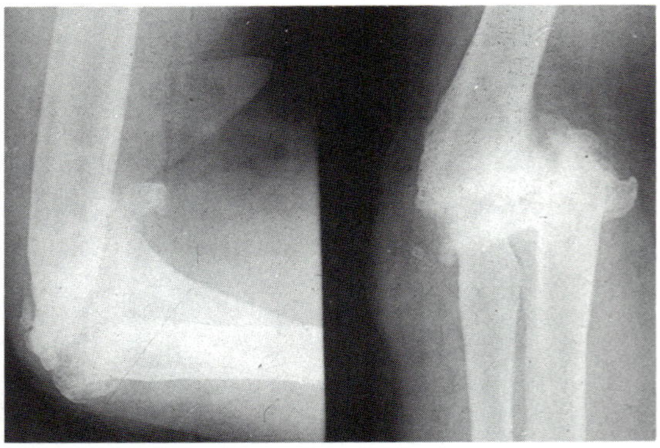

351 Radiograph of the same patient.

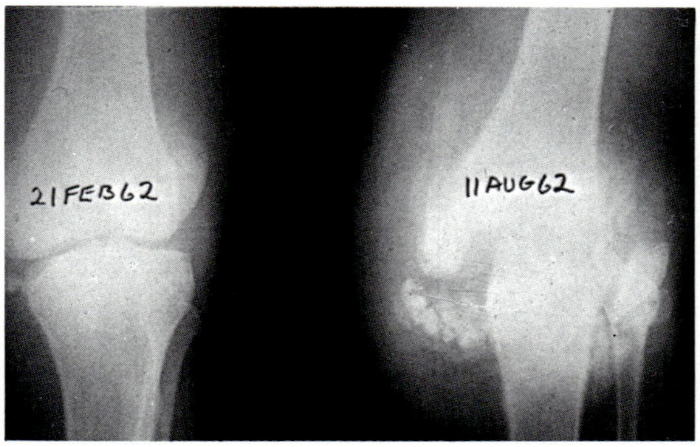

352 Tabes dorsalis. Secondary disorganisation of knee and foot joints, secondary to neurosyphilis.

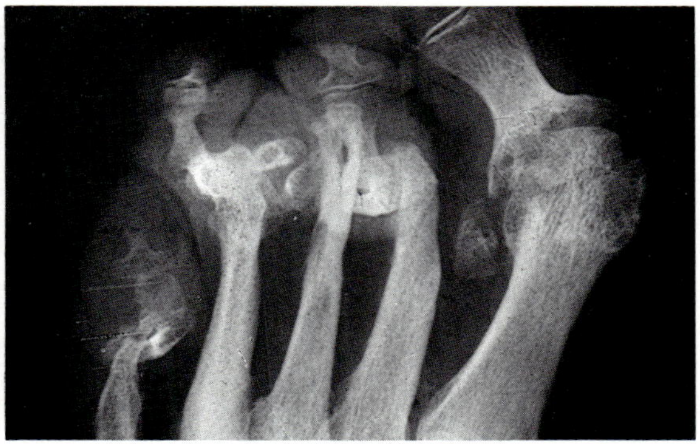

353 Radiograph of the same patient.

Hansen's disease

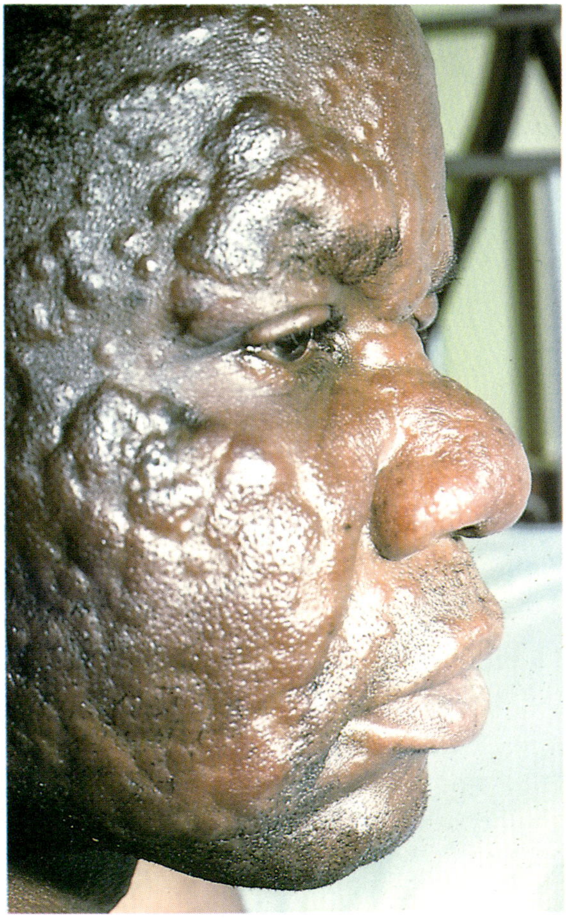

354 Lepromatous leprosy. The leonine facies.

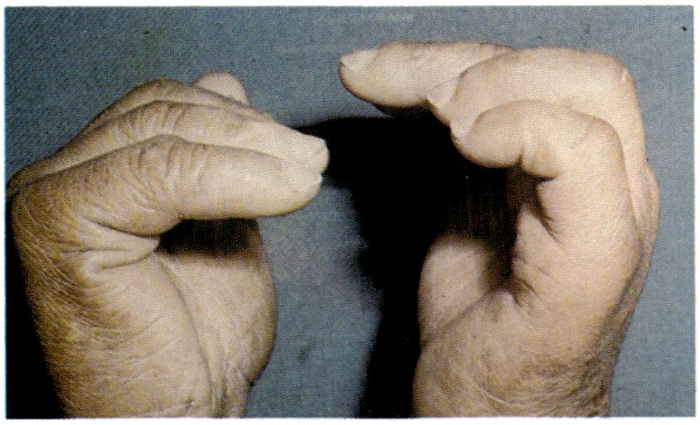

355 Infiltration of subcutaneous tissues of the hand by granulomatous masses.

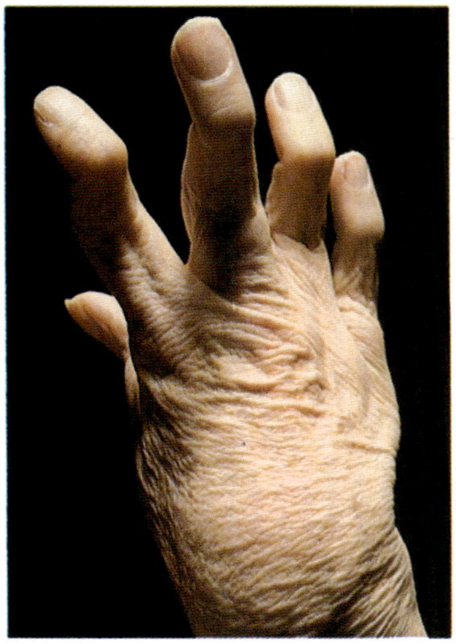

356 Intrinsic paralysis. Peripheral neuropathy leading to paralysis of the muscles of the hand and a consequent claw-hand.

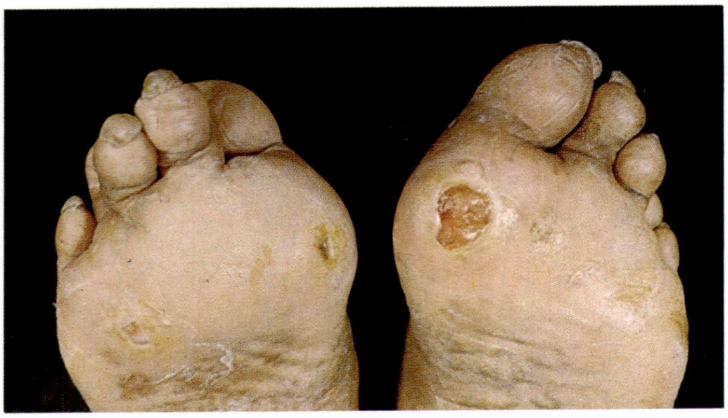

357 Anaesthetic foot: trophic ulceration.

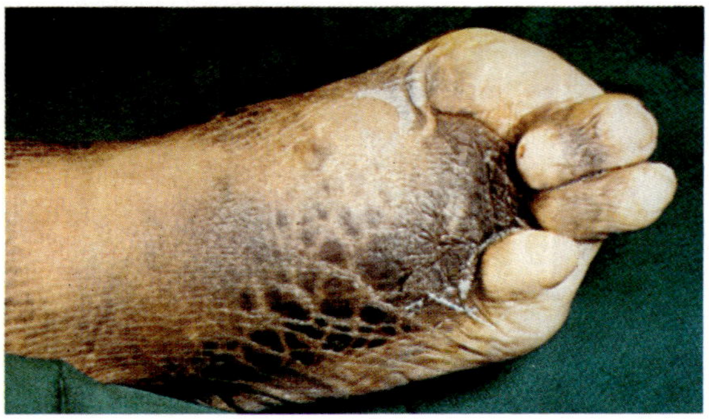

358 Anaesthetic foot. Progressive absorption of anaesthetic digits resulting from repeated minor injury.

Tumours of soft tissue, cartilage and bone

Benign soft tissue tumours

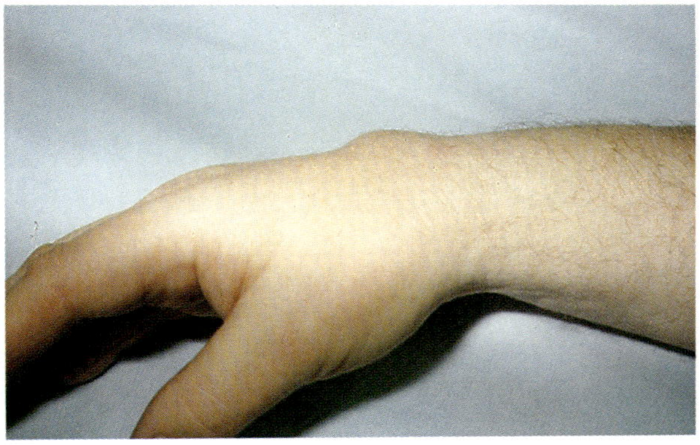

359 Ganglion. The commonest tumour seen in orthopaedic practice consists of a simple pseudocyst containing viscous fluid. It usually arises from the synovial membrane of a joint or tendon sheath.

The dorso radial and volar radial aspect of the wrist is the commonest site.

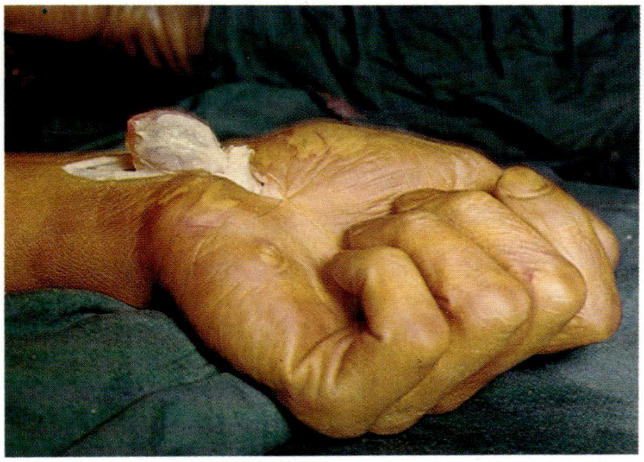

360 This ganglion arose from the sheath of flexor carpi ulnaris.

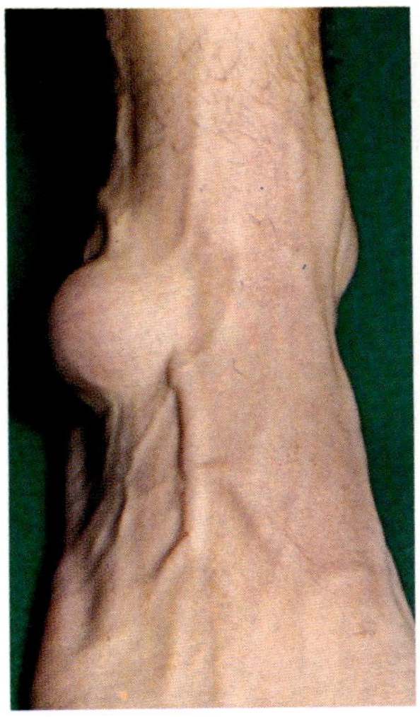

361 Simple ganglion arising from the ankle joint.

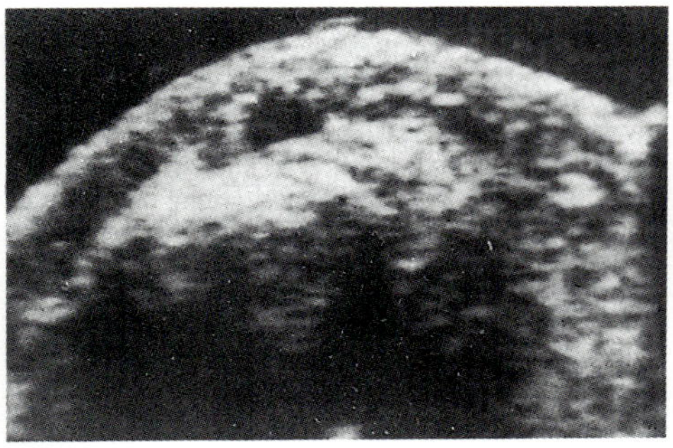

362 Small ganglia can be more painful than the typical larger varieties. This small occult scapholunate ganglion was the cause of undiagnosed wrist pain until located by ultrasound scan.

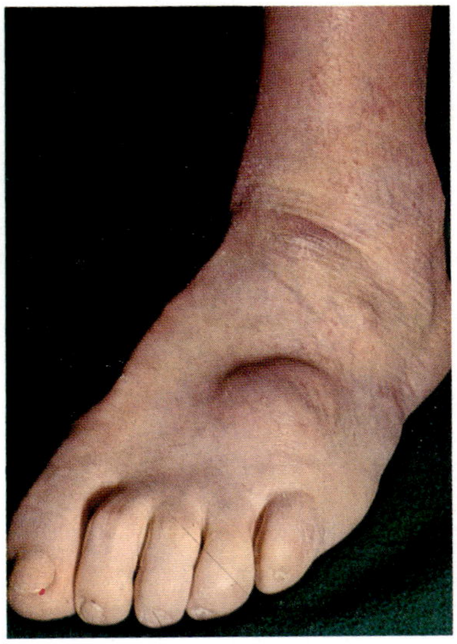

363 Lipomas are common benign subcutaneous tumours, seen here in the subcutaneous fat on the dorsum of the foot.

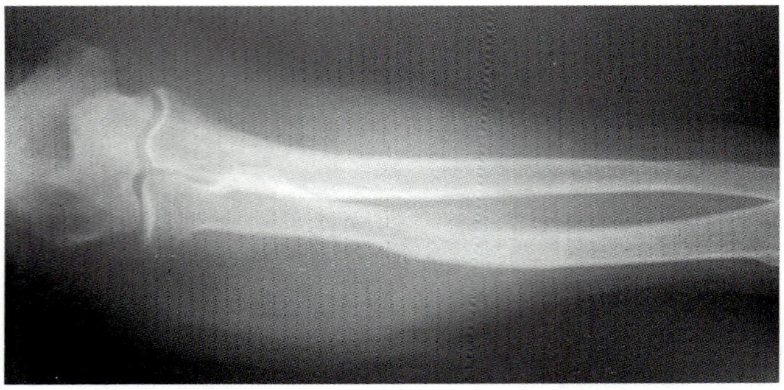

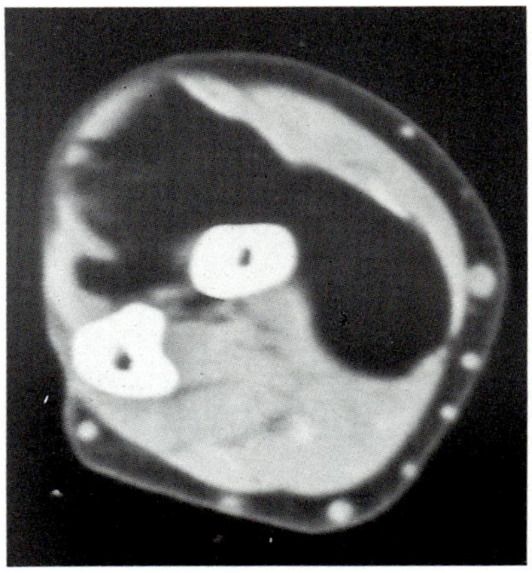

364 & **365** Large lesions can develop within muscular compartments. A CT scan demonstrates the extent of a lipoma deep within the extensor compartment of the forearm.

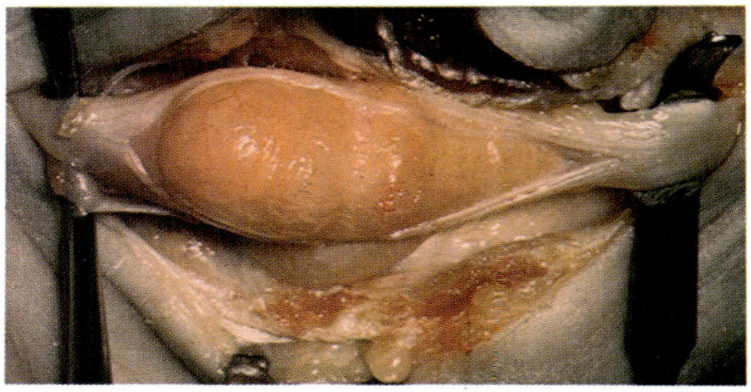

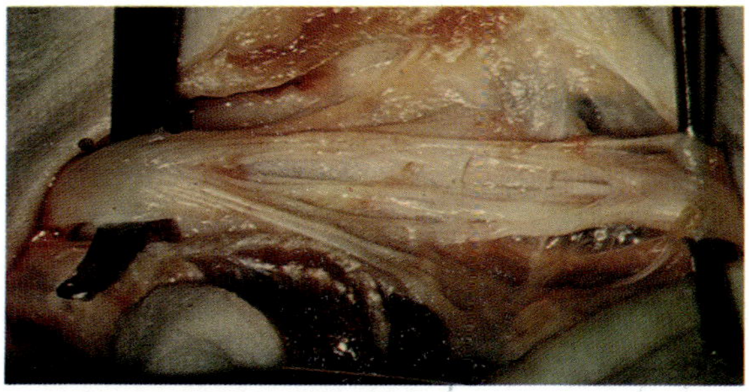

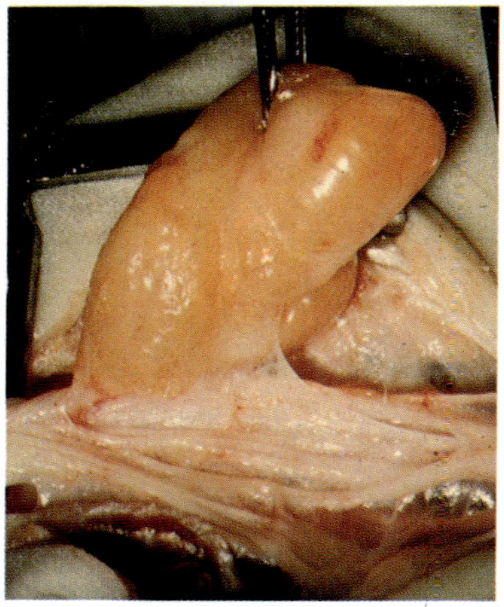

366–368 Intraneural lipoma is shelled out of the ulnar nerve at the wrist. It lies within the nerve sheath but does not penetrate the nerve bundles, which remain intact after removal.

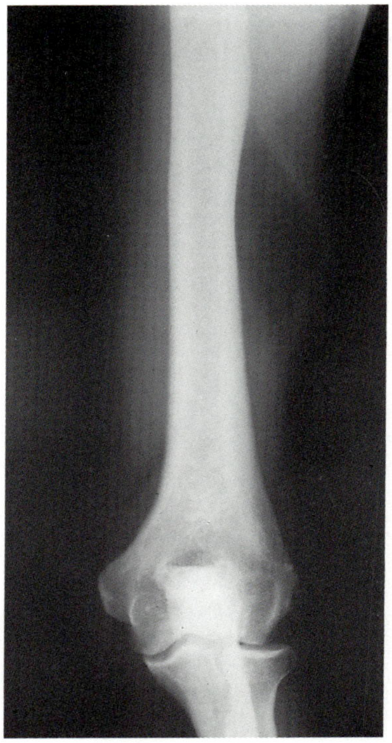

369 Sub-periosteal lipoma. The radiolucent tumour can be clearly seen. Pressure effects have indented the humeral shaft.

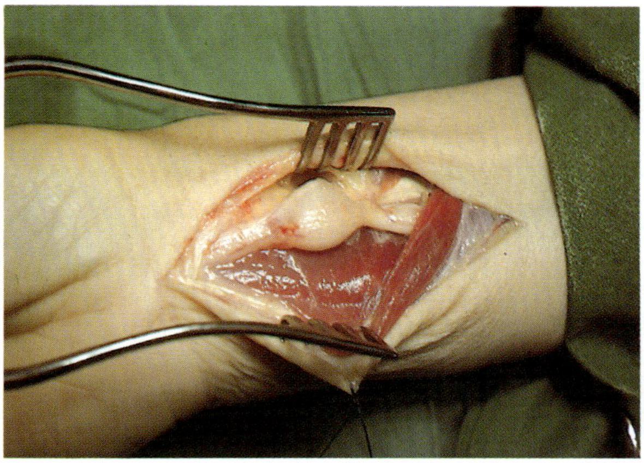

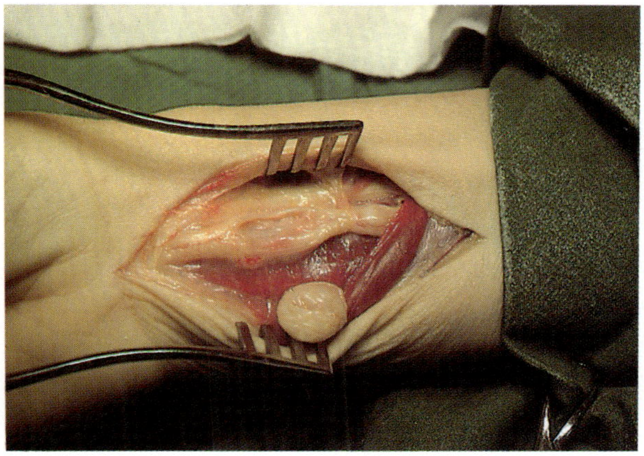

370 & **371** Neurilemmoma (Schwannoma). An innocent tumour arising from the Schwann cells of peripheral nerve and only very gradually affecting the nerve-conducting tissues by direct pressure. There is no infiltration and so the tumour can be shelled out without damaging the nerve fibres.

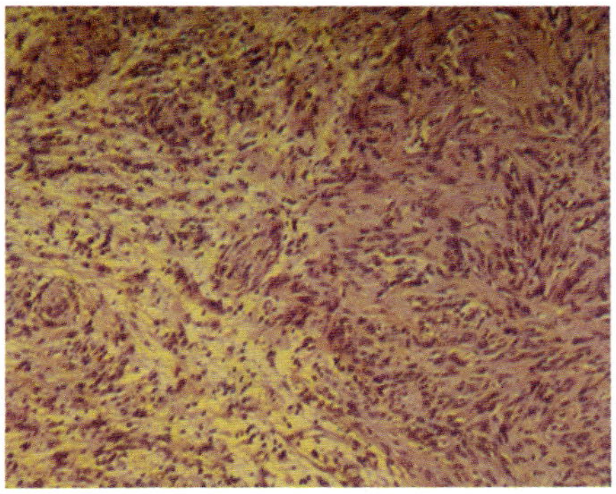

372 Neurilemmoma. Spindle cells arranged in compact groups separated by loose areolar tissue (Antoni type A and type B tissues).

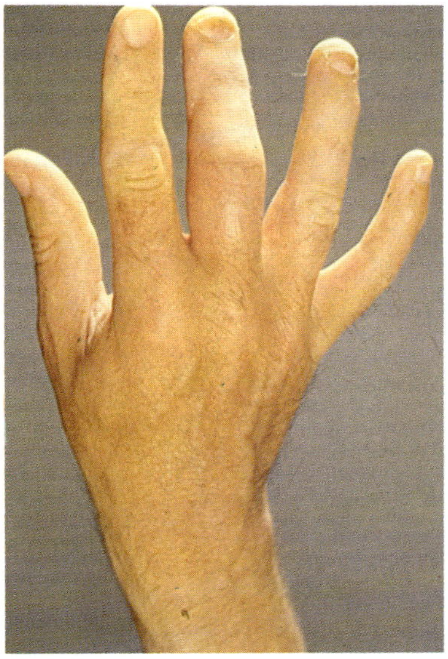

373 Giant cell tumour of tendon sheath. A giant cell tumour – almost always benign – occasionally arises from synovial tendon sheath. Here it has developed in the flexor tendon sheath of the right middle finger.

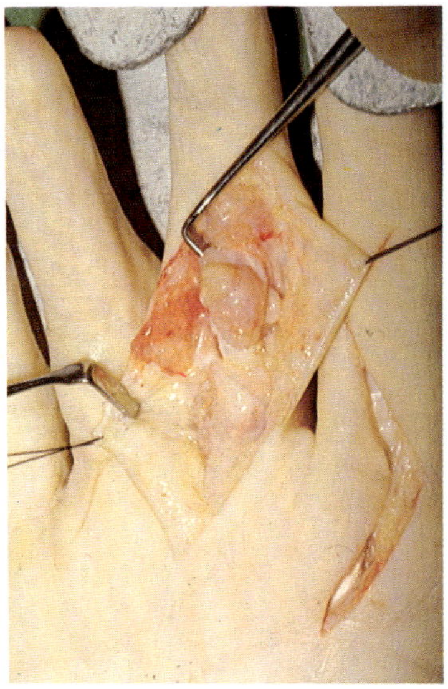

374 Displayed at operation, the tumour has a typical orange colour. Local recurrence of the lesion is not uncommon. The lesion is not a true tumour but a localised pigmented villonodular tenosynovitis.

Pigmented villonodular synovitis (PVNS)

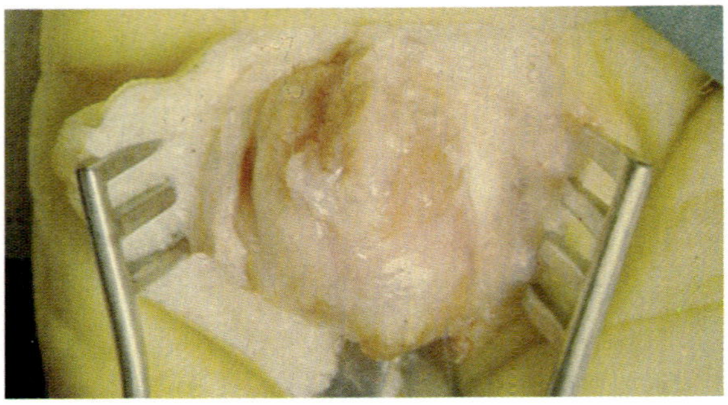

375 Pigmented villonodular synovitis (PVNS). This is a non-malignant but locally invasive condition arising from synovial membrane. It is commonest in the knee joint but is also seen in wrist, hand and other joints.

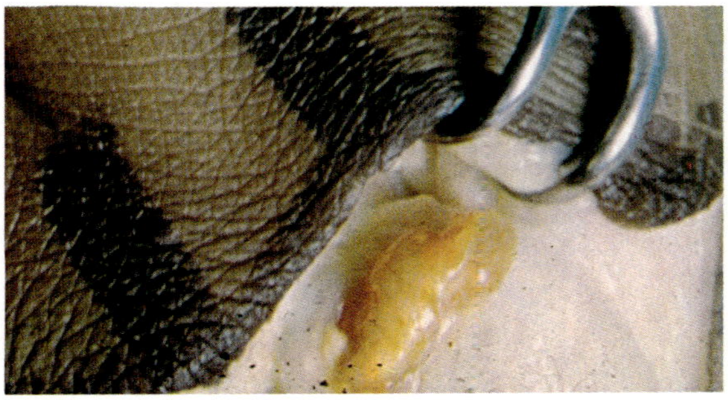

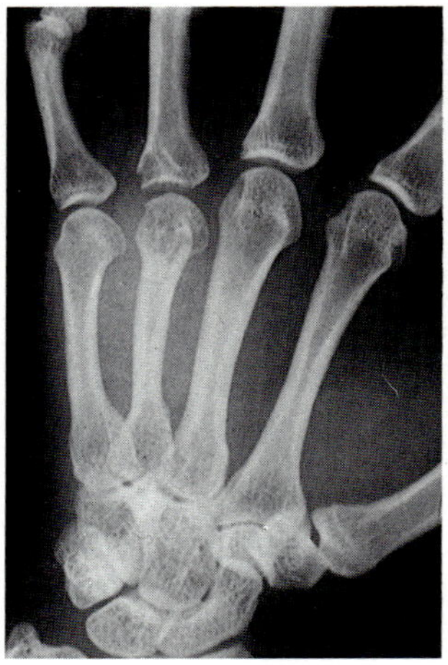

376 & **377** PVNS of the metacarpo-phalangeal joint of the ring finger extending through from palmar to dorsal surfaces. Careful inspection of the radiograph shows typical erosion of the base of the proximal phalanx of the affected joint.

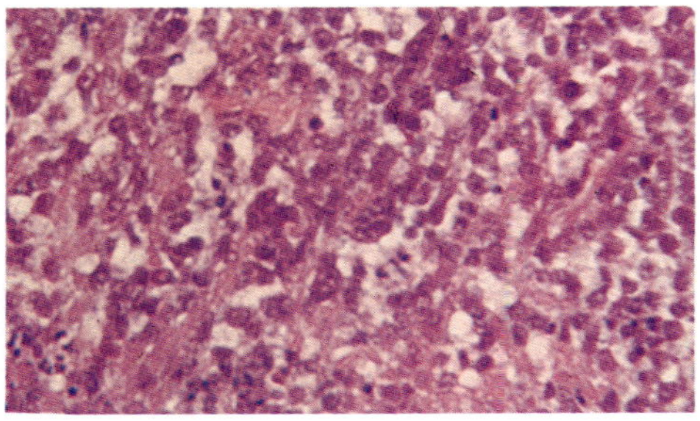

378 A mixed inflammatory cell infiltrate in which multinucleated giant cells are present and are scattered throughout the fibro-fatty connective tissue. Tiny fragments of iron-staining material are evident. (*× 200*)

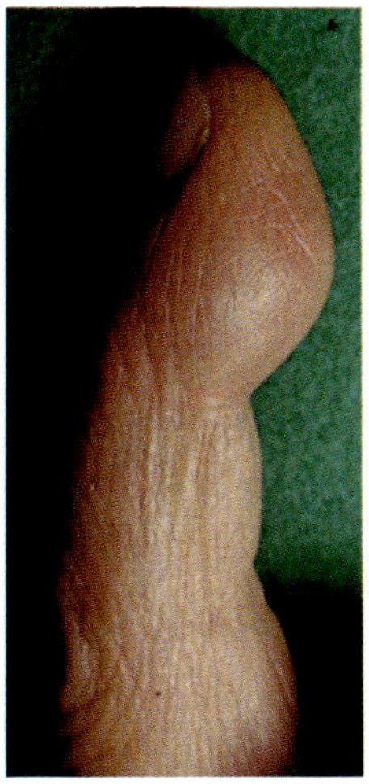

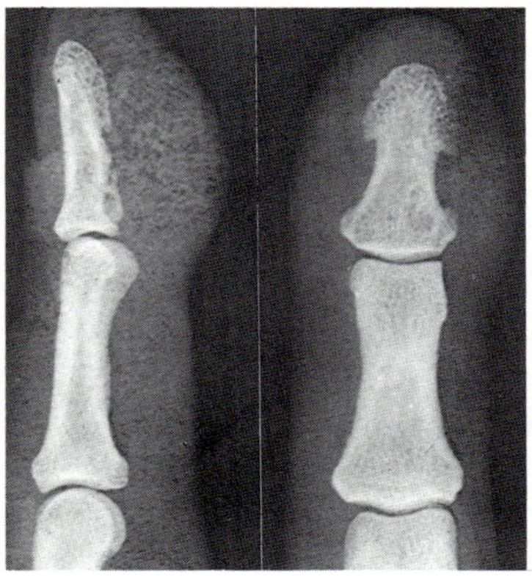

379 & **380** PVNS in the pulp of an index finger probably arising from the terminal IP joint.

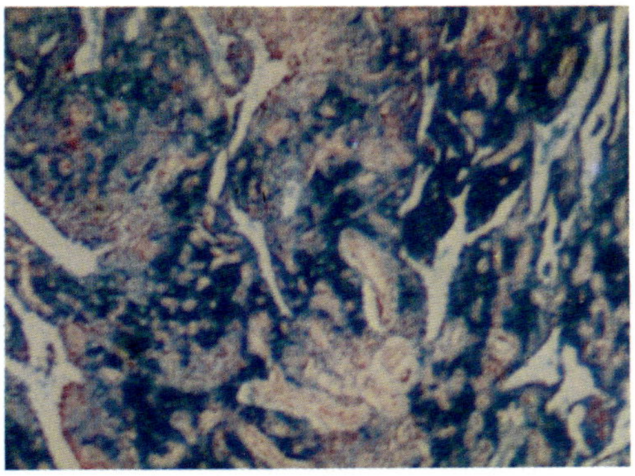

381 Tissue Perl stained for iron pigment; the lesion is more mature and the collagen tissue is more dense. (*x 50*)

Glomus tumour

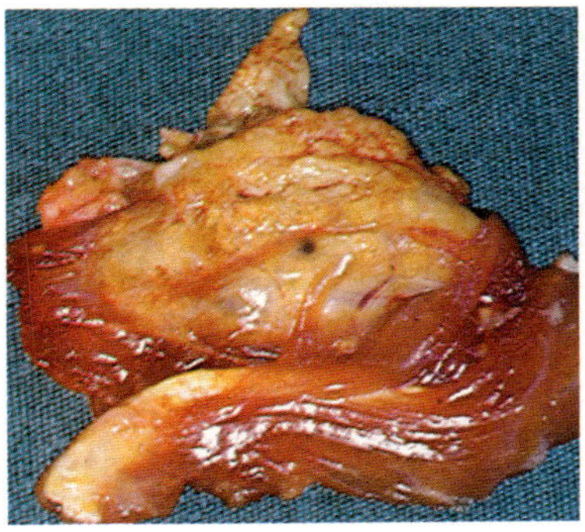

382 Glomus tumour. A rare but very painful tumour, characteristically found in fingers and toes, sometimes beneath the nail. The tissue shown is about 5 mm in diameter, but the tumour itself is only the very central portion of this, and is minute.

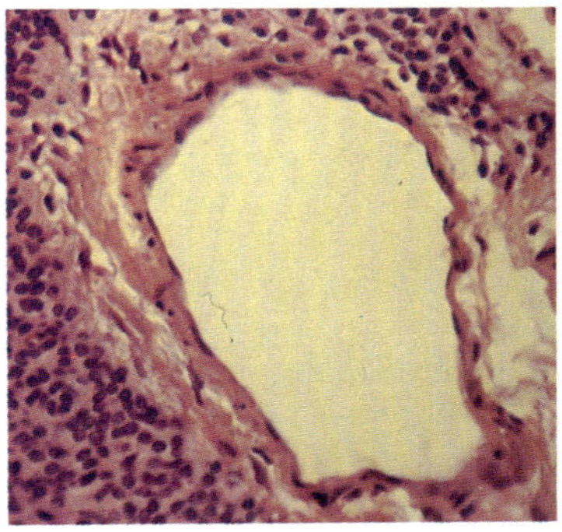

383 Round to oval cells of considerable uniformity surrounding a blood vessel. (*x 200*)

Congenital vascular malformation

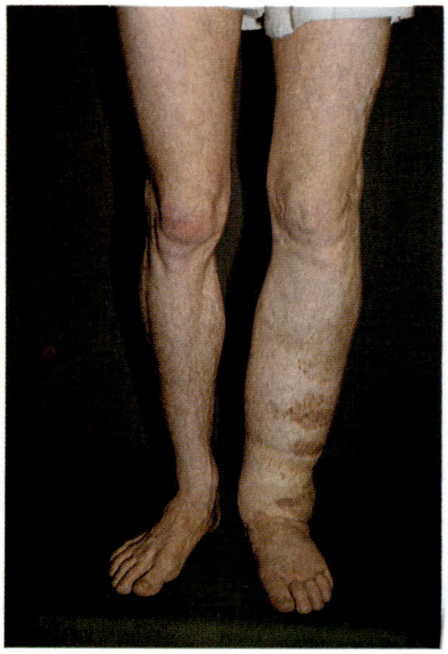

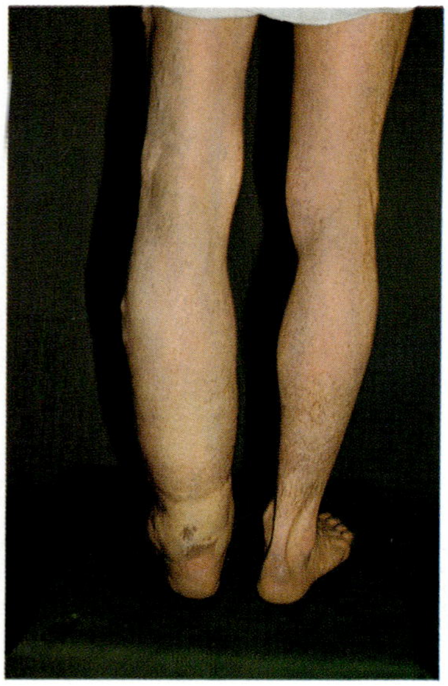

384 & **385** A network of veins and capillaries extending through the muscles, subcutaneous tissue and skin of most of the left leg. The increase in girth and the discolouration of the skin are evident. There was no increase in length in this case.

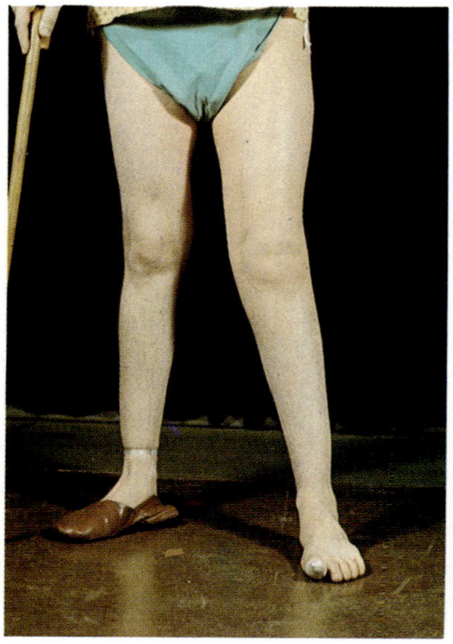

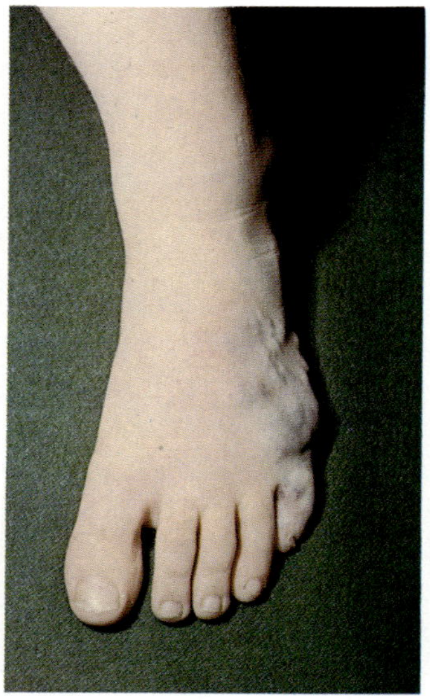

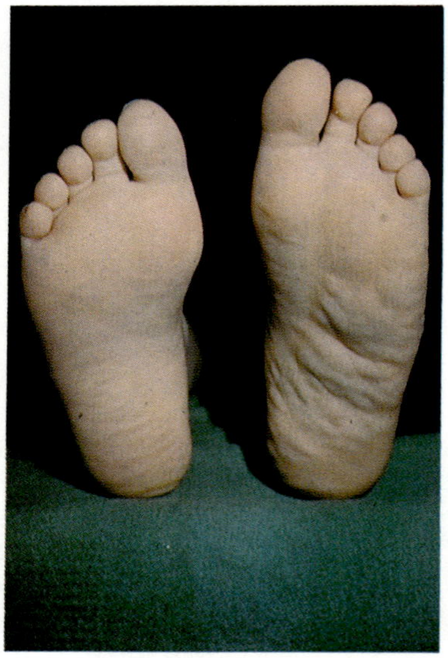

386–388 Congenital arteriovenous malformation affecting the whole of the left lower limb in a young man. In the thigh it was contained within the substance of the quadriceps muscle and in the foot it was evident on the dorsal and plantar surfaces. In addition to local swelling and obvious vascular malformation there was an increase in girth and length of the limb.

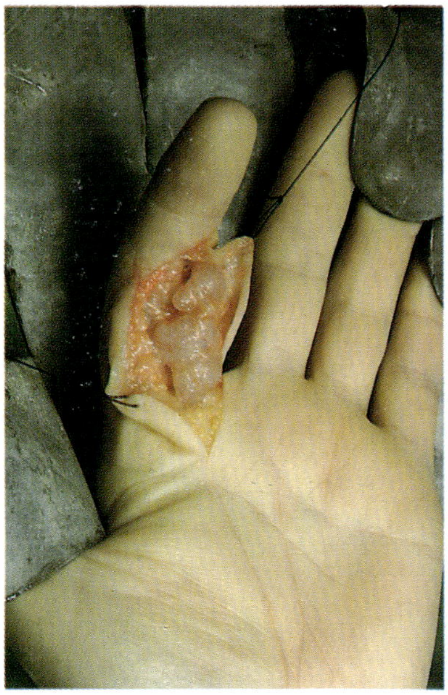

389 Benign tendon sheath chondroma. Soft tissue chondromas are rare, the hands and feet being the commonest sites. They are believed to arise from areas of synovial metaplasia. The lesion shown is within the flexor tendon sheath. Characteristically, the histology is aggressive when histological criteria for bony chondromas are applied; their behaviour, however, is benign although local recurrence is not uncommon.

Benign bone tumours

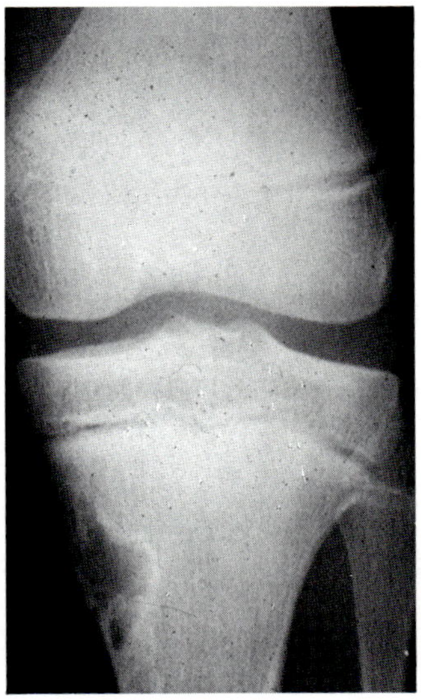

390 Non-osteogenic fibroma of bone: an incidental finding on a radiograph. This is possibly the only lesion of bone that can be diagnosed with certainty by radiographs alone. It is entirely benign.

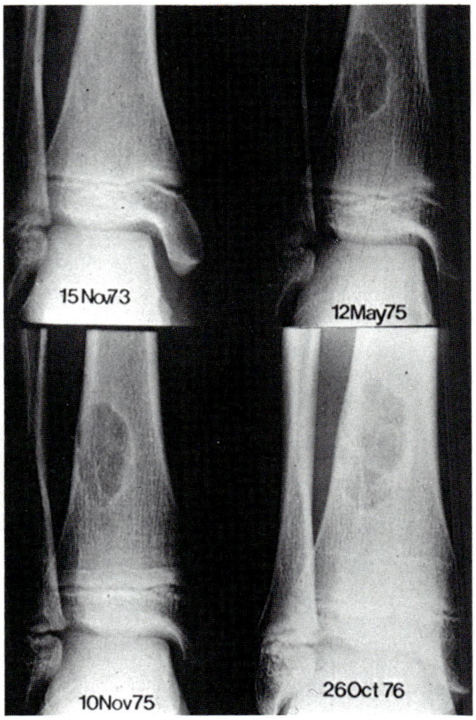

391 Non-osteogeneic fibroma at the lower end of the tibia. Within 3 years the lesion has altered in shape and size and is beginning to fade.

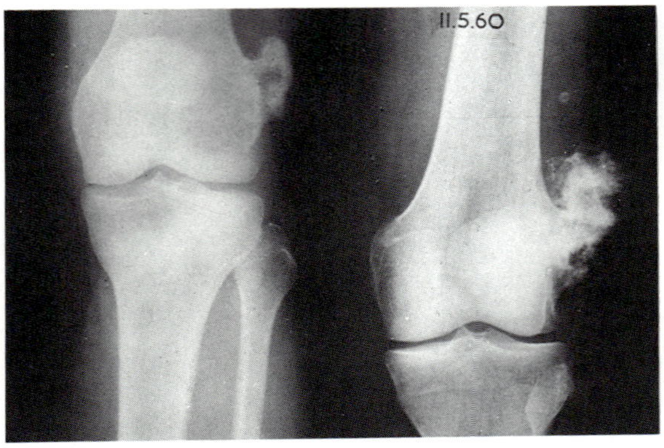

392 Osteochrondroma ('exostosis'). A mass is seen arising from the lower end of the femur pointing away from the growth-plate.

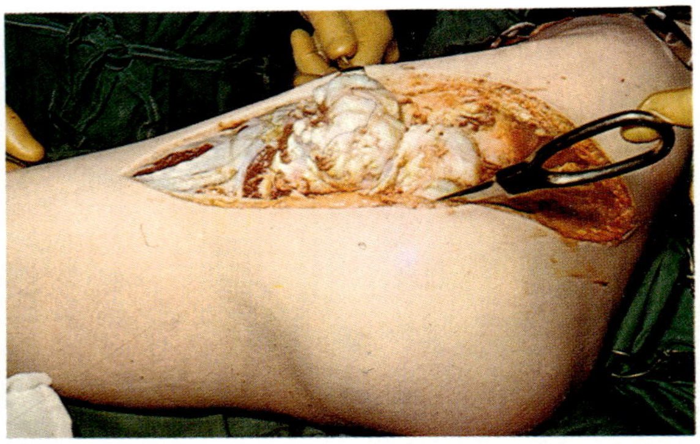

393 The osteochondroma is displayed at operation when its cartilage cap is clearly noted.

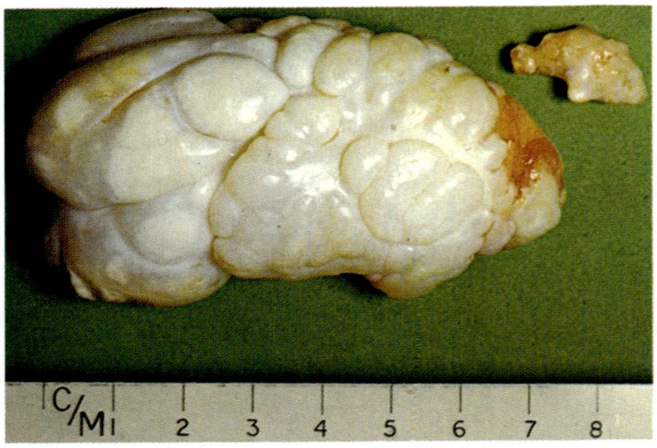

394 The resected osteochondroma.

Osteoid osteoma

This tumour most commonly presents from adolescence up to early adulthood, is most commonly seen in the lower limb bones the femur and tibia being the commonest sites. There is a male preponderance of 3:1. The tumour is small and causes an intense and characteristic pain that frequently disturbs sleep. In many cases the pain typically responds to salicylates. The tumour is often difficult to locate.

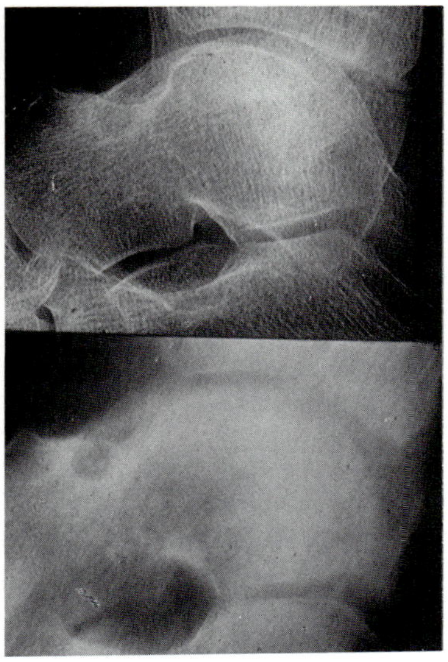

395 A typical osteoid osteoma in the neck of the talus. In the plain film above it is barely visible; in the tomograph below the characteristic nidus surrounded by a transplant moat is clearly visible.

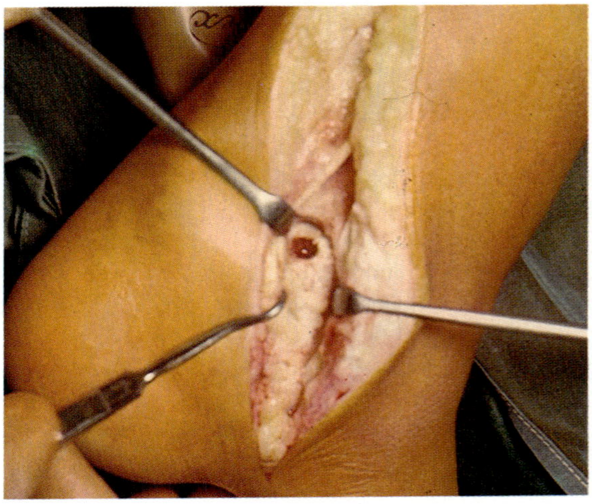

396 The pink soft tumour seen at operation.

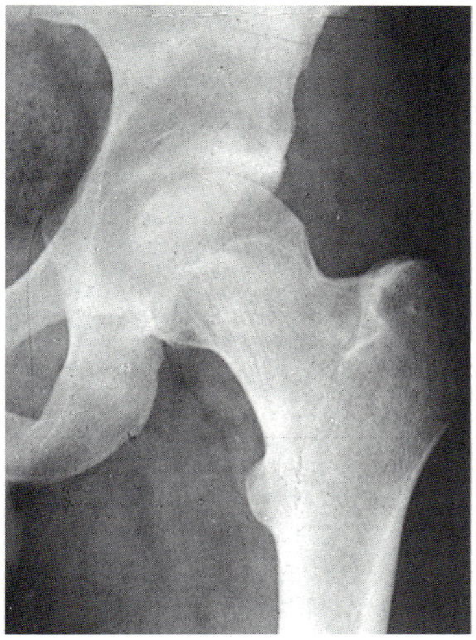

397 Osteoid osteoma at the base of the greater trochanter, which is visualised only with difficulty in the plain radiographs.

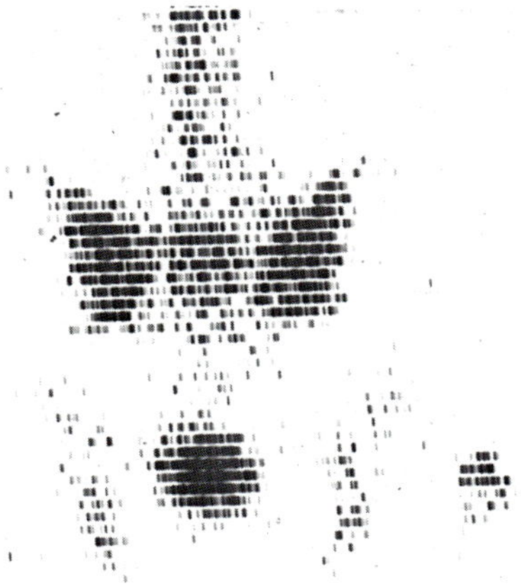

398 The bone scan shows a marked increase of uptake of radioactive Tc in the region of the greater trochanter.

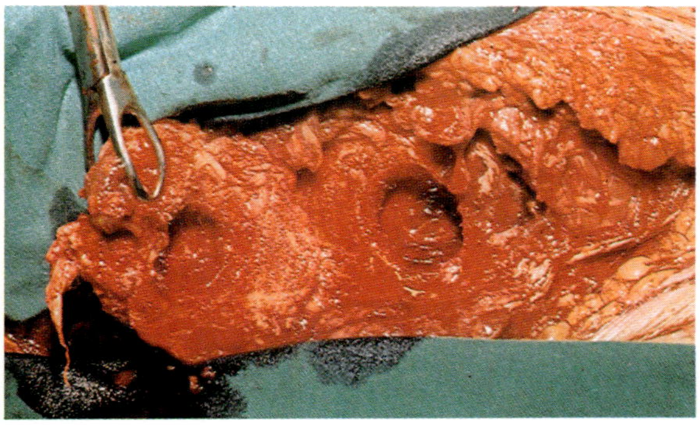

399 When the trochanter is lifted at operation the nidus containing the soft tumour is clearly visible.

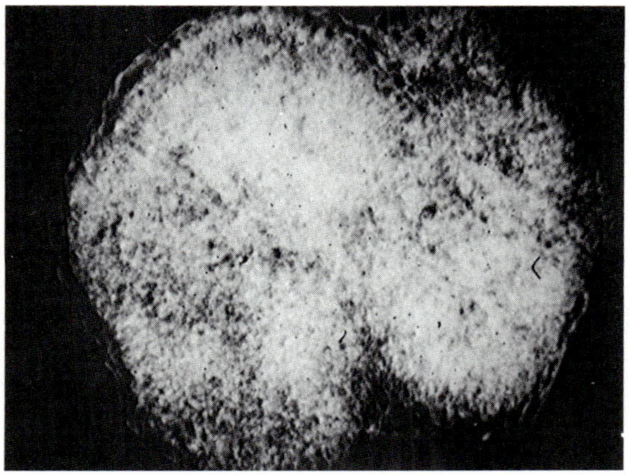

400 A slab radiograph of the material removed from **399**. The whole lesion has been lifted from its bed in the bone and in the centre of the cancellous bone lies a small soft mass.

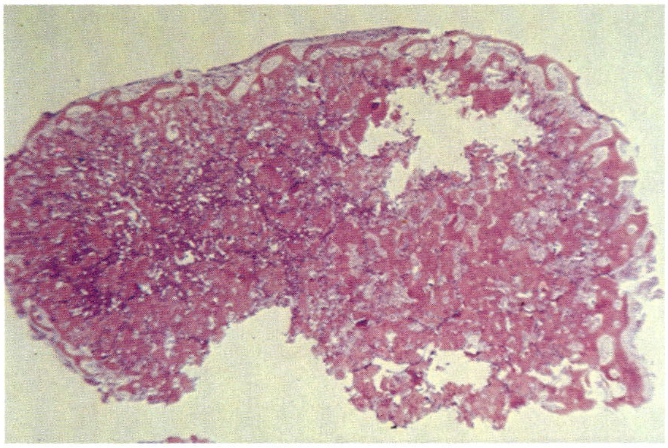

401 The tumour is composed of short irregular immature bone trabeculae in vascular fibrous tissue which contains some osteoclasts. (*x 5*)

Benign osteoblastoma

This is also classified as a 'giant osteoid osteoma' because it has many of the same characteristics, except for its size. There is male preponderance and the lesion commonly presents during the first three decades of life. There is a marked predilection for the vertebral column.

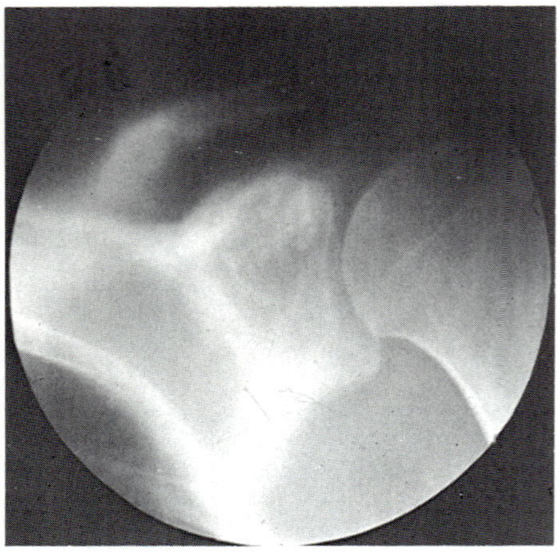

402 Pain in the shoulder region and loss of normal shoulder movements were the presenting features. Plain radiographs appeared normal, but tomography revealed a lesion in the neck of the scapula.

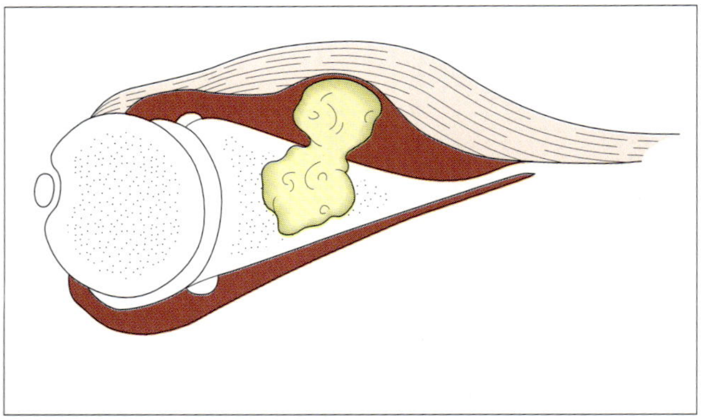

403 A diagram of the tumour as seen at operation. It arises from the neck of the scapula and bulges out backwards to lift the 'belly' of the supraspinatus muscle. This relation accounted for the fact that the patient was unable to abduct his shoulder prior to operation.

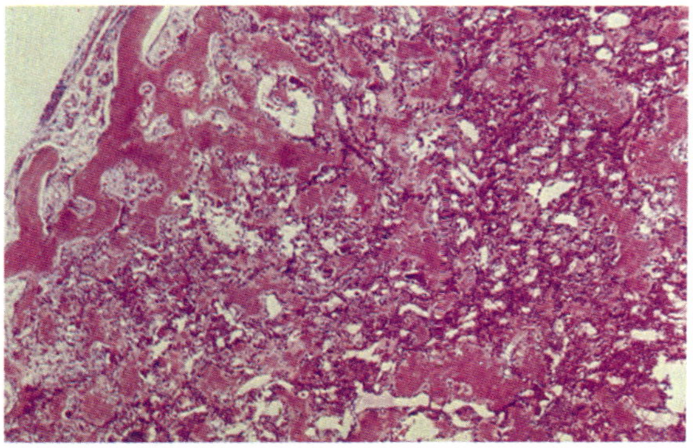

404 The lesion showing the same characteristics as an osteoid osteoma. (*x100*)

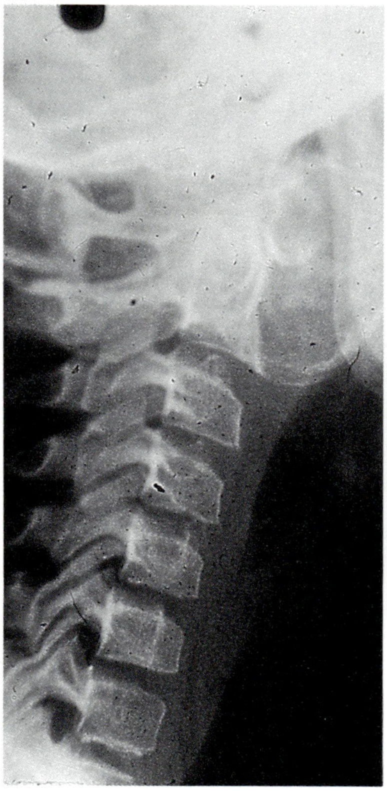

405 Osteoblastoma in the spinous process of C1.

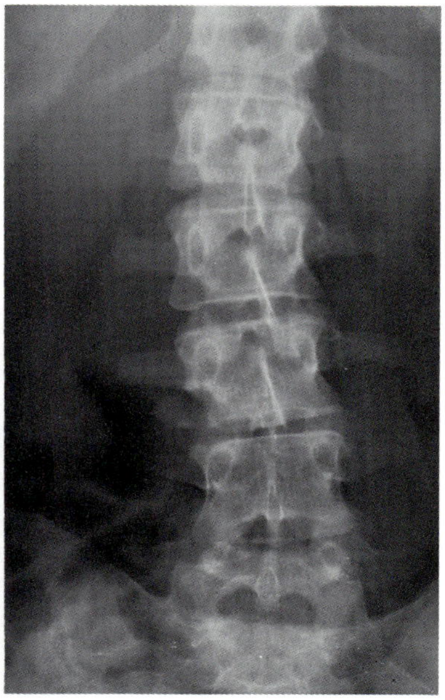

406 Osteoblastoma just below the pedicle of L3, causing a scoliosis.

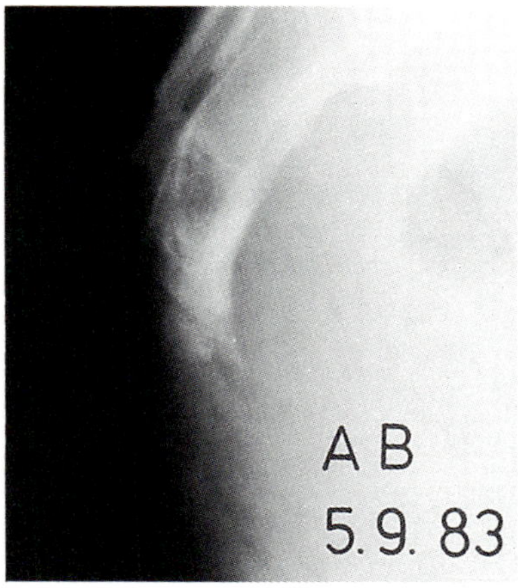

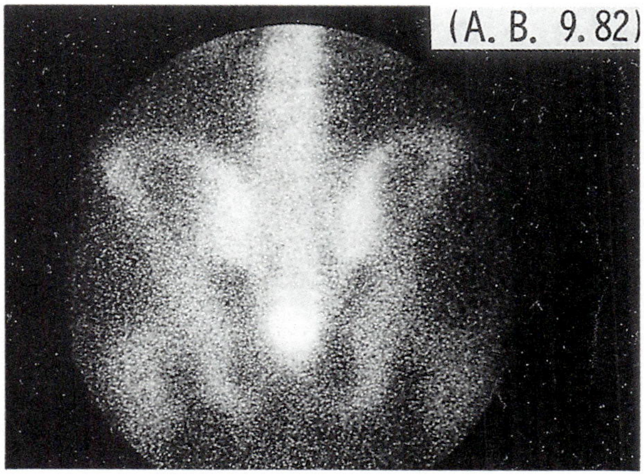

407 & **408** Osteoblastoma of the lower sacrum; the scan shows increased uptake at the site of the lesion.

Haemangioma of bone

Although this condition is benign, in the sense that it does not metastasize, it may be locally extremely destructive. It varies from a single relatively simple lesion, e.g. of a vertebral body, to an extensive destructive lesion of a long bone. An extreme example, as is depicted here, is of the 'vanishing bone syndrome' of Gorham.

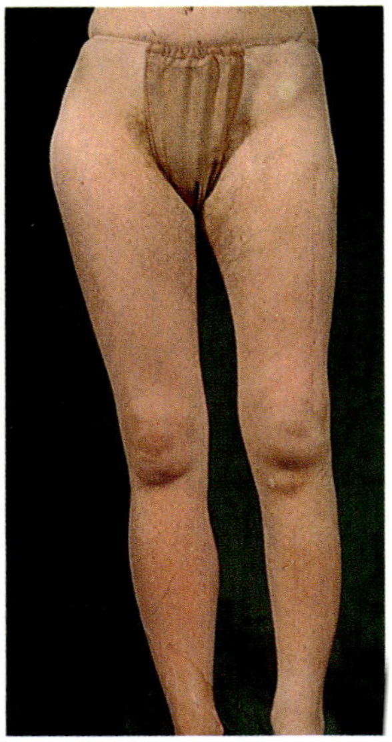

409 A 24-year-old girl with swelling, pain and deformity in the upper end of the right femur.

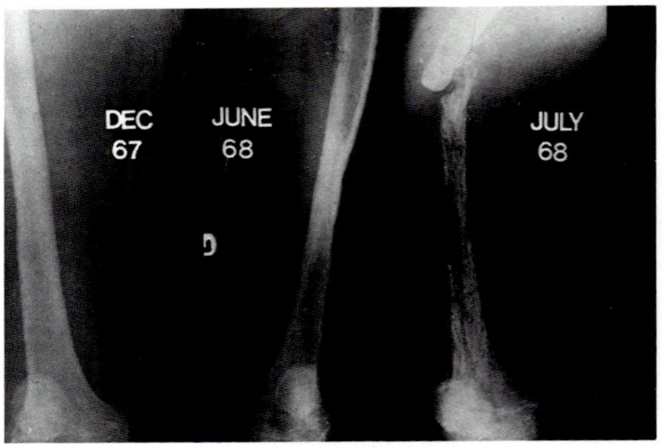

410 Serial radiographs of the femur. In the course of 8 months the lesion advanced very rapidly and a pathological fracture finally occurred.

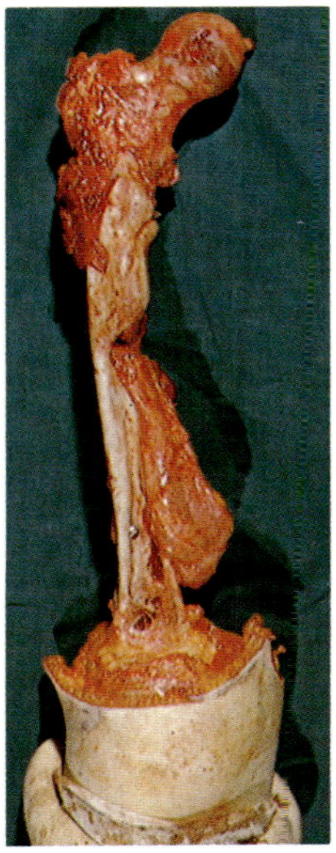

411 The specimen is resected for replacement by a prosthesis.

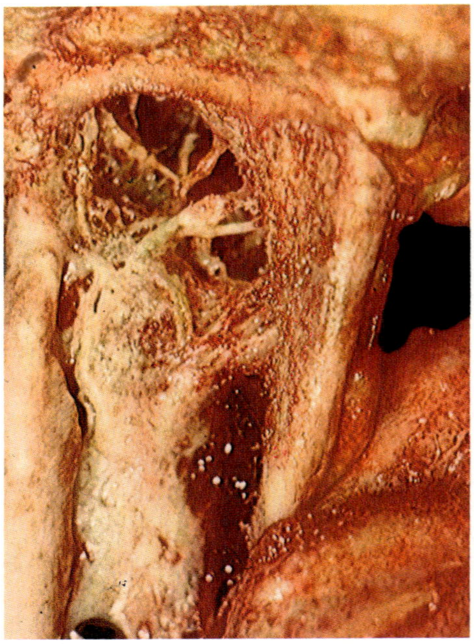

412 Enlargement of the specimen to show the considerable resorption of the osseous trabeculae, the remainder being very thickened and running vertically. The characteristic 'sunburst' reticulated appearance is well shown.

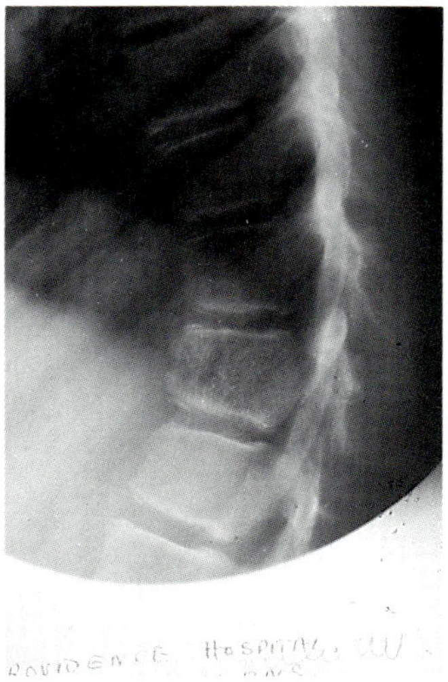

413 Haemangioma of a vertebral body showing typical striated appearance.

Aneurysmal bone cyst (ABC)

This is a tumour-like lesion within bone consisting of a cavity filled with blood. The lesion expands, thins and destroys the cortex. Radiologically, it can be confused with a giant-cell tumour. However, it is a less common lesion than giant-cell tumour and presents in a younger age-group. Eighty percent of giant cell tumours occur in individuals of 20 years or over; 80% of ABCs occur in individuals under 20 years of age. It is benign.

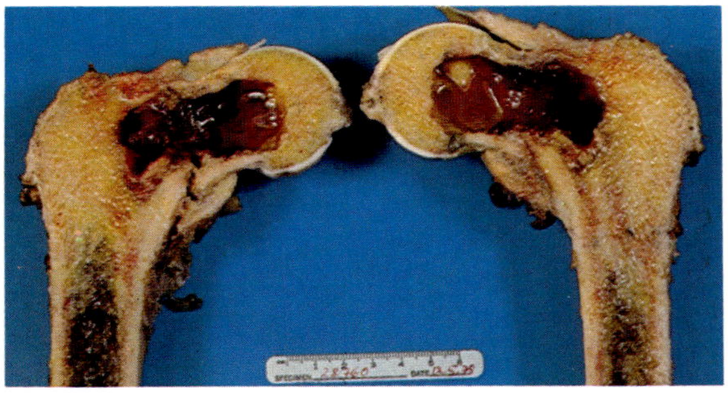

414 Aneurysmal bone cyst occupying the neck of a femur through which a pathological fracture has occurred.

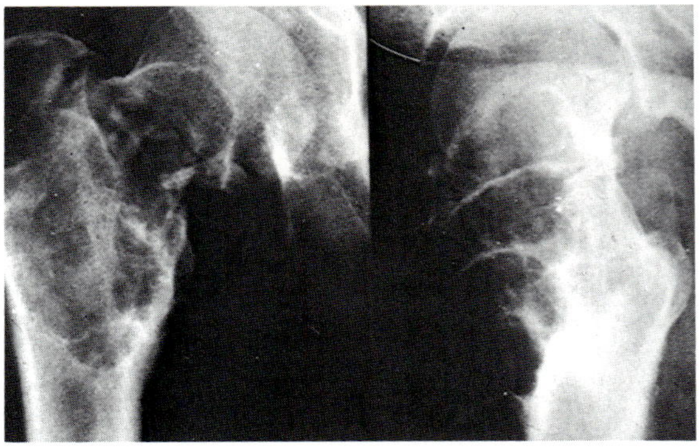

415 An aneurysmal bone cyst in a similar position.

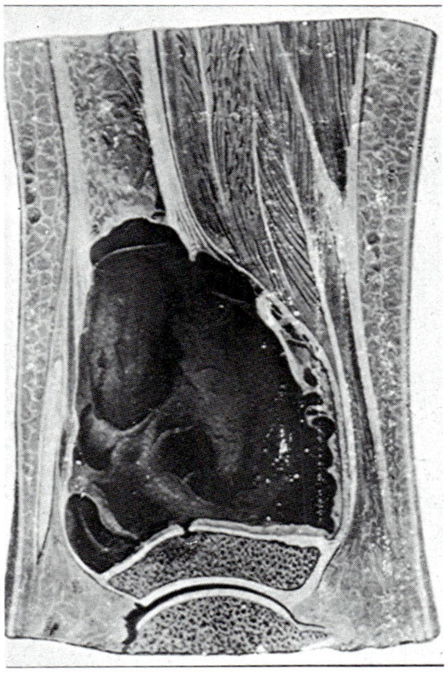

416 Pathological specimen of an aneurysmal bone cyst at the lower end of the tibia.

Simple (unicameral) bone cyst

Simple cysts are thought to arise from a disturbance of growth at the epiphysis. The commonest sites are upper humerus, diaphysis of femur and proximal diaphysis of tibia. They become apparent during the first two decades either owing to local pain or to pathological fracture. Occasionally, they are a coincidental radiological finding.

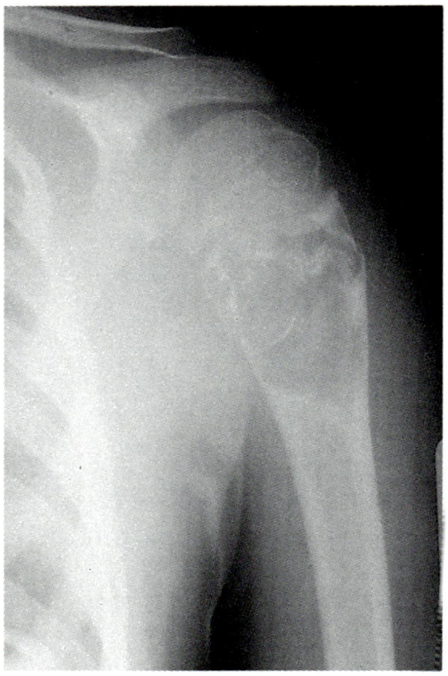

417 Typical features. Cortical expansion with thinning of cortical bone. The lesion may be seen to move from metaphysis to diaphysis as growth occurs.

Enchondroma

These are benign tumours of hyaline cartilage that are usually found centrally located in a bone. The commonest site is in the small bones of the hand and, indeed, chrondroma is the commonest bony tumour found in the hand.

Multiple enchondromatosis is a dysplasia that has already been discussed (see Ollier's Disease). Malignant change in isolated enchondromas is rare, being commoner in lesions affecting the flat bones. In multiple enchondromatosis malignant change may occur in up to one-third of cases.

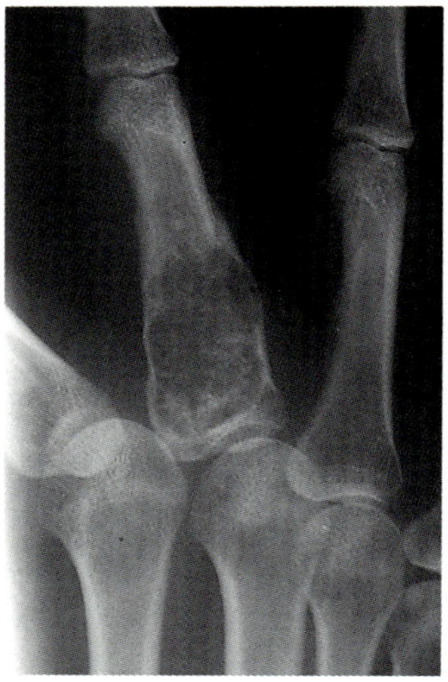

418 Many chondromas are asymptomatic being discovered coincidentally on radiography. Those in the hand commonly present after pathological fracture.

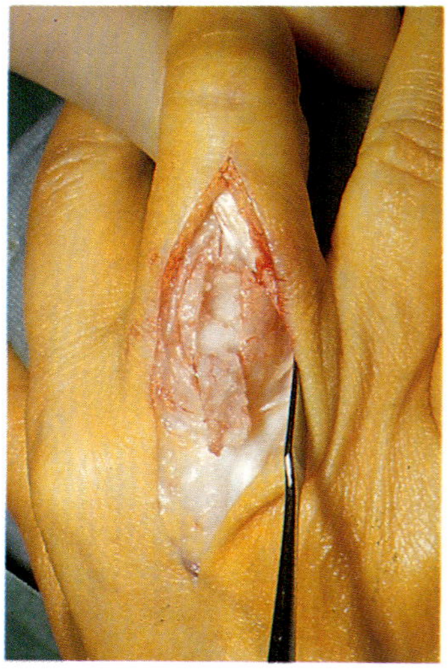

419 Treatment by curettage and grafting the cavity is frequently successful.

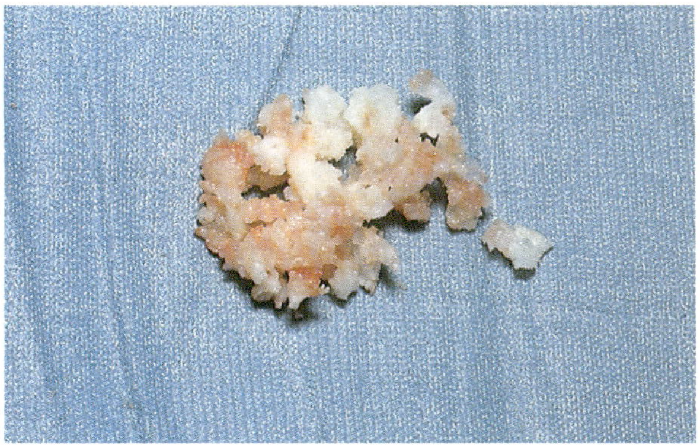

420 Curettings of lesion shown in **418** & **419**.

Giant-cell tumour of bone (osteoclastoma)

These tumours occupy a position between benign and malignant tumours. About 40% are entirely benign, about 40% are locally invasive and recurrent and the remainder metastasize. There is a slight female preponderance.

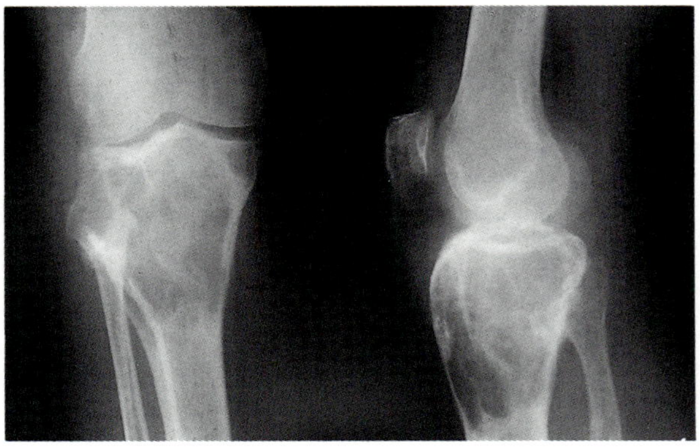

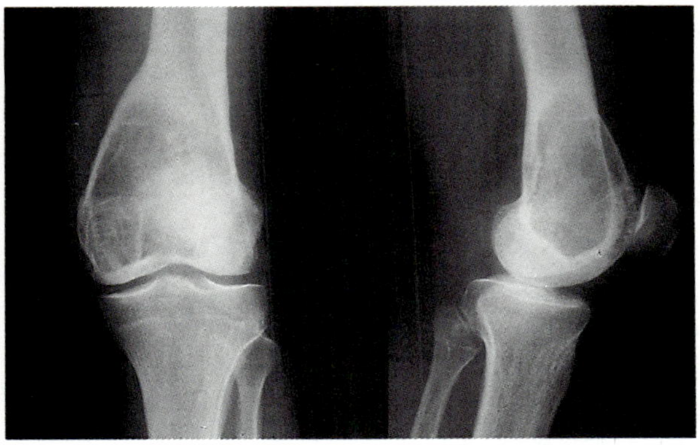

421 & **422** Giant cell tumours in the two commonest sites. There are no features that can be considered absolutely typical. Commonly, however, they appear as expanding rarefied lesions, almost invariably epiphyseal, abutting the adjacent joint surface. They frequently lie eccentrically with thinning of the adjacent cortex. Periosteal reaction and reactive sclerosis are unusual.

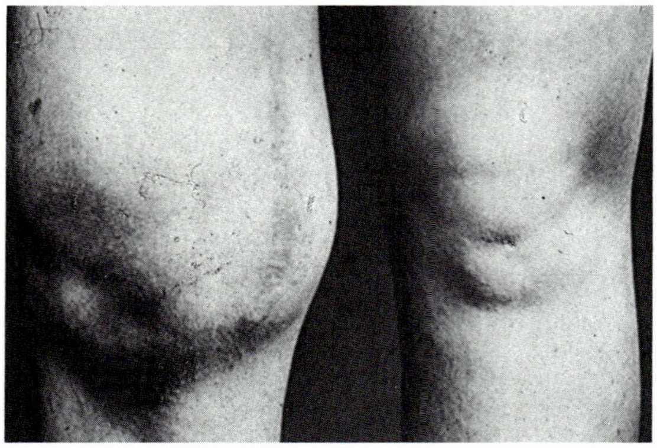

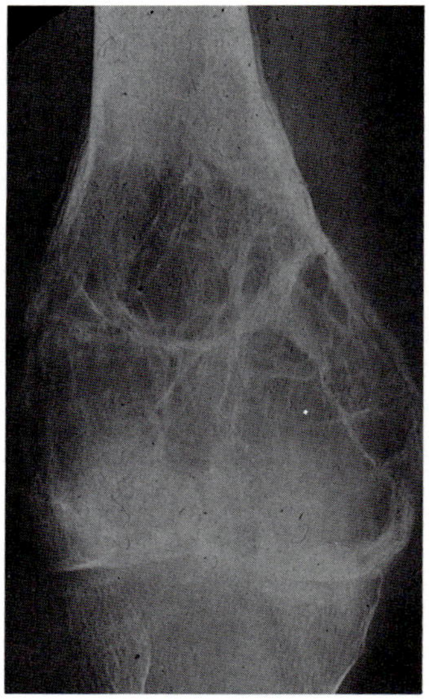

423 & **424** Fifty per cent of giant cell tumours occur about the knee. This case shows a recurrence in the lower femur.

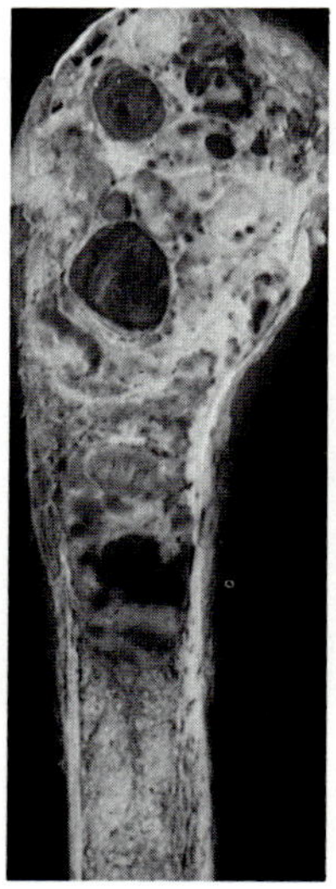

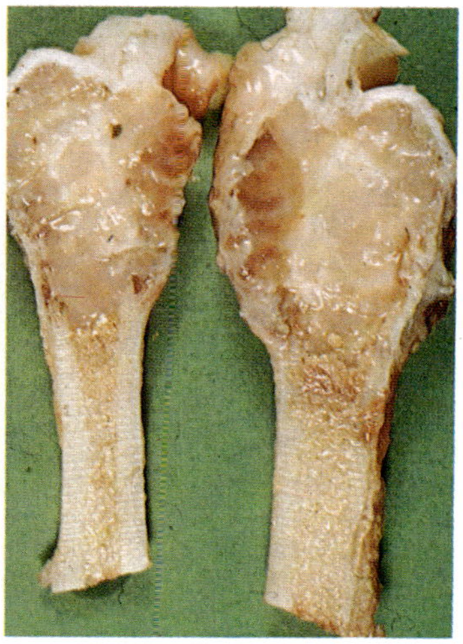

425 & **426** The macroscopic appearance of giant cell tumour. The tumour expands the involved bone with cortical thinning; extension of the lesion to the articular cartilage is characteristic of the tumour. Small areas of cystic or necrotic change with blood-filled cavities are not unusual, giving the tumour a variegated appearance.

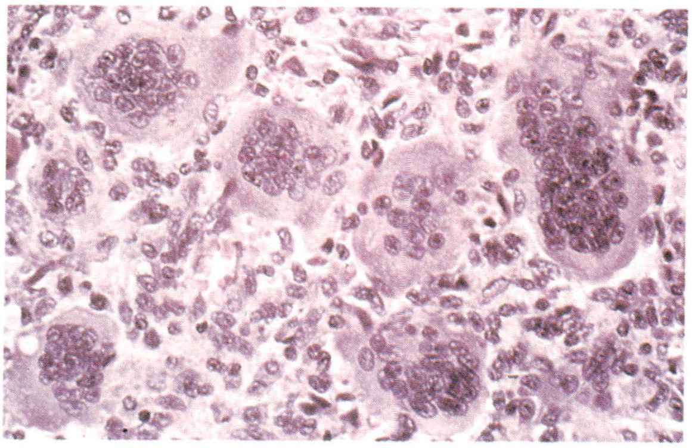

427 The tumour's cell of origin is unknown. Microscopically, it consists of a stroma of mononuclear cells among which are numerous multinucleate giant cells. The giant cells very likely arise from fusion of the proliferating mononuclear cells.

Giant cells are a feature of a number of benign conditions of bone and are not exclusive to giant cell tumours 'proper'. Inclusion of these benign 'giant cell variants' in published works on giant-cell tumours has led to false optimism regarding the true nature of this sometimes agressive tumour.

Giant cell 'variants':
- Non-ossifying fibroma.
- Chondroblastoma.
- Chondromyxoid fibroma.
- Aneurysmal bone cyst.
- Simple bone cysts.
- Fibrous cortical defects.
- Brown tumours.
- Giant cell reparative granuloma.

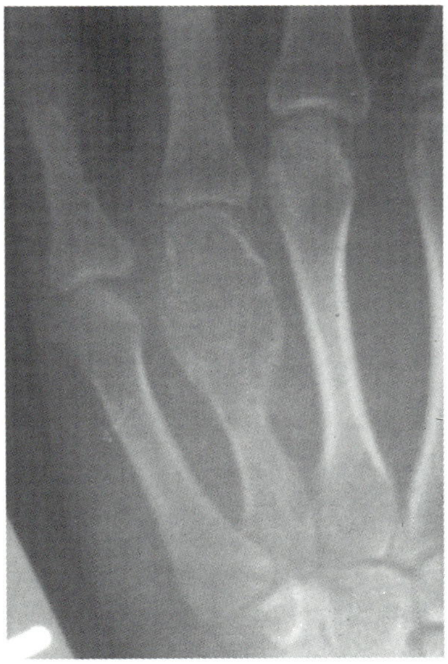

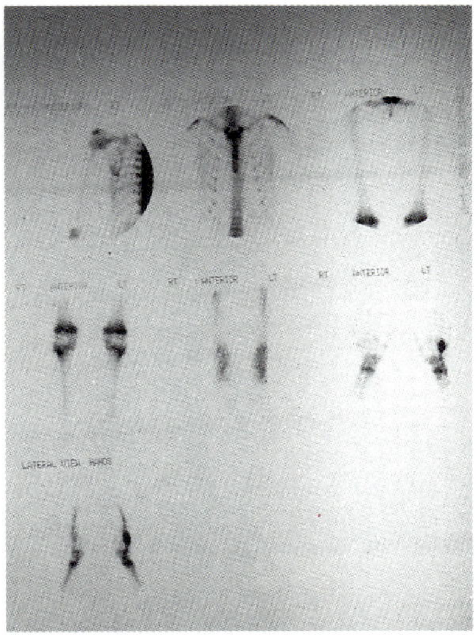

428 & **429 Multicentric giant cell tumours**. Although uncommon, if the 'primary' lesion is in the hand or the wrist an 18% chance of a multicentric lesion has been reported. A bone scan is therefore essential before considering treatment. In this case the lesion was in the fourth metacarpal, there was no multicentric lesion.

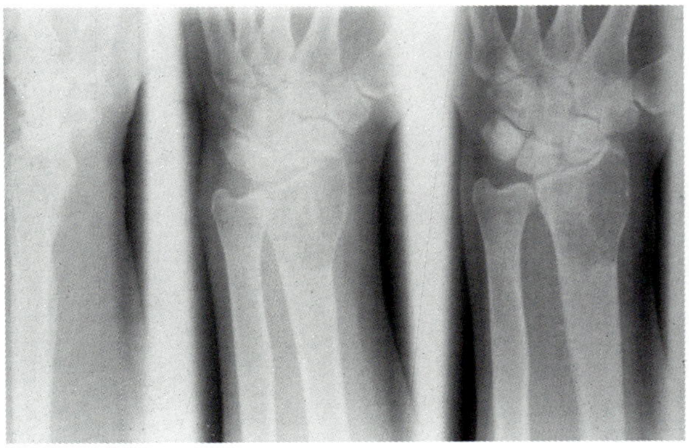

430 Giant cell tumour in the distal radius, the third commonest site.

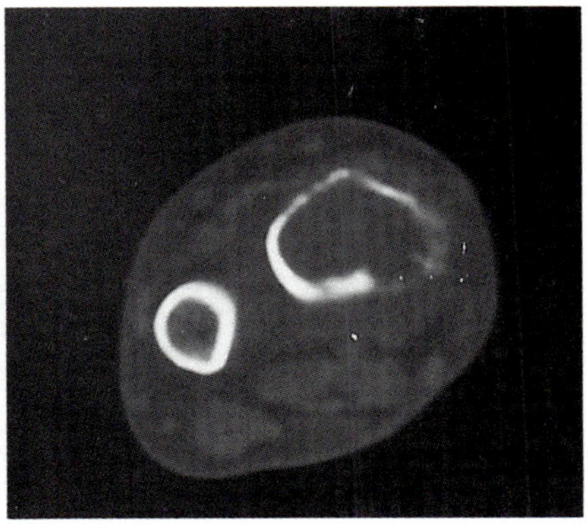

431 CT scan of the lesion showing the extent of cortical loss.

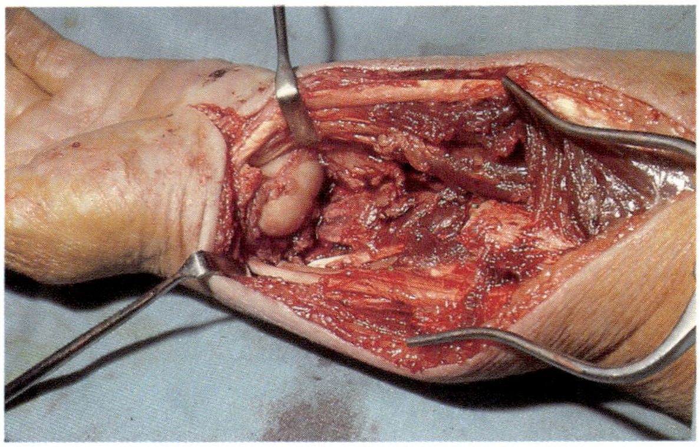

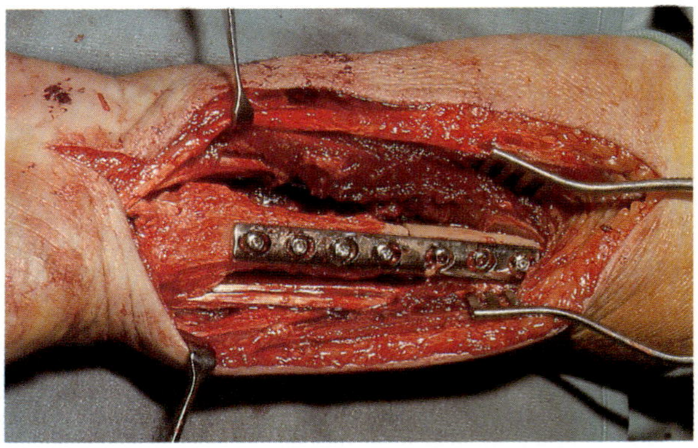

432 & 433 Operative pictures after excision of distal radius and replacement with a non-vascularised, ipsilateral upper fibular graft.

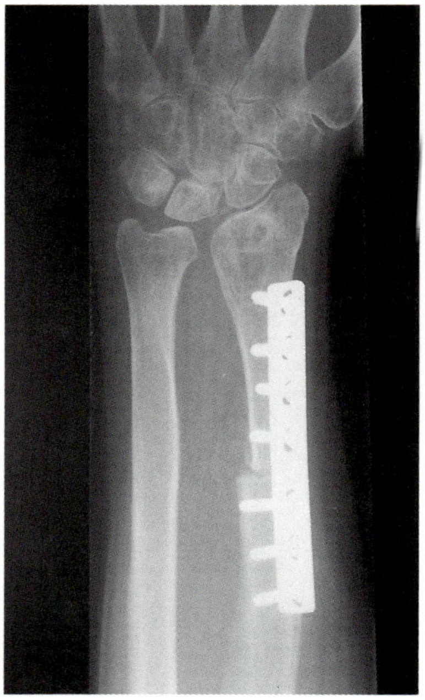

434 Post-operative radiograph.

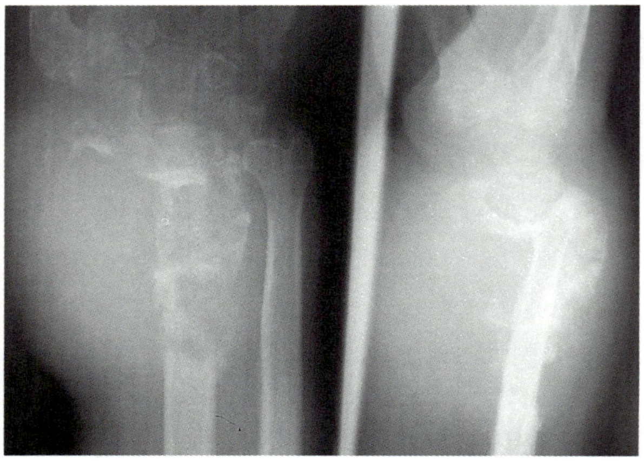

435 Sarcomatous change in recurrent giant cell tumour of the distal radius over 30 years after initial curettage.

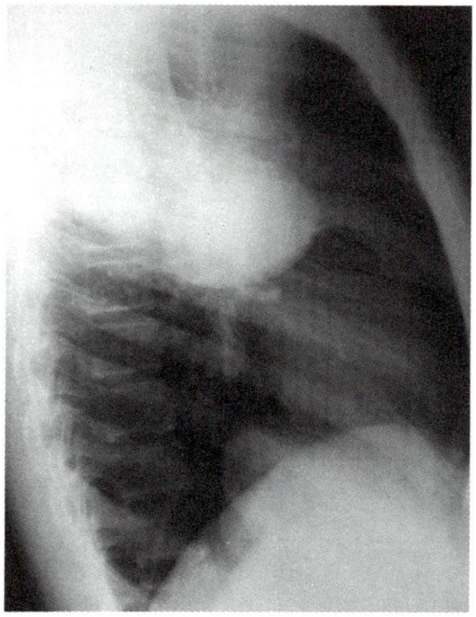

436 The lung is the commonest site for secondaries from a metastasising giant cell tumour.

Primary malignant tumours of soft tissue

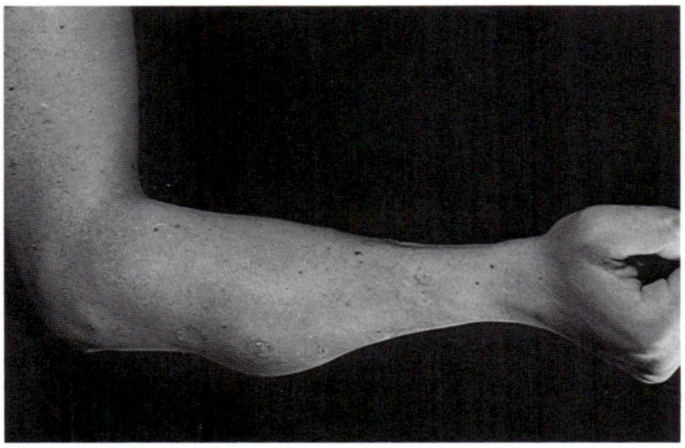

437 Fibrosarcoma. A mass in the forearm of a young man which was solid and attached to deep structures but not to skin.

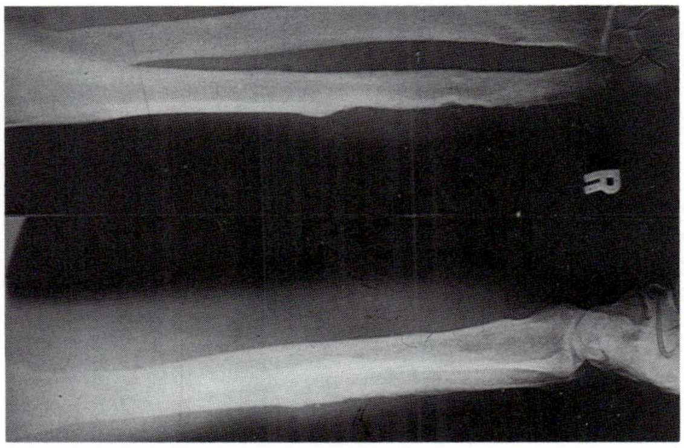

438 The ulna has become eroded from without.

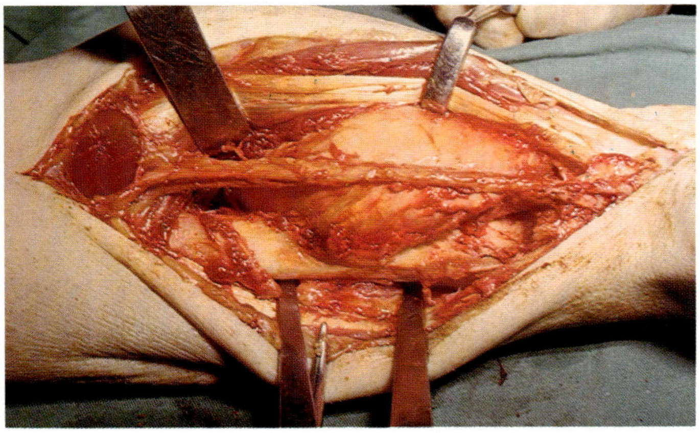

439 The tumour mass displayed at operation.

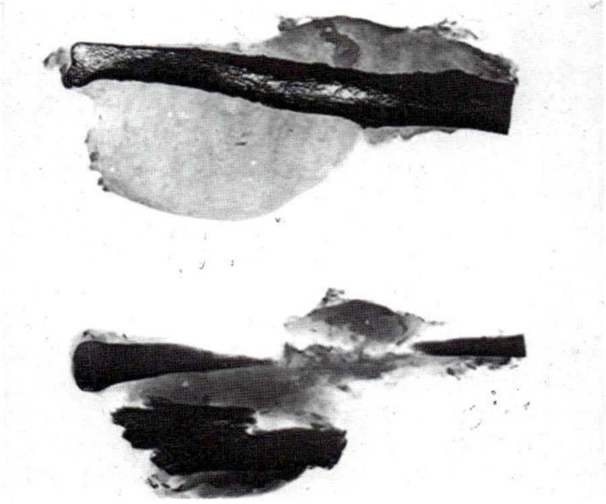

440 A slab radiograph of the resected ulna.

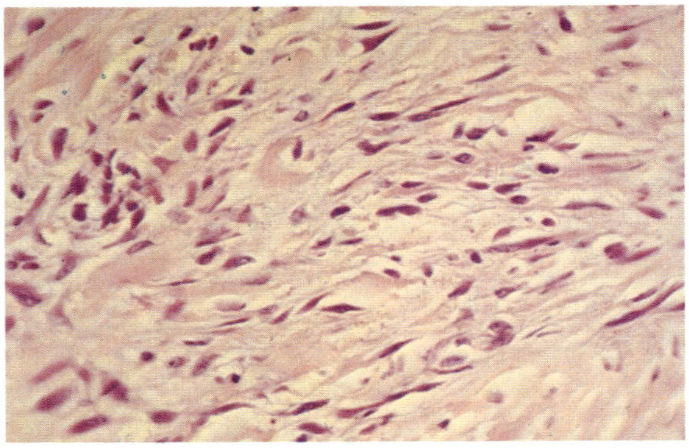

441 Bundles of fibroblasts interspersed by collagen. *(x 350)*

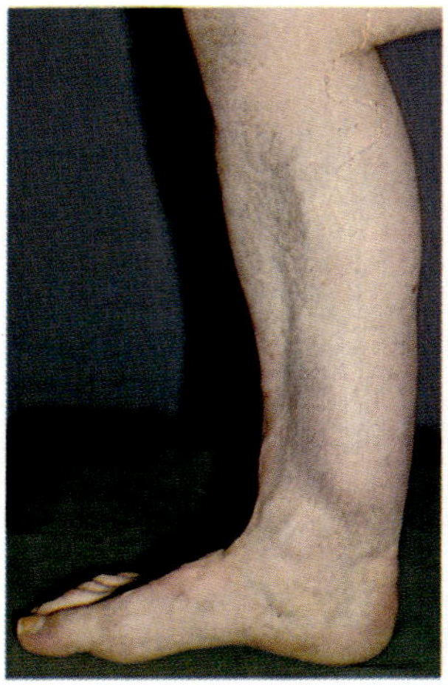

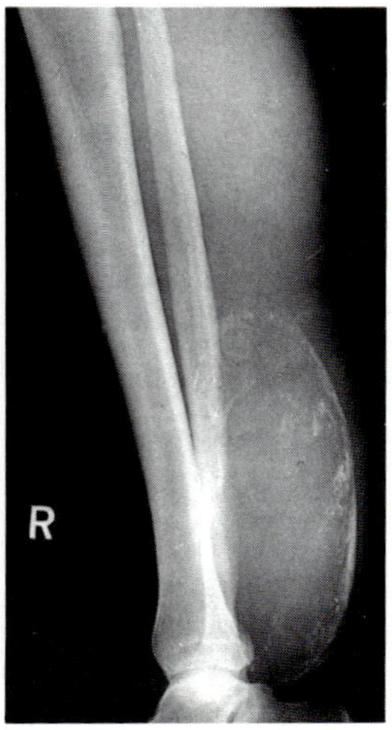

442 & **443**
Myxosarcoma. A solid mass arising in the postero-medial aspect of the lower half of the right leg of a middle-aged man. Radiograph shows an apparently encapsulated soft tissue mass with specks of calcification and new bone formation.

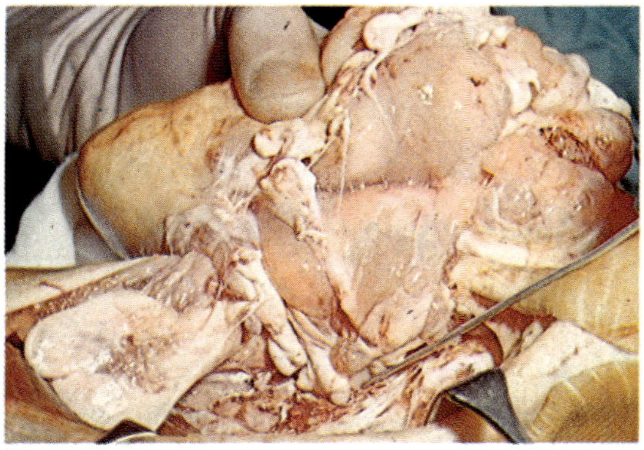

444 The large tumorous mass is excised.

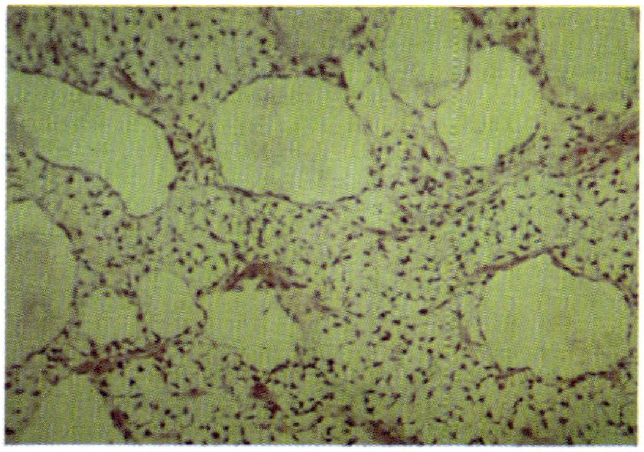

445 The tumour has many unusual features. It is composed of stellate myxoid cells with pools of mucin. It was considered to be a myxosarcoma. The patient died of pulmonary metastases 3 years later. (*× 200*)

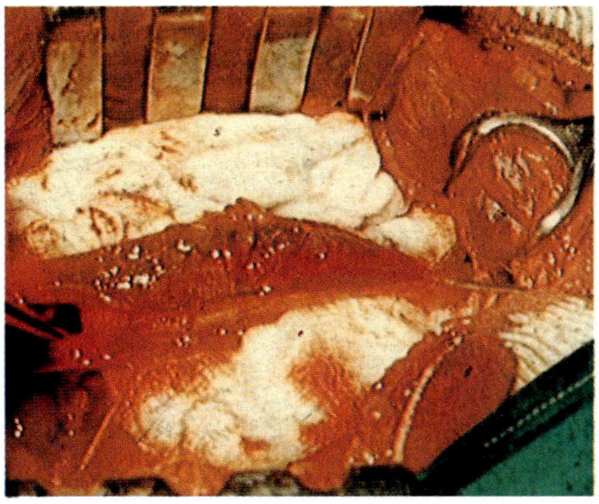

446 Malignant tumour of the sciatic nerve. This patient presented with one simple symptom: when the back of his thigh was pressed upon he experienced tingling in his big toe! There were absolutely no other abnormal symptoms or signs. At operation a fatty tumour was found to lie within the substance of the sciatic nerve in the upper third of the thigh, and extended intraneurally upwards.

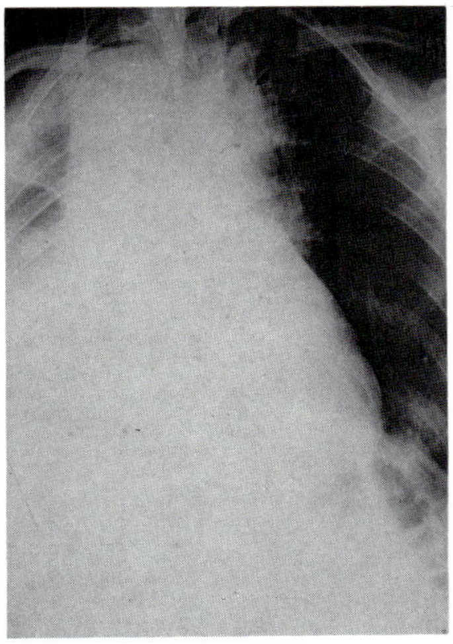

447 The patient died 18 years later of massive mediastinal secondary deposits.

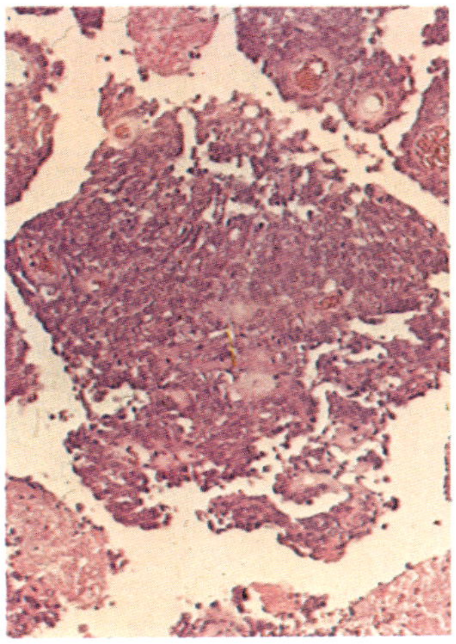

448 The tumour had the same appearances at the primary and secondary sites. The cellular tumour showed extensive areas of necrosis. It is an undifferentiated malignant neoplasm located within a nerve, classified as a neurosarcoma. (*x 100*)

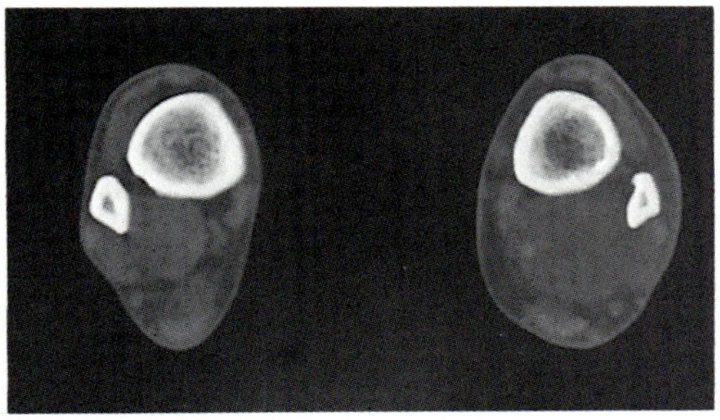

449 MRI has become an important preliminary investigation into the extent of soft tissue sarcomas. The extent to which a lesion is contained or has burst out of a fascial compartment has major implications for treatment. This lesion, a leiomyosarcoma shown here on a CT scan, lies in the space between the Achilles' tendon and the tibia, an extracompartmental site. Amputation was felt to be the treatment of choice.

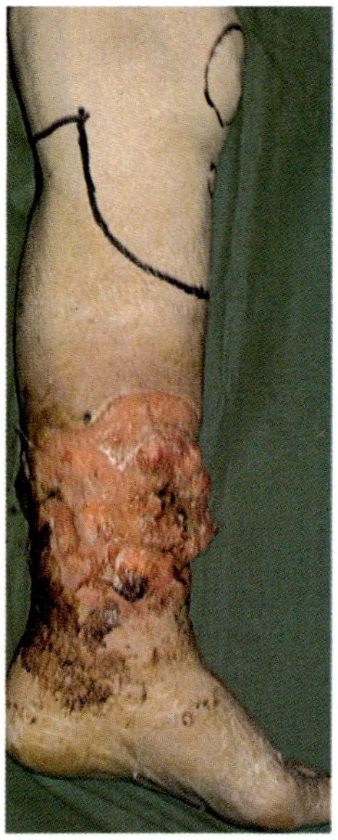

450 Diagnosed as Yaws. This patient had an ulcer on the medial aspect of her right lower leg for many years. A sudden increase in the extent of the ulcerated area and the increase of pain caused her to seek medical advice.

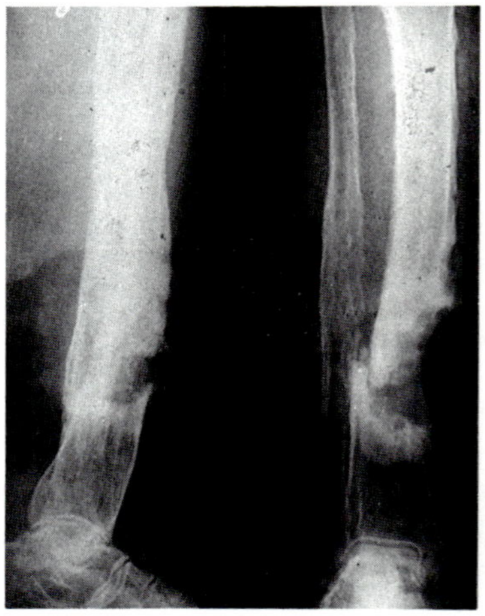

451 The tibia has been eroded by the soft tissue disease surrounding it.

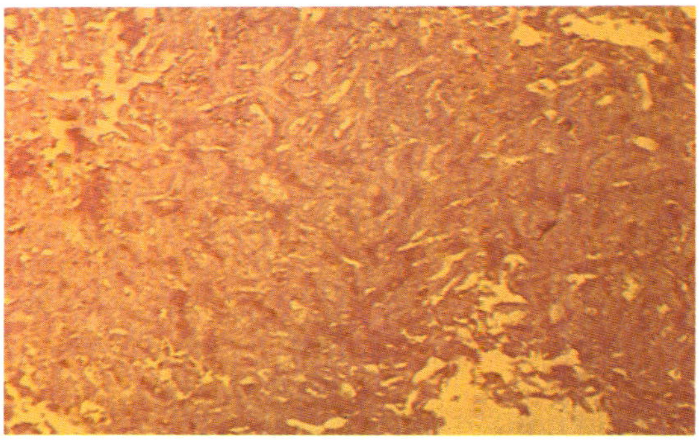

452 Biopsy showed that epithelioma had developed in the Yaws ulcer. The leg was amputated.

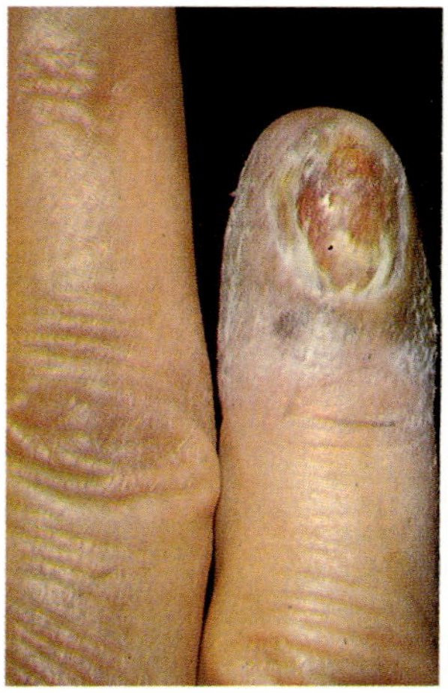

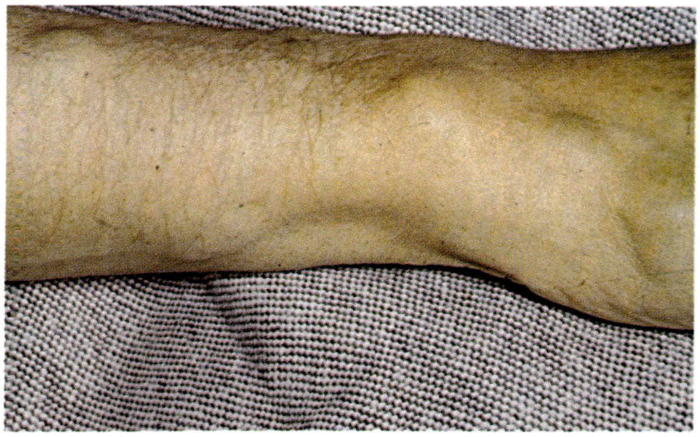

453 & **454** Malignant melanoma arising from the nail-bed of the little finger. The malignant melanoma has spread along the lymphatics and a secondary tumour has developed on the dorsum of the lower forearm.

Malignant tumours of bone

Chondrosarcoma

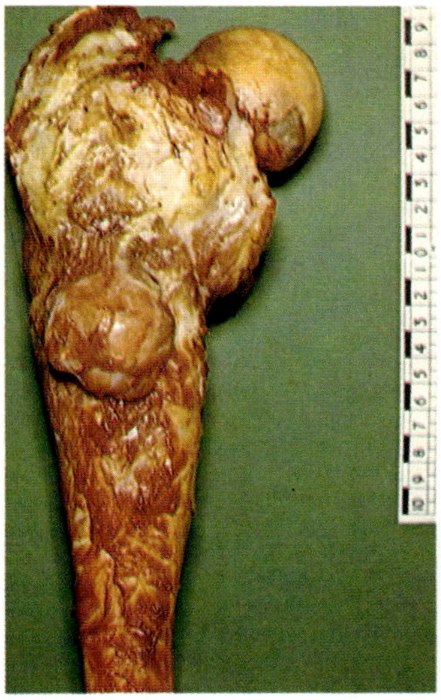

455 Chondrosarcoma of the upper end of the femur, which has enlarged and distorted the bone.

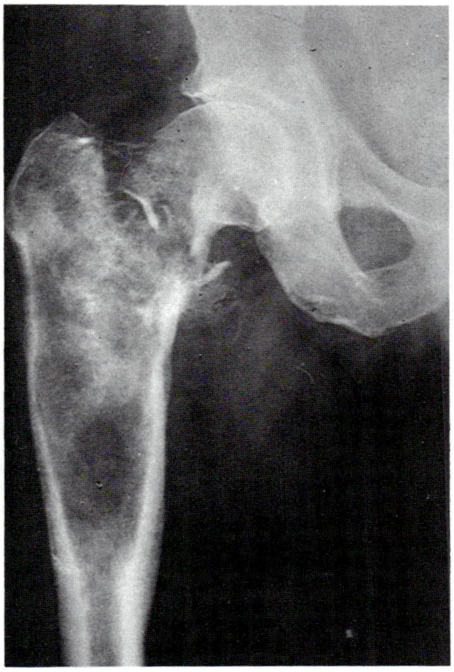

456 Radiograph showing that a pathological fracture has occurred at the base of the neck of the femur.

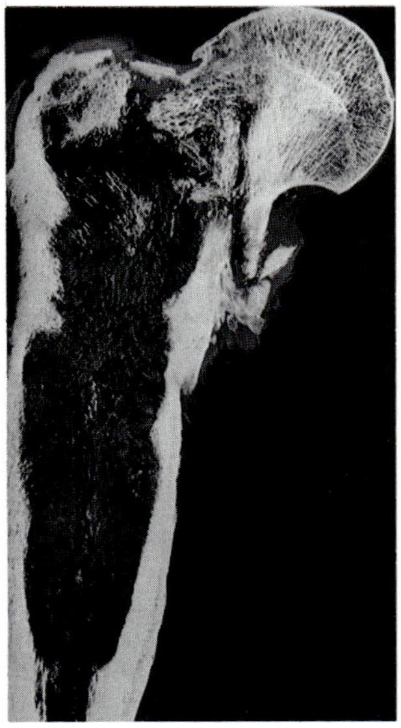

457 Slab radiograph of the specimen which delineates its extent and also confirms the pathological fracture.

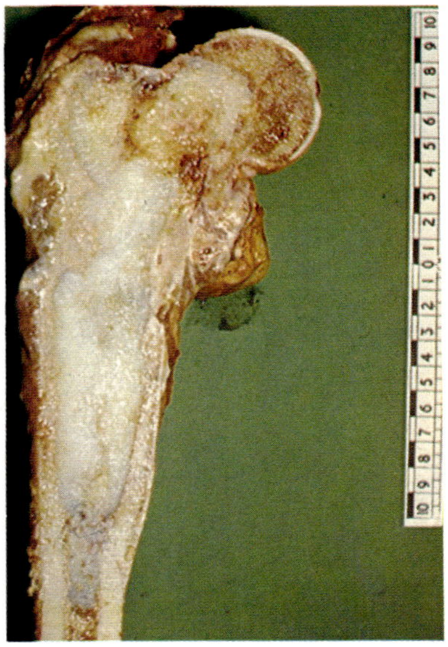

458 Hemisection of the specimen to show tumour cartilage occupying and expanding the bone.

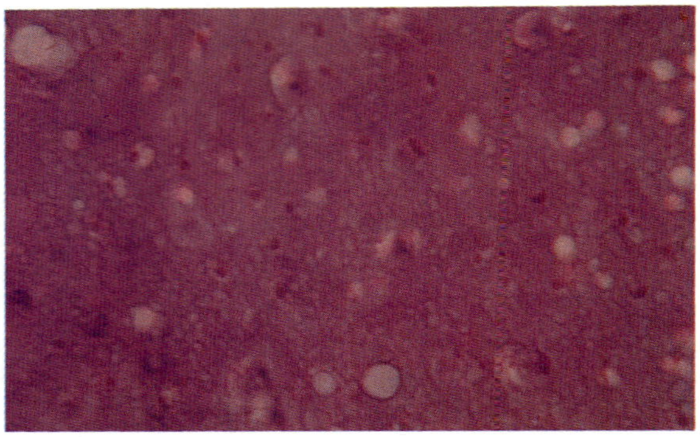

459 The specimen shows a mass of immature cartilage cells with multiple mitotic figures. (*x 400*)

Osteosarcoma

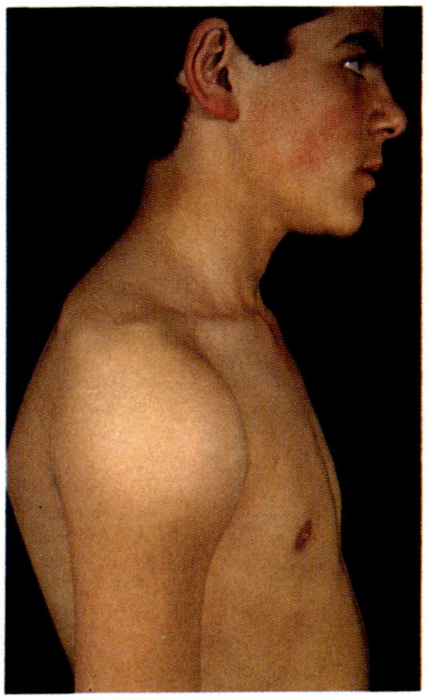

460 A large painful swelling in a 15-year-old boy at the proximal end of the right humerus. It had appeared in only a few weeks. At least half of the cases of osteosarcoma are situated around the knee joint, but any bone may be affected. It can simulate osteomyelitis.

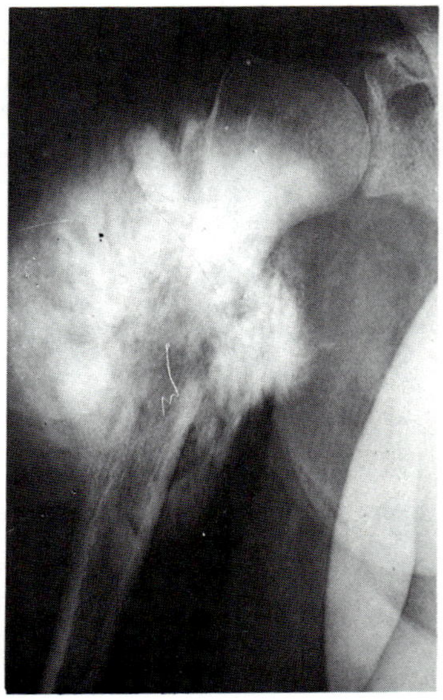

461 Radiograph shows the lytic defects within the bone, periosteal new bone formation, and the characteristic 'sunray' spiculation.

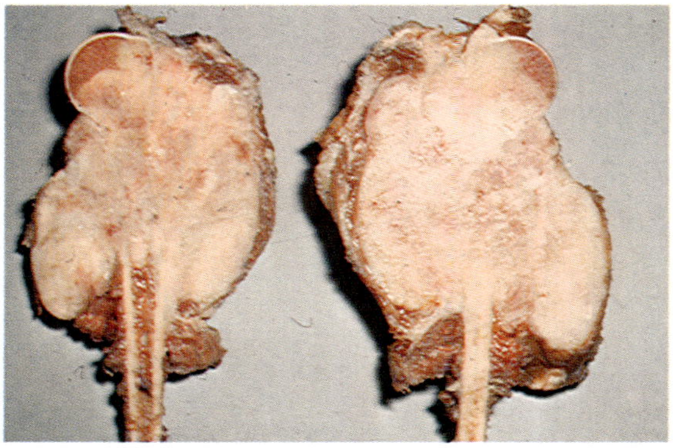

462 The specimen removed by disarticulation at the shoulder.

Ewing's tumour

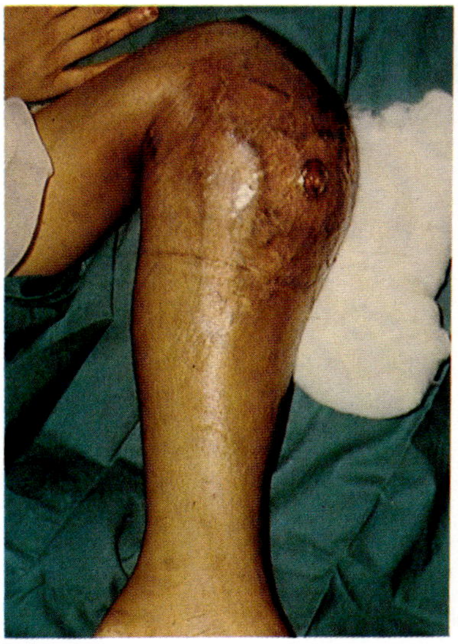

463 Ewing's tumour: an advanced case of the upper end of the tibia in a teenage boy, which has not responded to radiotherapy. Severe pain and constitutional disturbances are a feature.

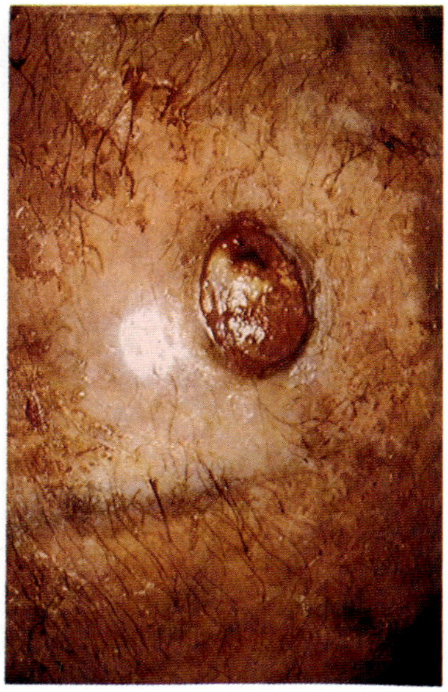

464 The centre of the tumour has ulcerated through the skin. Dilated veins are seen in the lower half of the tumour.

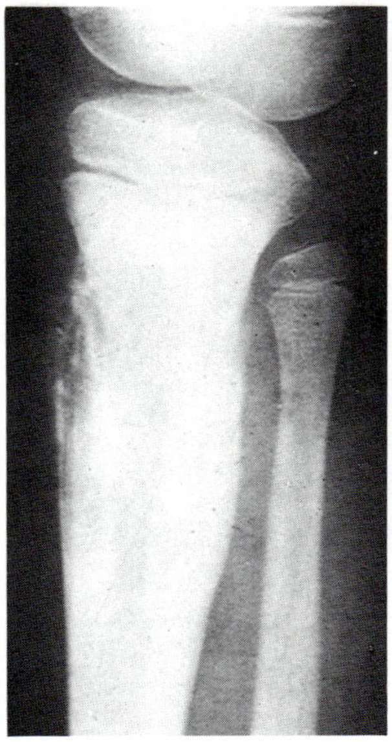

465 Radiograph of the tumour shows a mottled destructive pattern, without any clear zone of transition, involving the medulla of the bone and permeating the anterior cortex.

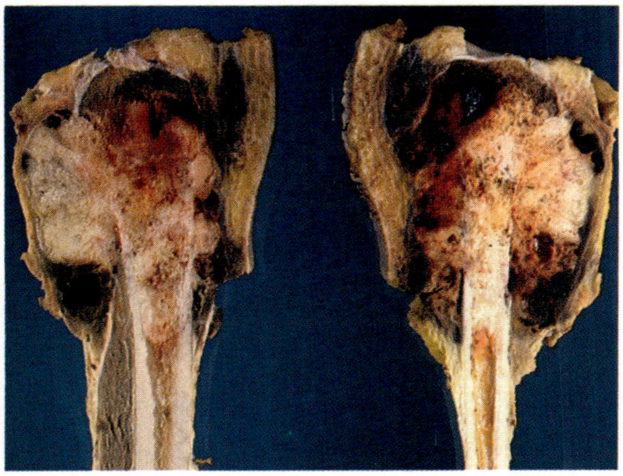

466 Tumour specimen recovered at amputation.

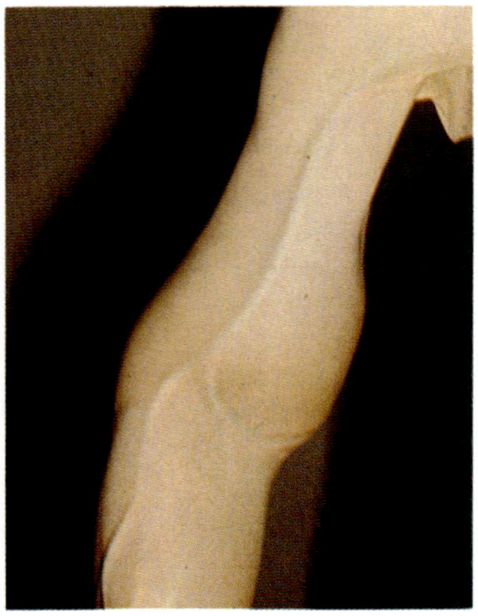

467 Paget's sarcoma of the humerus.

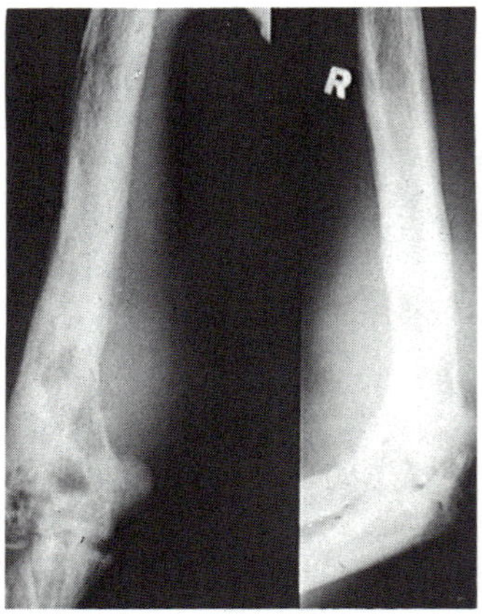

468 The radiograph appearances are characterised by a destructive type of lesion with relatively irregular new bone formation.

Malignant tumours of marrow elements

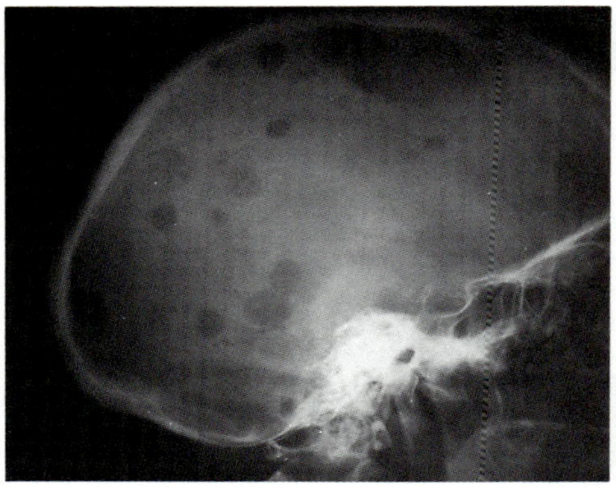

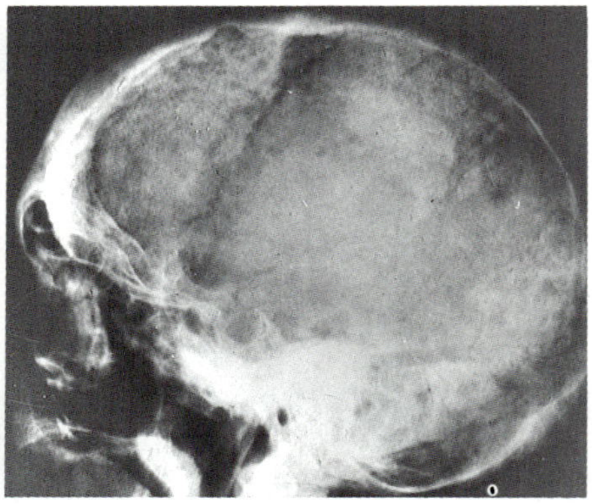

469 & **470** Multiple myeloma is a malignant infiltration of plasma cells. The osteolytic lesions have a classical punched-out appearance, seen here in the skull. Confluence of these lesions gives an osteoporotic appearance to the skull.

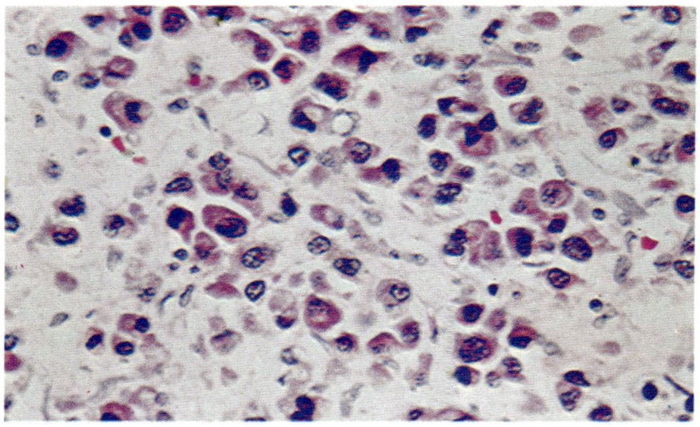

471 Microscopically, the principal component is the mature plasma cell. This typically has a basophilic cytoplasm with an eccentric nucleus whose densely stained chromatin clumps are arranged radially around the nuclear membrane. (*H&E × 250*)

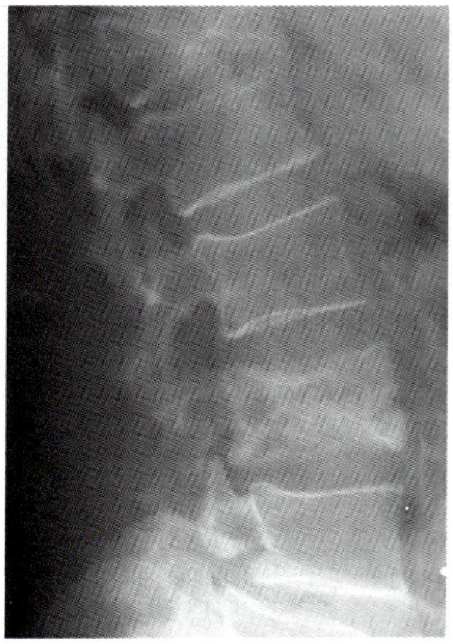

472 Spinal involvement is a common orthopaedic presentation of multiple myeloma with pain, vertebral collapse and sometimes sudden paralysis.

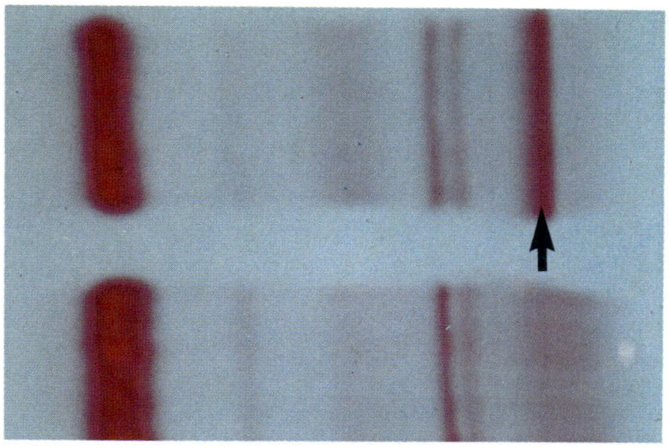

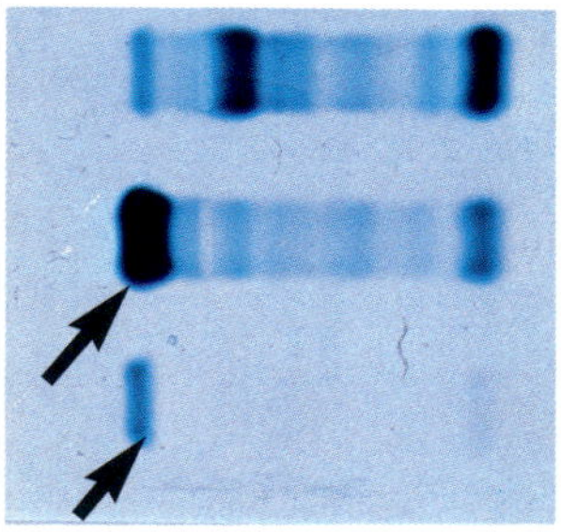

473 & **474** In myeloma, plasma protein electrophoresis demonstrates an abnormal protein band (myeloma band), this is the monoclonal gamma-globulin produced by the malignant plasma cells. The presence of these abnormal proteins in the blood causes an elevation of the ESR, usually above 100. Leakage of immunoglobulin small chains into urine produces the abnormal Bence–Jones protein.

Histiocytosis X

A mixed group of conditions ranging from 'tumours' of cholesterol-filled cells, to widespread deposition of granulomata in bone.

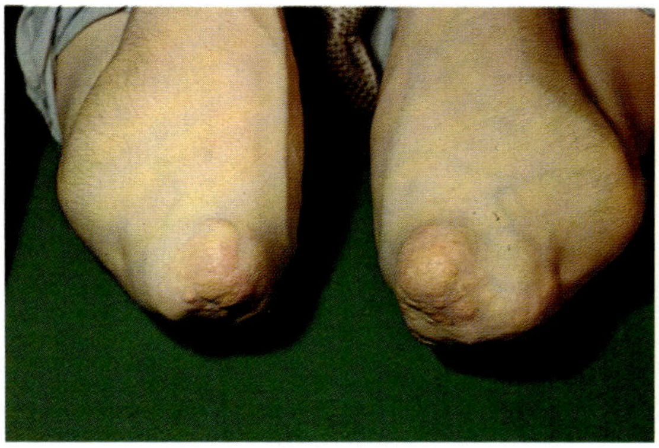

475 Simple xanthomatosis of the olecranon bursa.

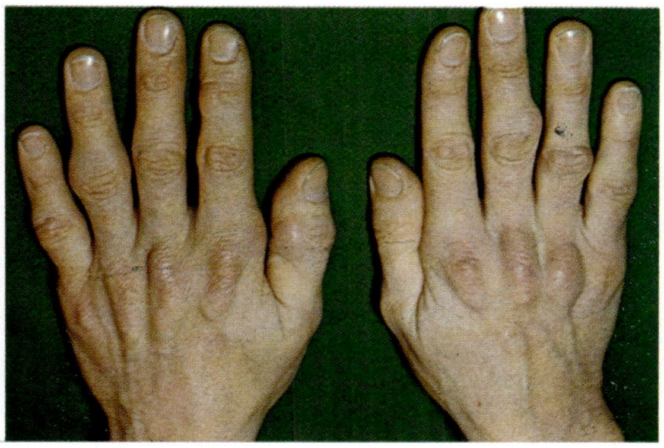

476 Hand–Schuller–Christian disease. Widespread histiocytic granulomatosis.

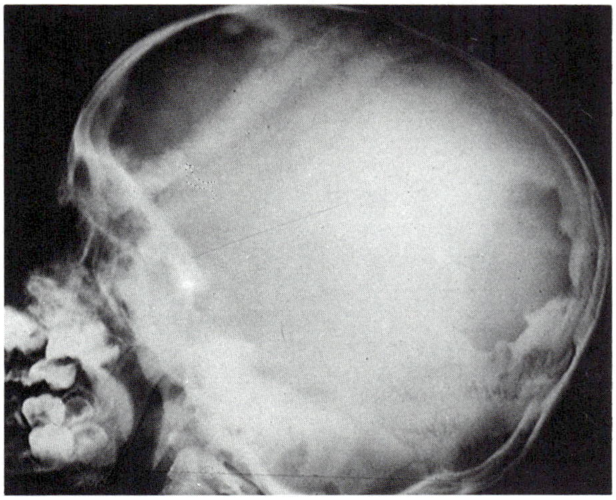

477 Radiograph of the skull in Hand–Schuller–Christian disease.

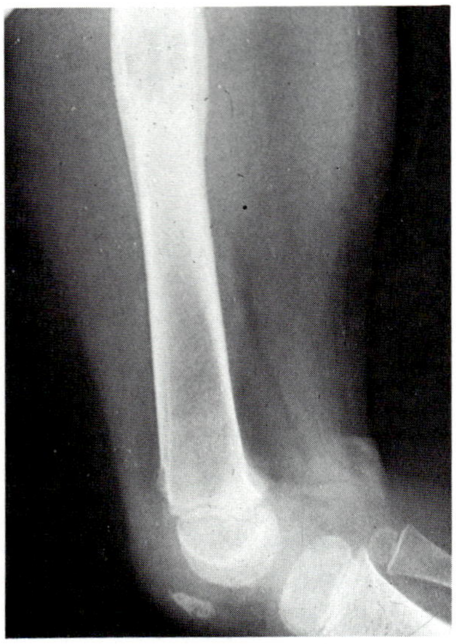

478 Eosinophilic granuloma of bone. The deposits may be single or multiple and usually resolve without treatment.

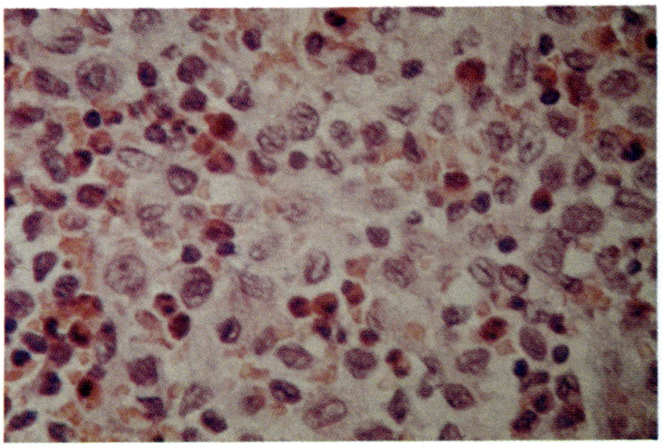

479 Eosinophilic granuloma of bone. Eosinophils dominate in the section, which also contains plasma cells, lymphocytes, histiocytes and other mononuclear cells. (x *400*)

Secondary malignant tumours of bone

Secondary malignant tumours of the skeleton are very much more common than primary malignant tumours. The typical primary sites from which secondary deposits occur are bronchus, kidney, breast, thyroid, large intestine and prostate. A few examples are shown here.

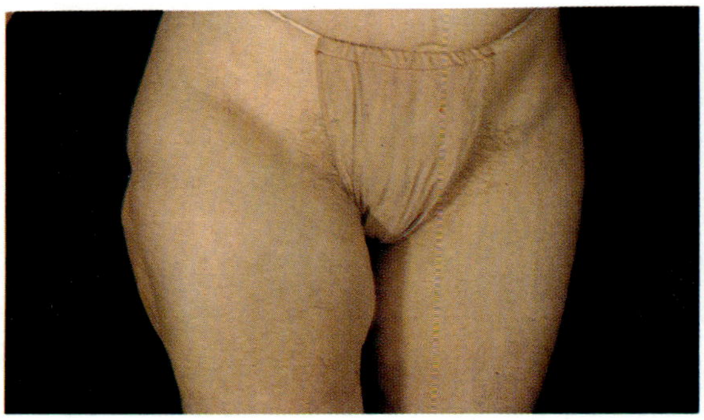

480 Thyroid. This 52-year-old lacy had pain and swelling in the upper aspect of her right thigh. Two years previously a malignant adenoma had been removed from her thyroid.

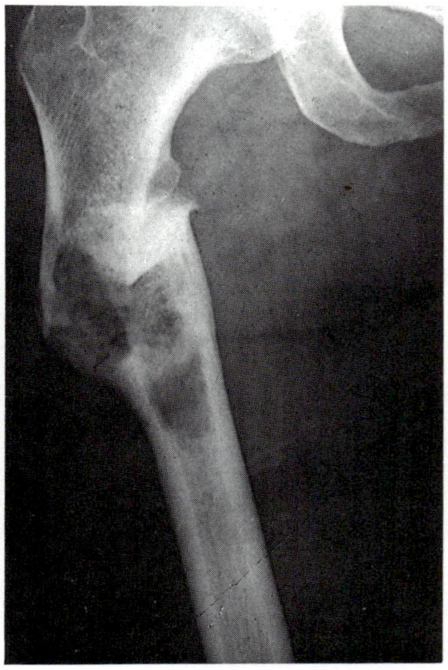

481 An isolated translucent deposit with very little bone reaction is seen: a pathological fracture has occurred through the malignant secondary deposit from the primary in the thyroid gland.

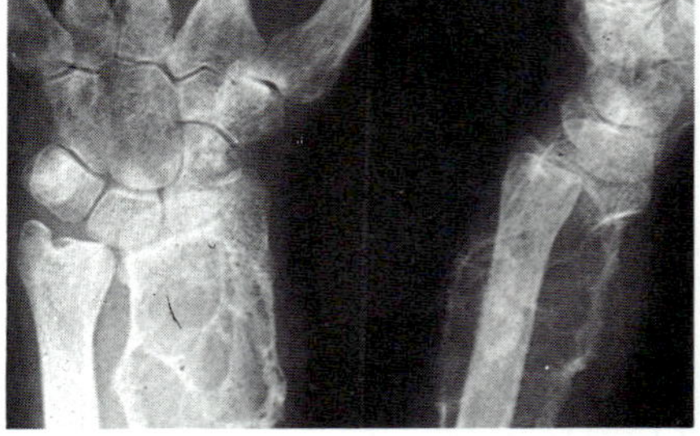

482 Kidney. Enlarged lower end of radius. There was increased warmth of the overlying skin and a vascular bruit could be heard. The honeycombed appearance of the expanded lower end of the radius with considerable thinning of the cortex is noted. The appearances are characteristic of a secondary hypernephroma.

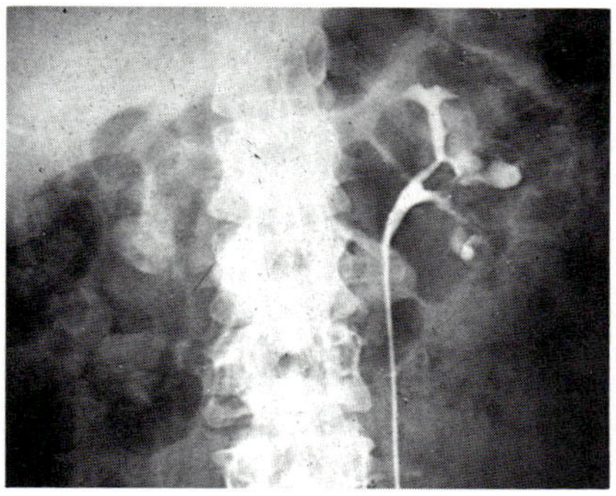

483 The primary tumour in the right kidney is confirmed by pyelography.

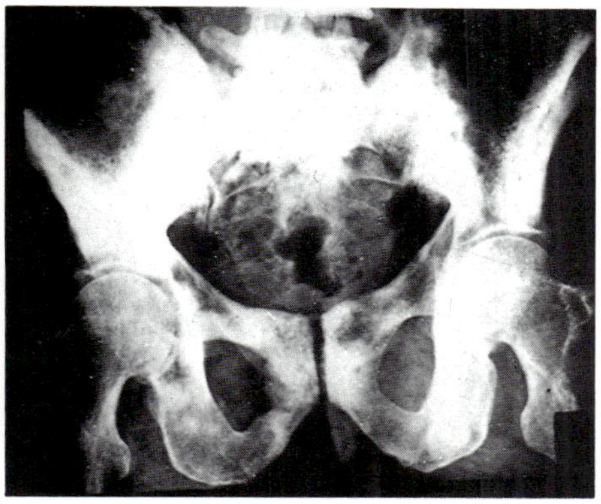

484 Prostate. Carcinoma of the prostate may produce widespread skeletal deposits which have a characteristically dense osteoblastic appearance.

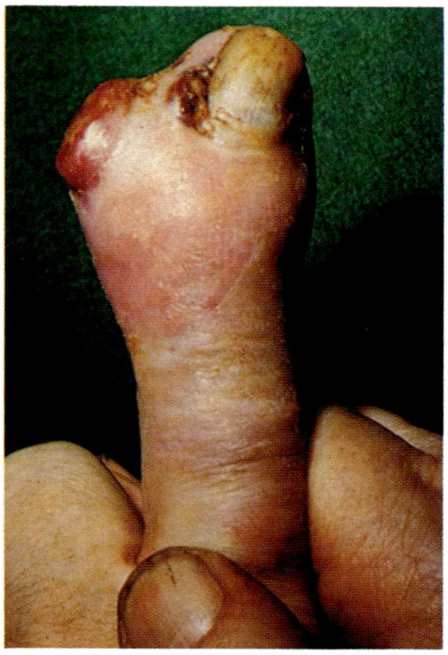

485 Rectum. An ulcerated tumour of the enlarged tip of an index finger caused by a secondary carcinoma. The primary tumour was in the rectum.

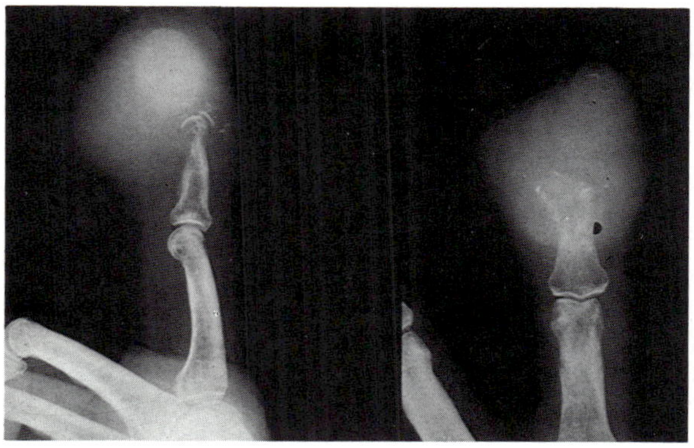

486 Radiograph of the tumour.

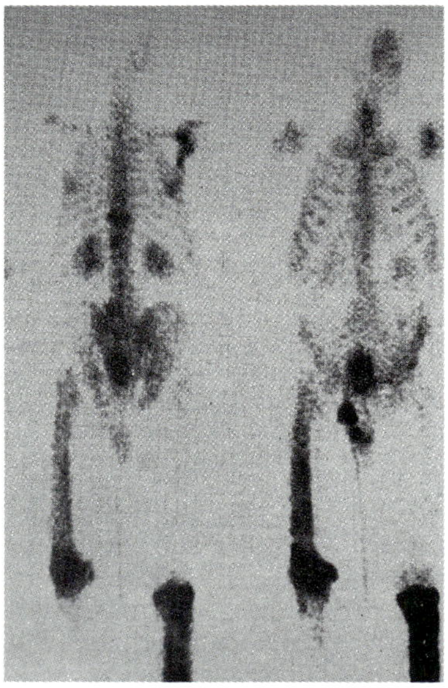

487 Multiple areas of increased isotope uptake on a body scan is a typical indication of metastatic disease.

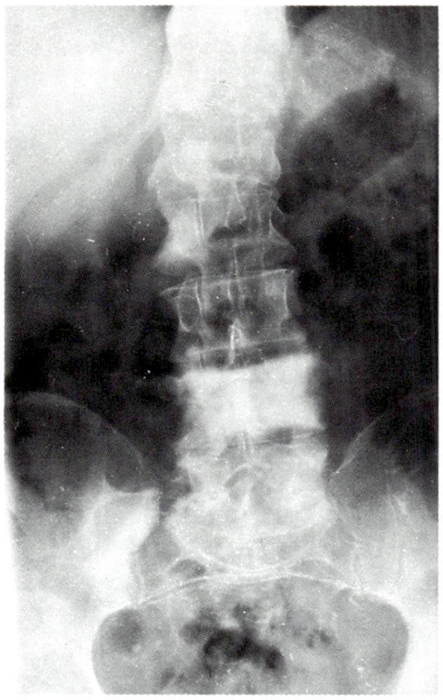

488 Vertebra nigrans. An isolated dense osteosclerotic vertebral body in this case due to prostatic secondaries. Other causes includes Paget's disease and lymphoma.

2 Regional section

Most orthopaedic problems present as a disorder of some localised part of the body, usually a joint. Before proceeding to a detailed clinical study of the local lesion one must first be satisfied that the presenting feature is not a localised manifestation of a generalised musculoskeletal disease. In this context the individual's general demeanour, facial appearance, stance and gait may be important pointers to generalised disorders and disease. In the pages which follow some examples of localised physical disorders commonly met with in clinical orthopaedic practice are presented but where some of these regional disorders are an expression of a more generalised disease this will again be stressed.

Facies

Facies

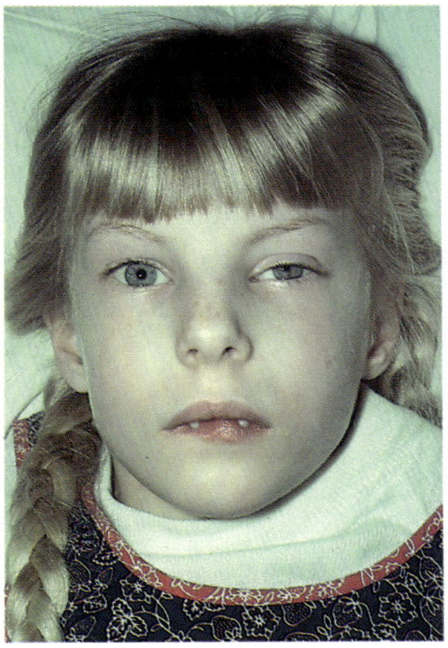

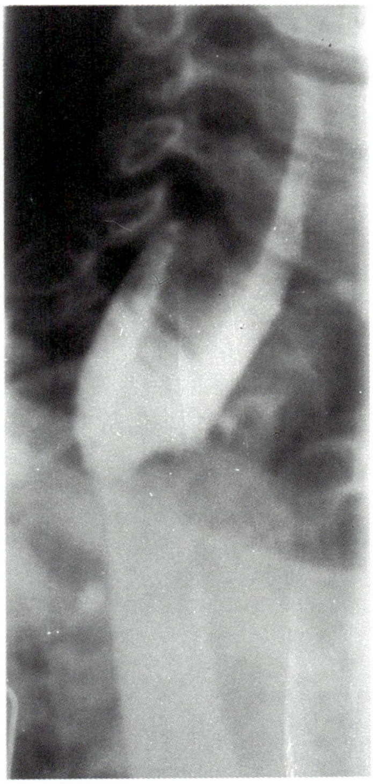

489, 490 Horner's syndrome. The ptosis and enophthalmos on the left side was caused by pressure from a neurofibroma on the lower cervical sympathetic ganglion.

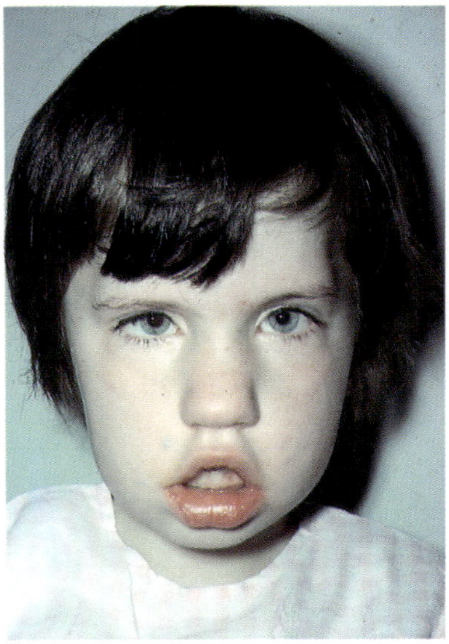

491 Myotonia congenita. This intelligent girl exhibits the classical 'rose bud' mouth and facial muscle drooping of this generalised inherited condition.

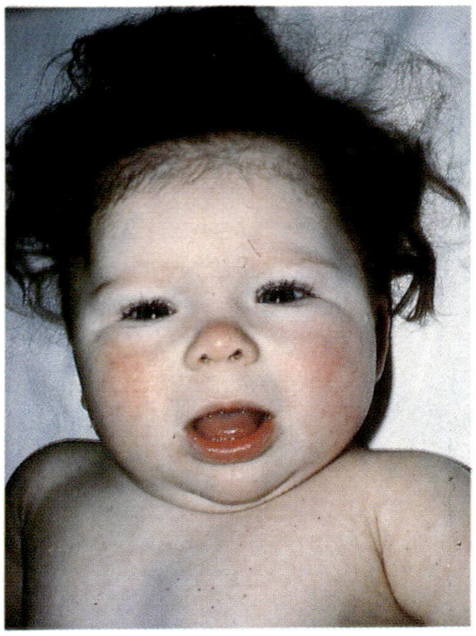

492 Congenital hypothyroidism. This infant shows the large tongue, coarse hair and bloated appearance of cretinism. She presented orthopaedically because of delayed locomotor development and poor ossification of the femoral head nuclei.

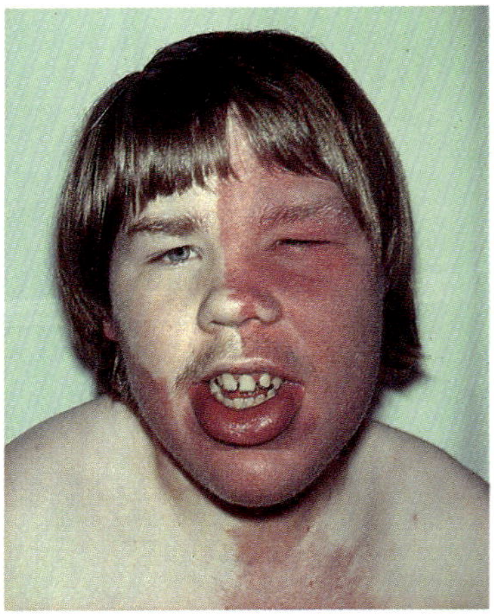

493 Sturge–Weber syndrome. Facial and cerebral vascular naevi resulting in a hemiplegia.

Neck, thoracic cage and shoulder girdle

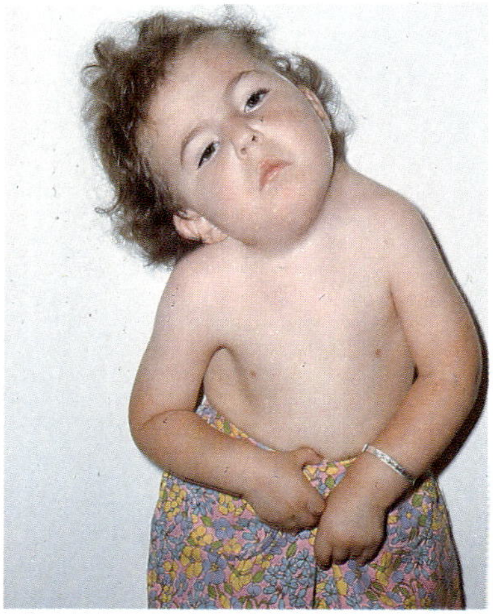

494 Congenital bony torticollis. The girl has associated brevicollis, deafness and branchial arch defects.

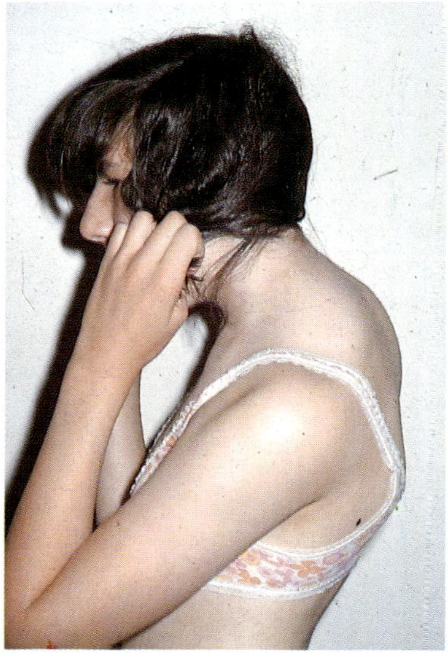

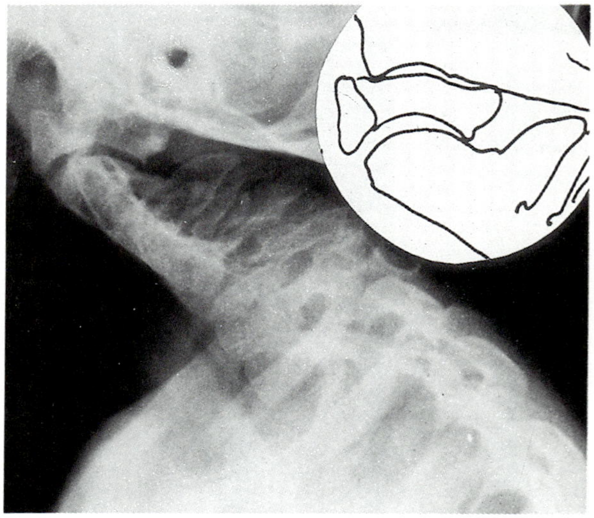

495 & **496** Klippel–Feil syndrome. Note the forward inclination of the neck. Radiologically, there is synostosis of multiple vertebral segments and, in this case, a hypoplastic odontoid.

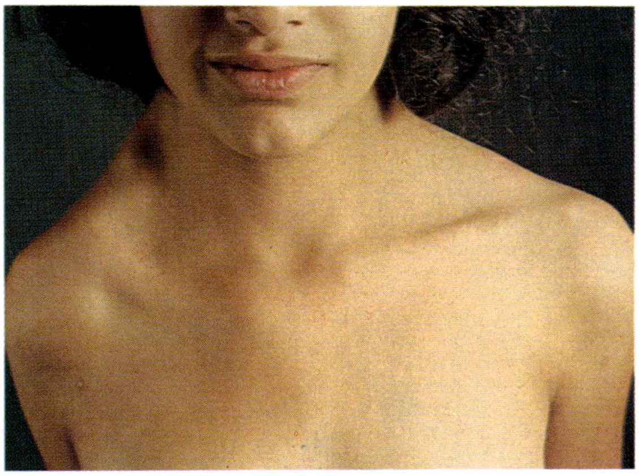

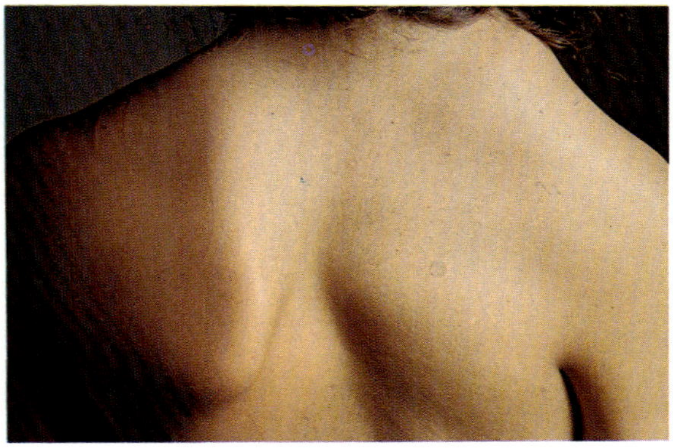

497 & **498** Klippel–Feil syndrome. There may also be failure of scapular descent, again associated with considerable abnormality of the cervical spine. The neck is often short and webbed, with a low hair line.

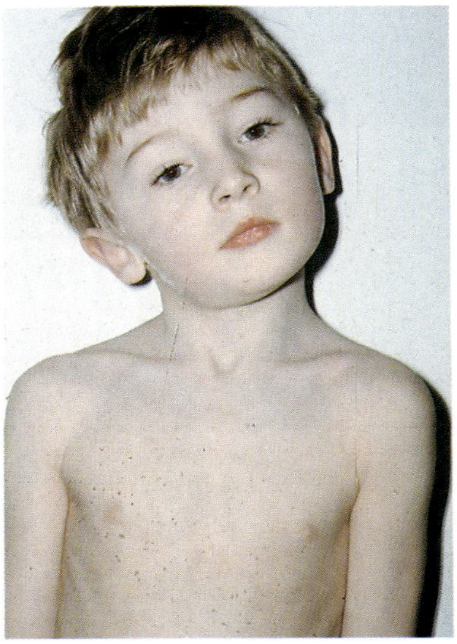

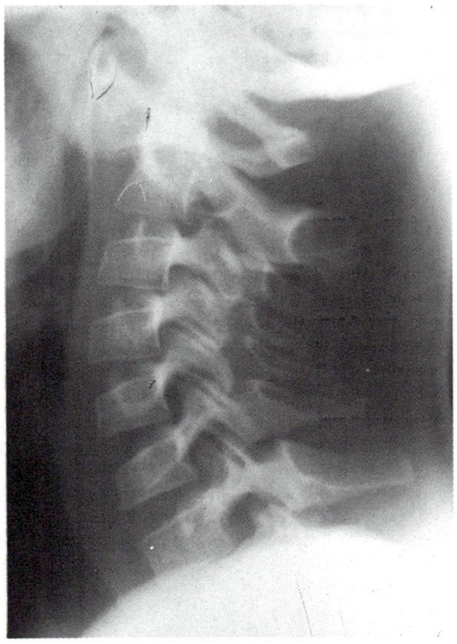

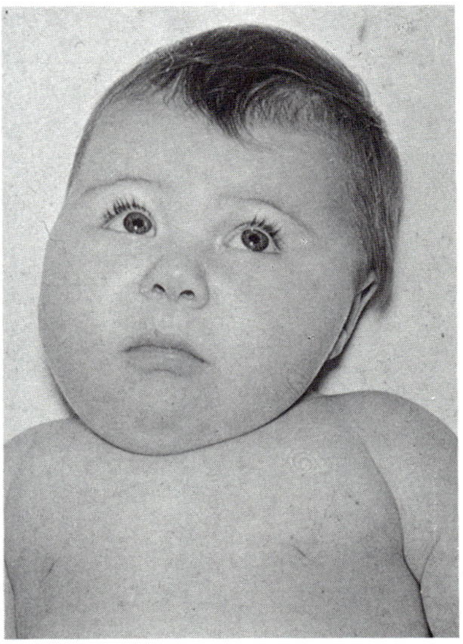

499 & **500** Atlanto-axial instability. This gives rise to a rotational type of torticollis due to asymmetrical forward subluxation of the atlas on the axis. Such instability can arise from a number of causes, e.g. post-infective laxity of the transverse ligament, trauma and Down's syndrome.

501 Myogenic torticollis (wry neck). The sternomastoid muscle on the left side of this child's neck is contracted so that his head is tilted to the left and rotated to the right. In 20% of cases a transient 'sternomastoid tumour' can be felt in the affected muscle.

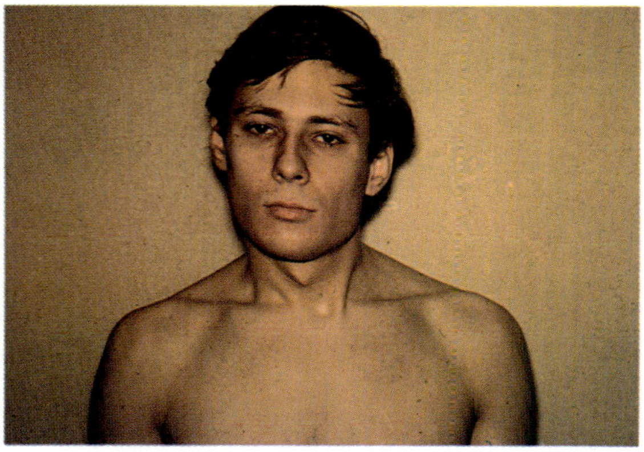

502 The deformity may persist into adult life. The tilting and rotation of the head become established and the eyes remain at different levels. The prominent manubrial head of the left sternomastoid muscle is clearly shown.

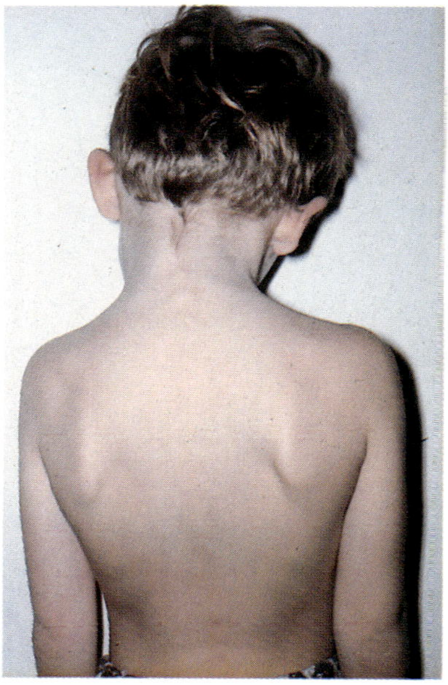

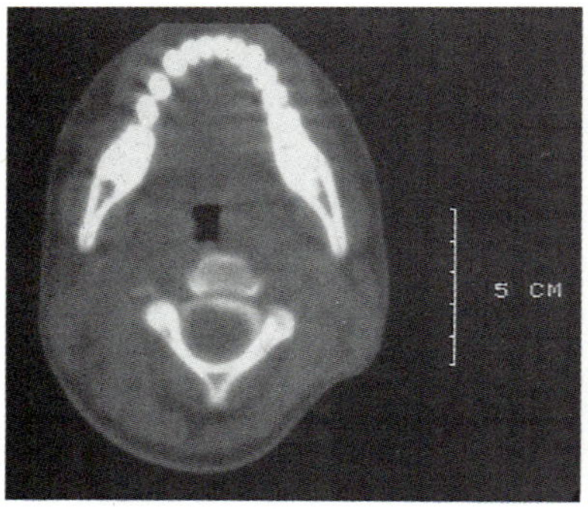

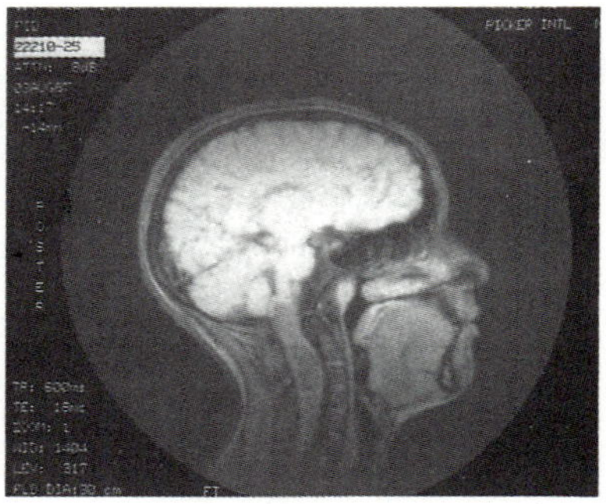

503–505 Recurrent torticollis. This child, in addition to the deformity, has variable neck pain arising from a cystic lesion in the cervical cord shown on both the CT and MRI scans.

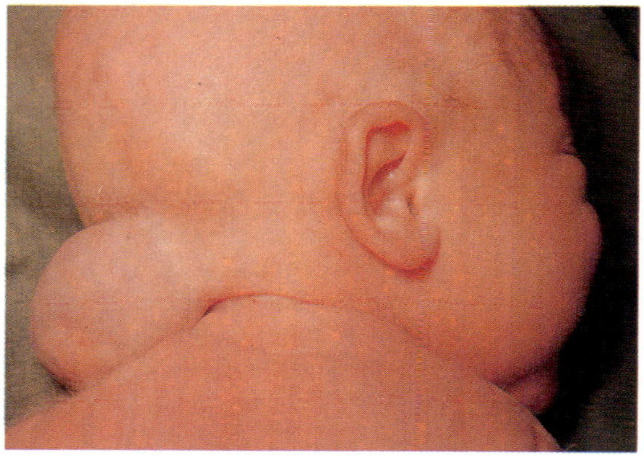

506 Cervical meningocele. The baby is otherwise normal, except for the brevicollis. As there is no spinal cord involvement there is no neurological deficit.

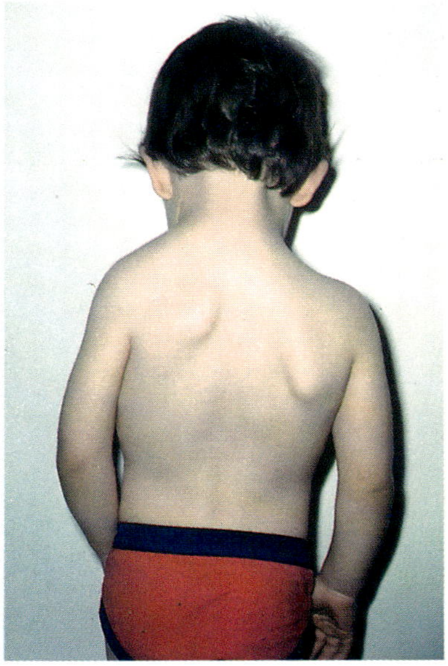

507 Sprengel's shoulder. This child's left scapula has failed to descend from its embryonic position.

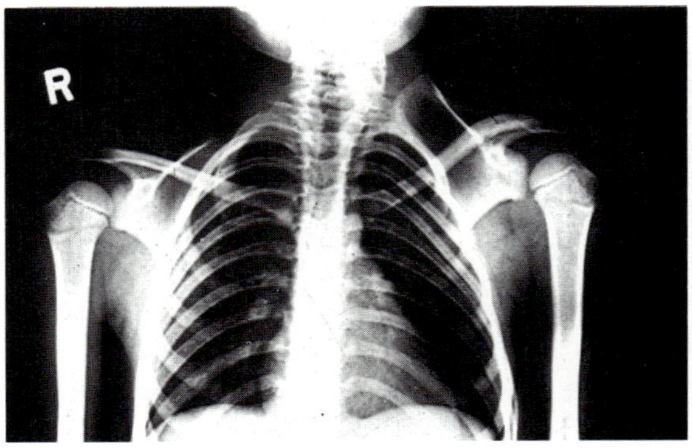

508 Radiograph to show the high, cervical position of the scapula.

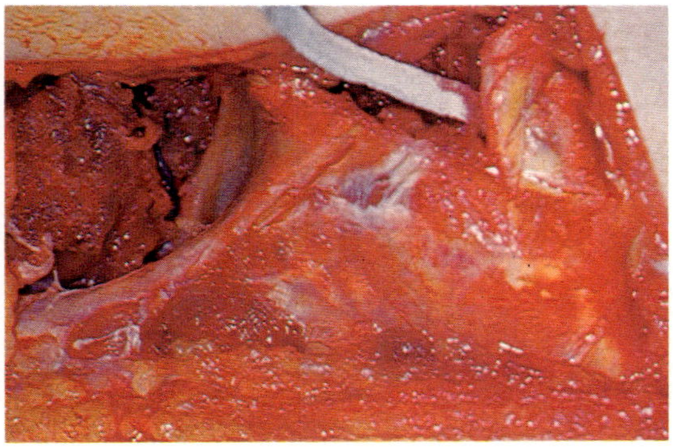

509 A fibrous band extends between the upper border of the scapula and the cervical vertebrae. This band may become ossified (omovertebral bone). The band is displayed at operation by the upper retractor.

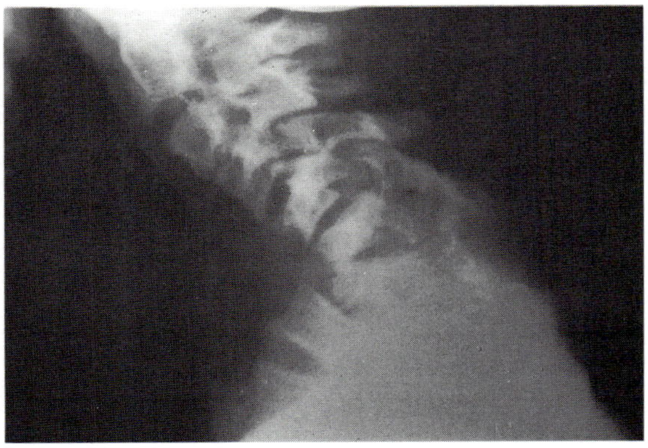

510 Progressive cervical kyphosis. There are numerous possible causes for this condition. The cause in this case was generalised neurofibromatosis.

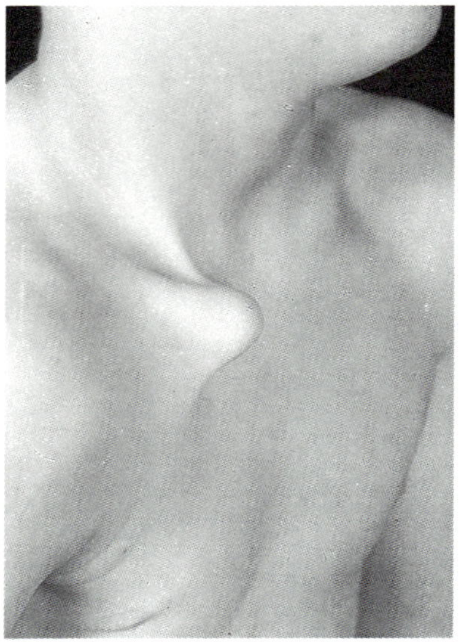

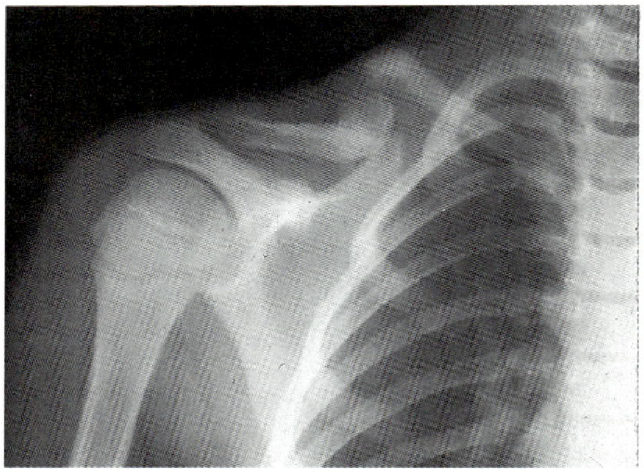

511 & **512** Congenital pseudoarthrosis of the clavicle. This is a rare entity which can be confused with non-union of a fracture. It may give rise to cosmetic problems and disability owing to discomfort. The lesion is almost invariably on the right side.

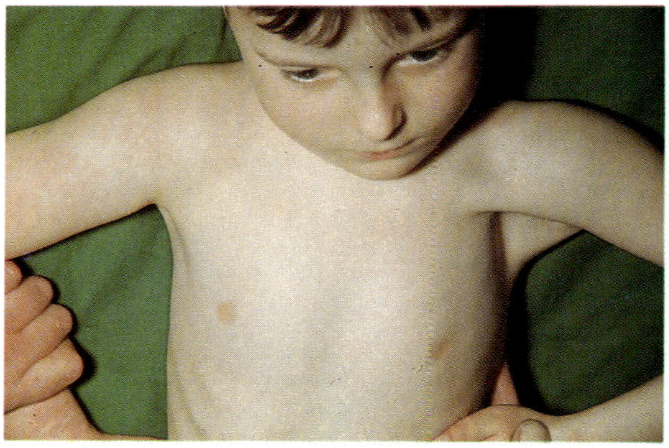

513 Partial absence of pectoralis major. This is generally an isolated anomaly with no disability arising.

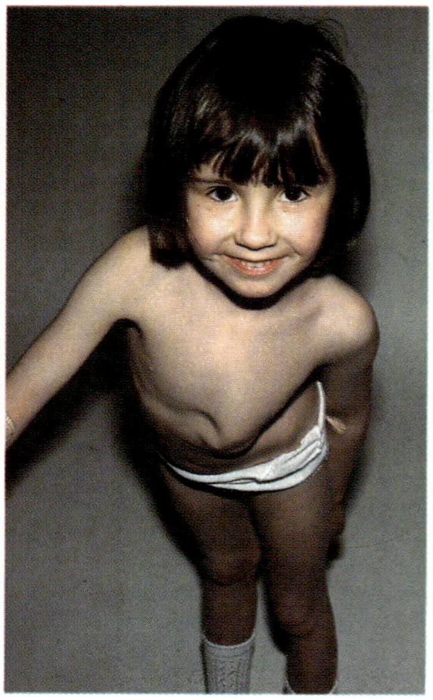

514 Pectus carinatum. The pigeon chest deformity is of cosmetic importance only. It may be accompanied by rib defects or fusions.

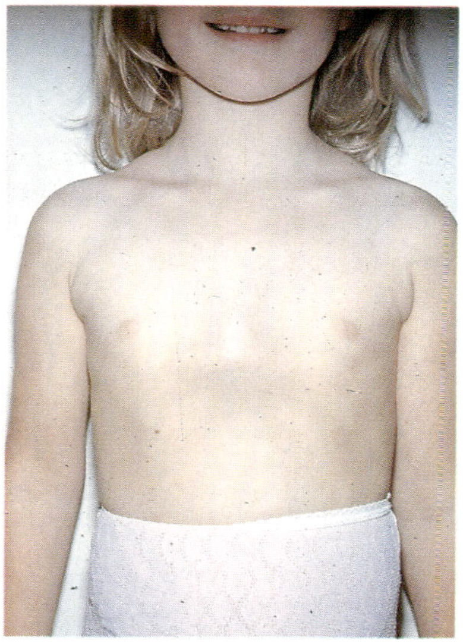

515 Pectus excavatum. This deformity is normally harmless but occasionally may be associated with mild cardiorespiratory embarrassment.

Cervical spondylosis

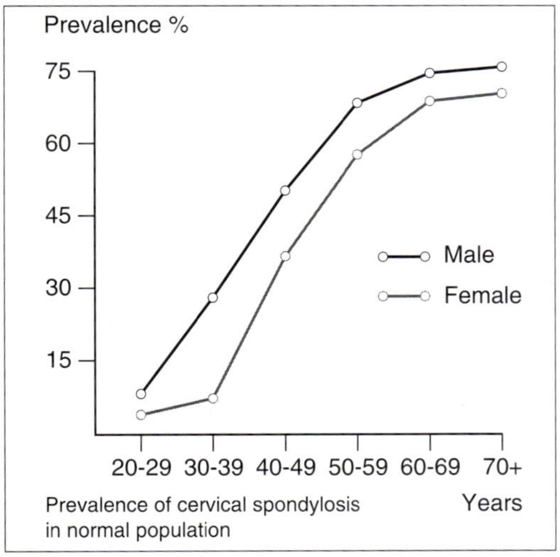

516 Degenerative arthritis of the cervical spine is such a common condition that it is considered a normal feature of biological ageing. The fact that cervical spondylosis is demonstrated on a radiograph does not necessarily indicate a disease process responsible for the patient's symptoms. The histograph shows how commonly radiographic cervical spondylosis appears in the general population.

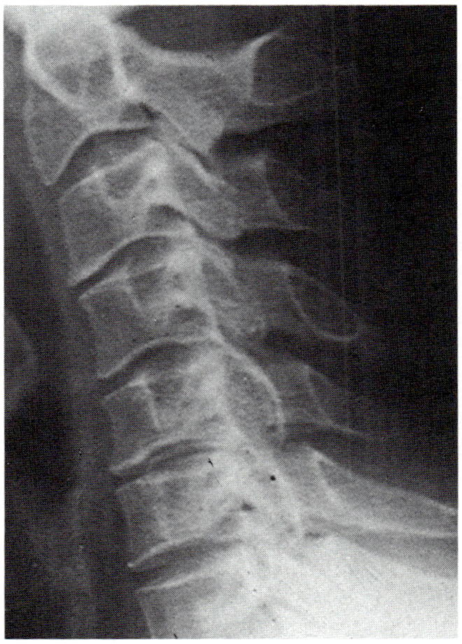

517 Acute cervical intervertebral disc protrusion. Often the only abnormality seen is the loss of normal cervical lordosis in the lateral radiographs. It is caused by muscle spasm. The bone and joint structure may be otherwise entirely normal in early cases.

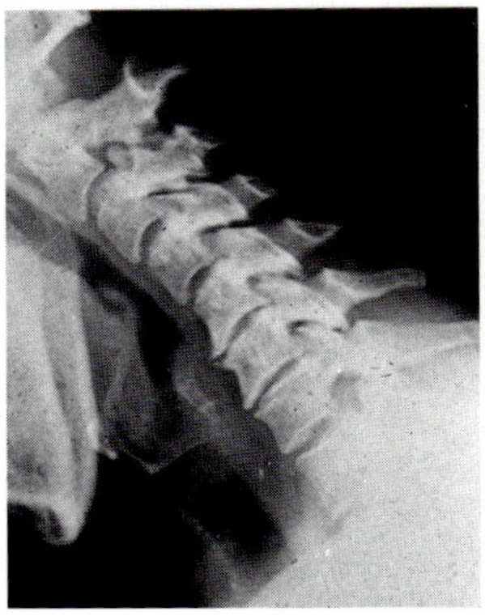

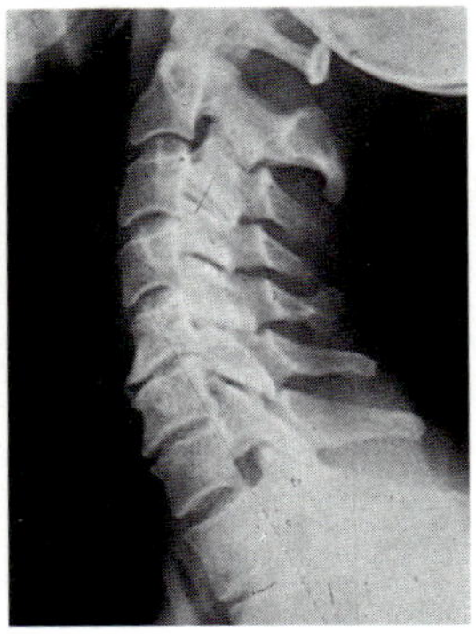

518 & **519** Radiographs of the cervical spine taken in full flexion and extension showing marked spondylosis at the commonest level, C5/6, symptomless in this case.

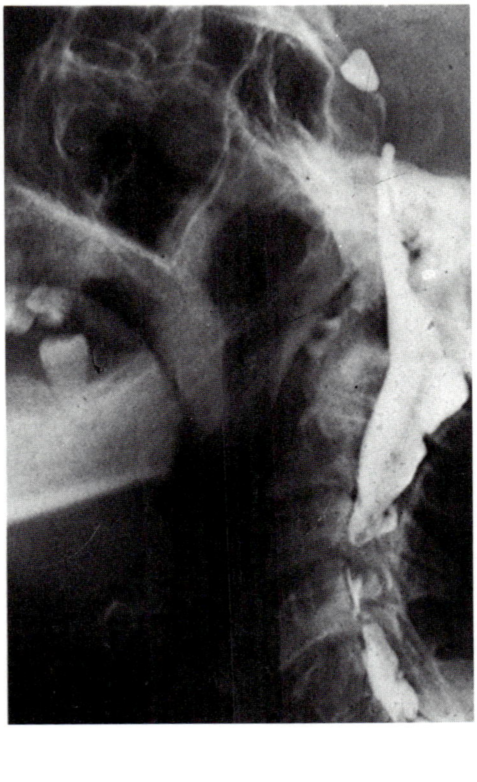

520 Cervical myelography. Interruption of the myodil column; in rare occasions this is caused by the pressure of osteophytes and disc material in cervical spondylosis.

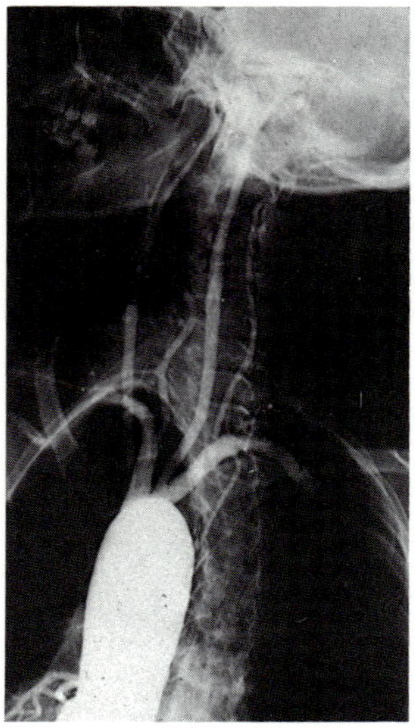

521 Angiography. Unexplained intermittent syncope. On turning her head to the left, the flow of contrast medium through the patient's left vertebral artery is interrupted.

Thoracic outlet (cervical rib) syndrome

A vascular syndrome with objective clinical findings due to vascular obstruction or thromboembolic phenomena is a well recognised entity (**525, 526**). A neurological syndrome, however, rarely has convincing objective signs (**527**). Complaints of vague discomfort, fatigue and subjective weakness of the upper limbs in middle aged women is frequently attributed by some to a thoracic outlet compression, but surgical decompression in such cases is often unrewarding and sheds doubt on the diagnosis.

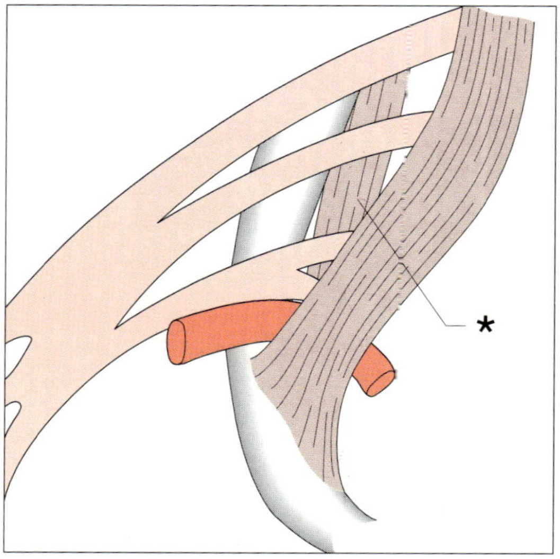

522 The subclavian artery and the lower trunk of the brachial plexus (C8, T1) lie, as it were, suspended in a sling formed by the scalenus anterior insertion in front and the first rib behind. An extra rib arising from C7, its fibrous equivalent, or an abnormal scalenus medius muscle, can sharpen the angle and embarrass the nerve and artery. The asterisk marks the position of such an anomalous structure.

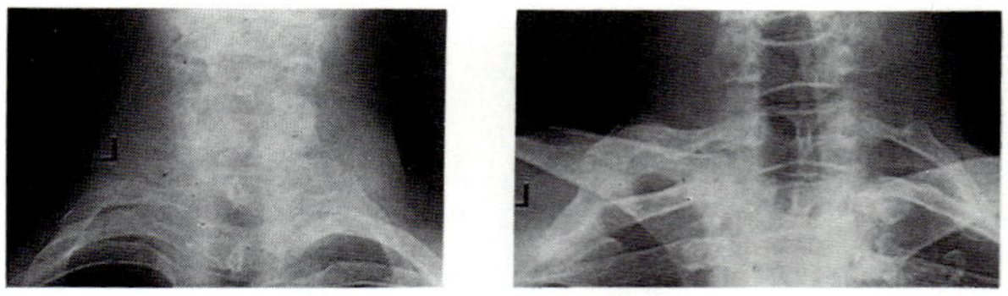

523 & **524** Bilateral cervical ribs. On the left the standard projection just shows the abnormal ribs; on the right a tilted projection of the same patient displays the ribs more clearly.

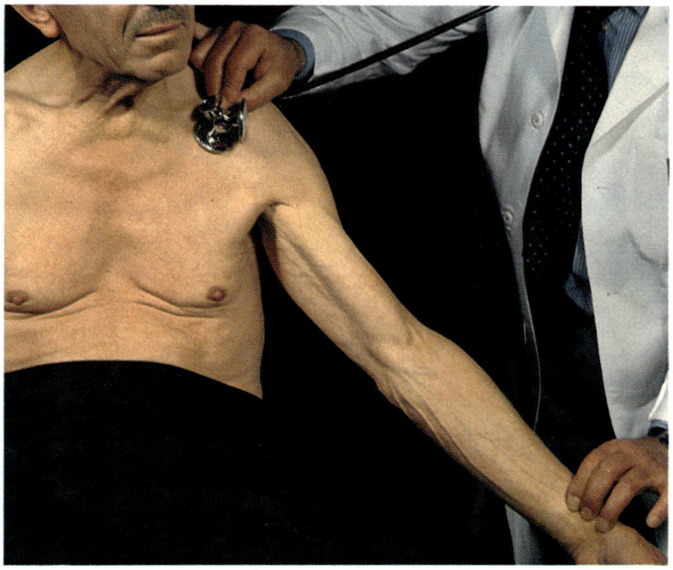

525 Adson's test. The patient's arm is pulled upon while his head turns towards and tilts away from, the affected side. The earliest sign of a thoracic outlet syndrome may be partial obliteration of the subclavian artery giving rise to a bruit and diminution or obliteration of the radial pulse.

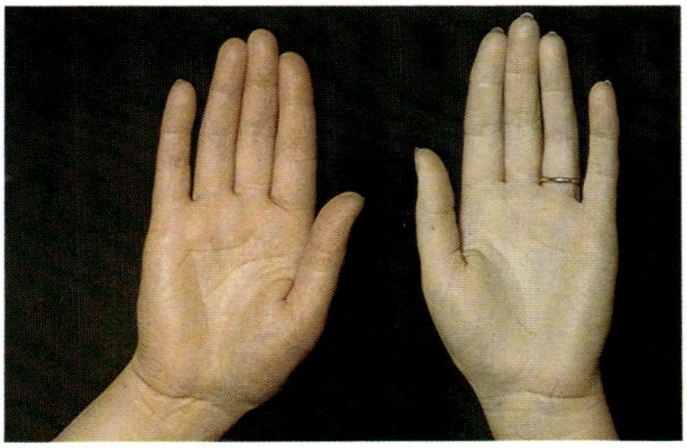

526 The cervical sympathetic nerve fibres are concentrated in the lower part of the trunk of T1. Irritation of these fibres by a cervical rib or abnormal band may cause blanching of the skin of the hand and fingers.

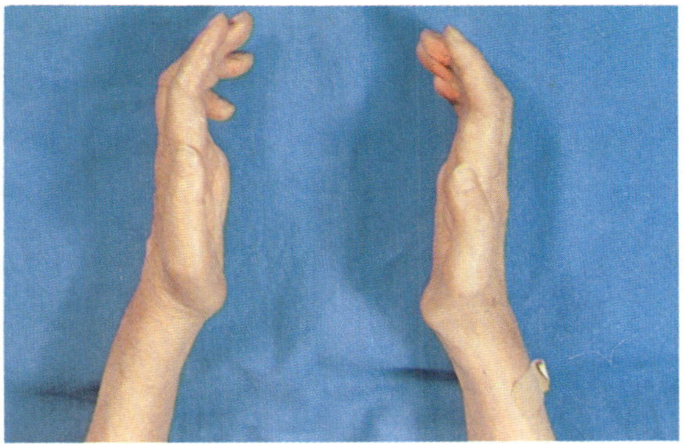

527 At a later stage, interruption of conduction of the fibres of T1 may cause wasting of the intrinsic muscles of the hand. The hypothenar muscles are shown here to be severely wasted.

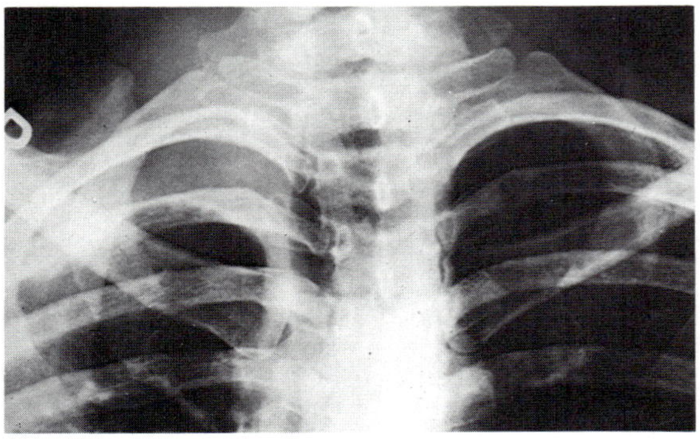

528 Occasionally no cervical rib is seen in the radiographs but an elongation of the transverse processes of the lowest cervical vertebra is noted. Probably, a fibrous band extends from the tip of this to the first or second ribs.

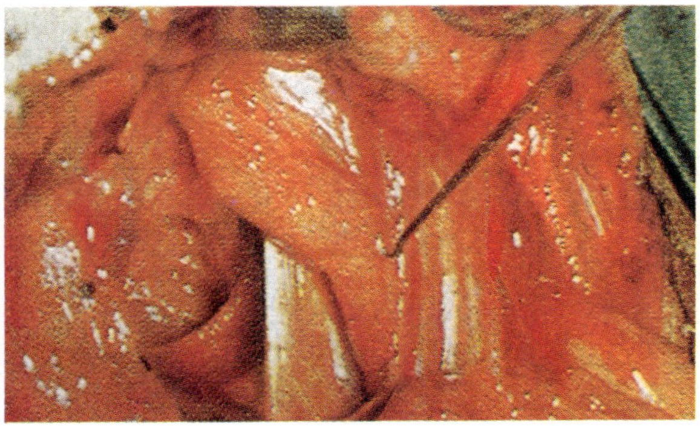

529 A well-developed fibrous band seen at operation in the position of scalenus medius lying behind the first thoracic nerve root and impairing its normal conduction.

Dorsal spine

Congenital kyphosis

This is due to a disturbance in segmentation of the embryonic spine anteriorly resulting in block vertebral bodies with wedging.

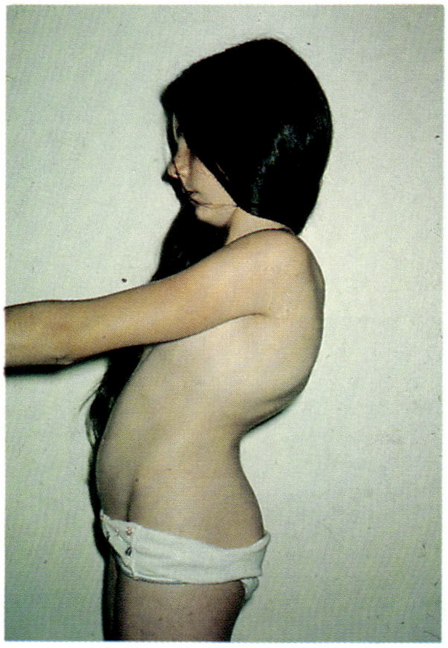

530 A young girl with congenital dorsi-lumbar kyphosis.

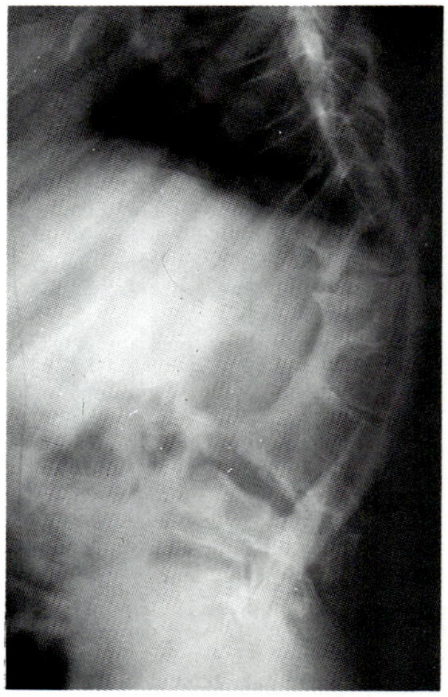

531 Lateral radiograph showing block vertebrae.

Acquired kyphosis

This may be due to developmental, infective, metabolic, neoplastic or paralytic lesions.

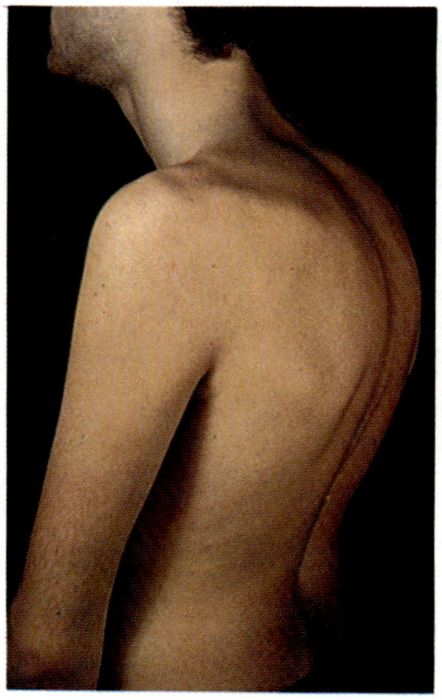

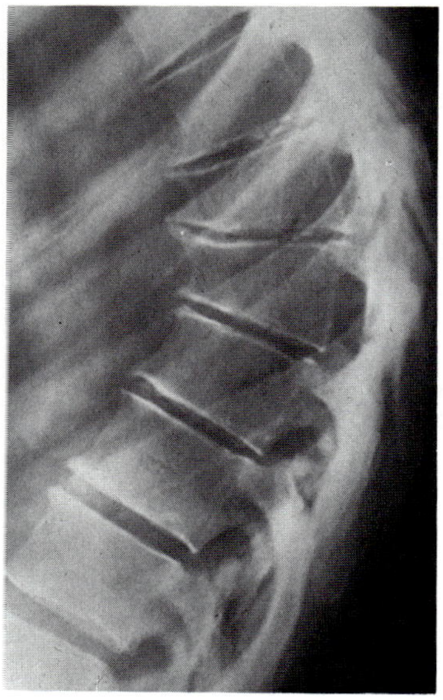

532 & **533** Scheuermann's disease (adolescent kyphosis). An adolescent becomes 'round shouldered', and he may or may not have accompanying pain in the early stages. The curve is rigid and not correctable. Several segments of the spine are involved so that the angle is not an acute one, i.e. it is a long-segment kyphosis. There is no disturbance of general health.

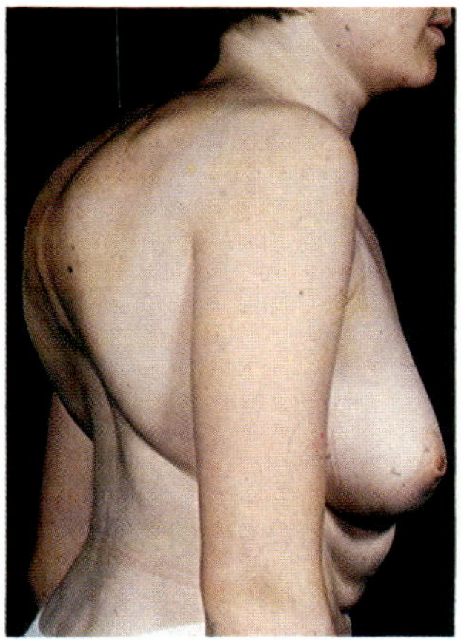

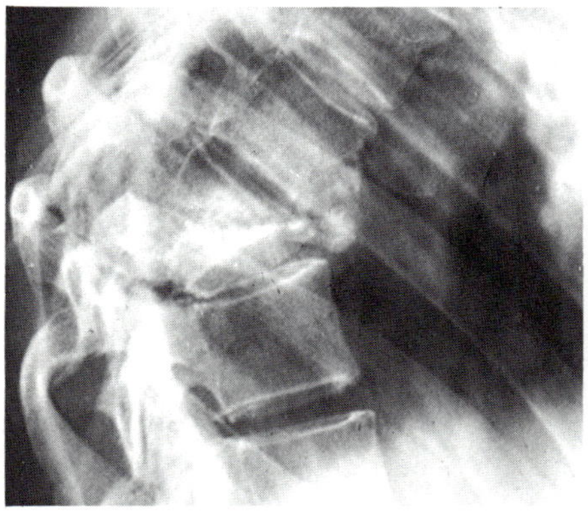

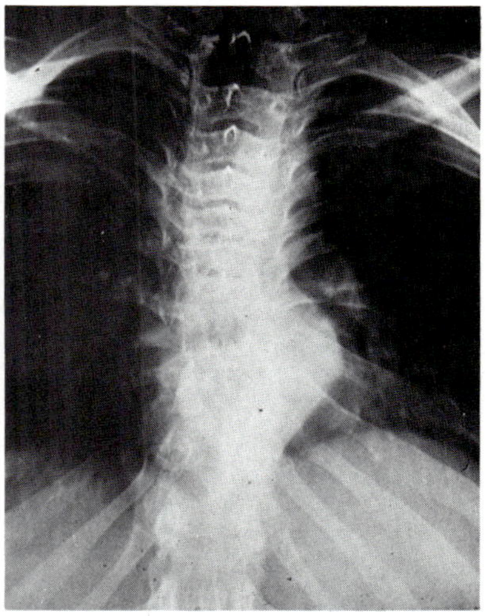

534–536 Tuberculosis of the spine (Pott's disease). In addition to the general disturbance of health, local pain, abscess formation and other important complications, the curve itself is distinguished by its more acute angle, owing to the fact that only one or two vertebrae are usually involved. It is a short-segment kyphosis.

The lateral radiograph (**535**) shows that the infection in the spine probably started between two mid-thoracic vertebrae and that the lower one has almost completely collapsed. The antero–posterior radiograph (**536**) shows a left-sided paravertebral abscess.

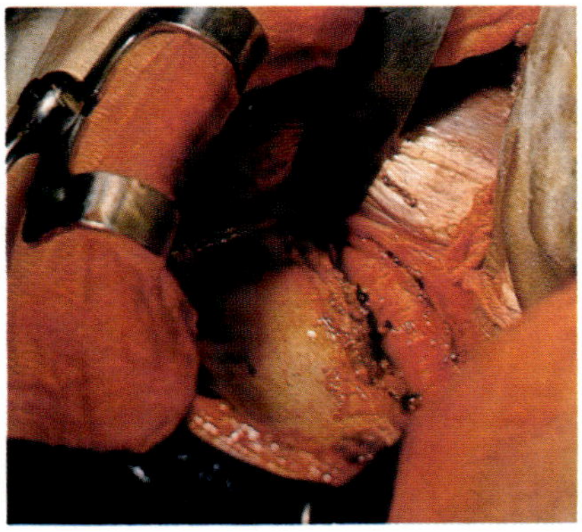

537 The abscess displayed immediately to the left of the thoracic aorta at operation.

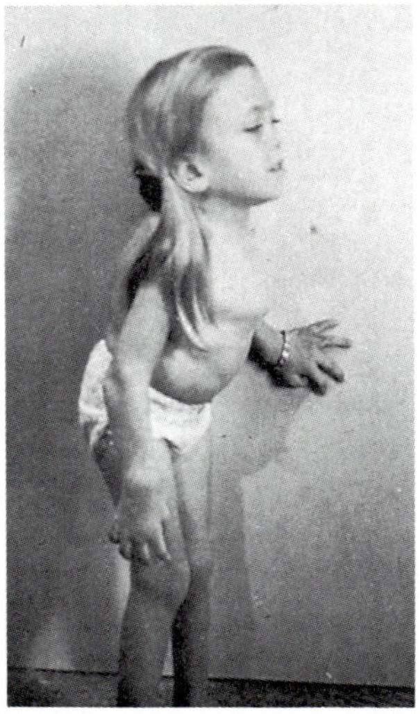

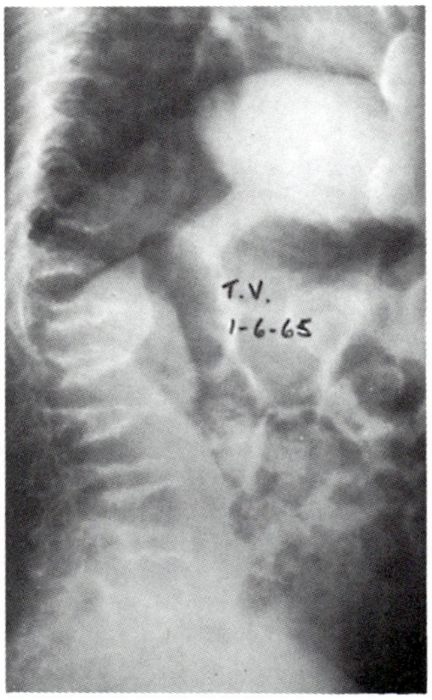

538 & **539** A young girl with Morquio–Brailsford's disease showing a diffuse kyphosis. Radiographs show the classical 'slipper'-shaped vertebral bodies.

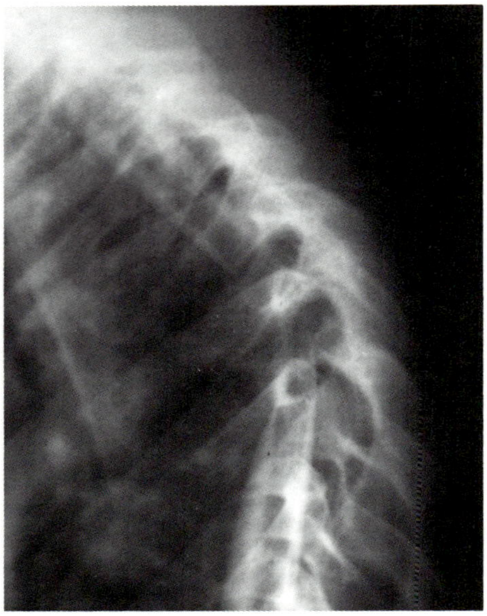

540 Lateral radiograph of dorsal vertebral body collapse and myelographic blockage caused by secondary neoplasia.

Spina bifida

Spina bifida is caused by the failure of the two halves of the neural arch to fuse in foetal development. It varies in severity from a simple incidental finding on a radiograph, spina bifida occulta, to protrusion of elements of the spinal cord with complete paralysis below the level of the lesion, spina bifida aperta. Some examples are given here.

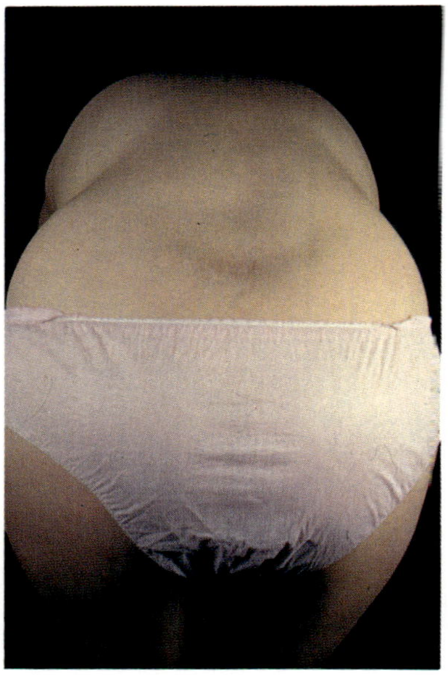

541 Fine cutaneous capillaries and a slight depression over the lower part of the lumbar spine. Occasionally there may be tufts of hair.

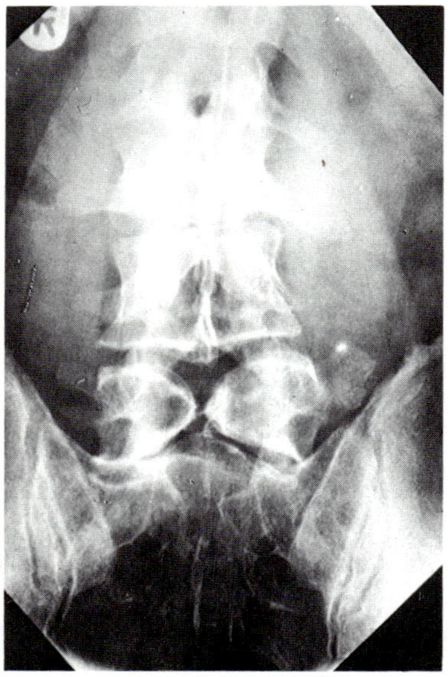

542 The radiograph shows that the 5th lumbar and 1st sacral vertebrae have failed to fuse posteriorly in the midline.

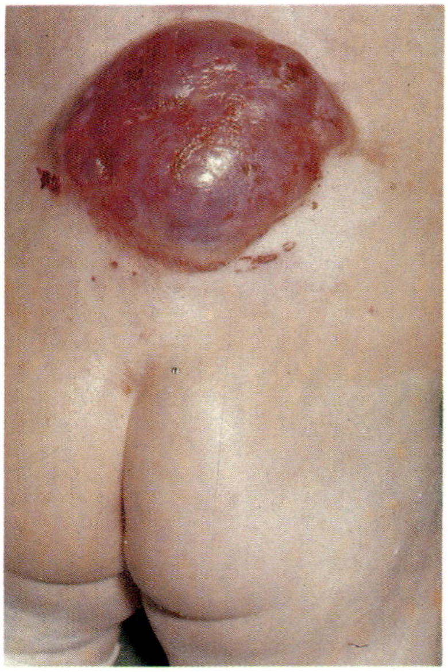

543 An example of an open meningomyelocele at birth, prior to closure.

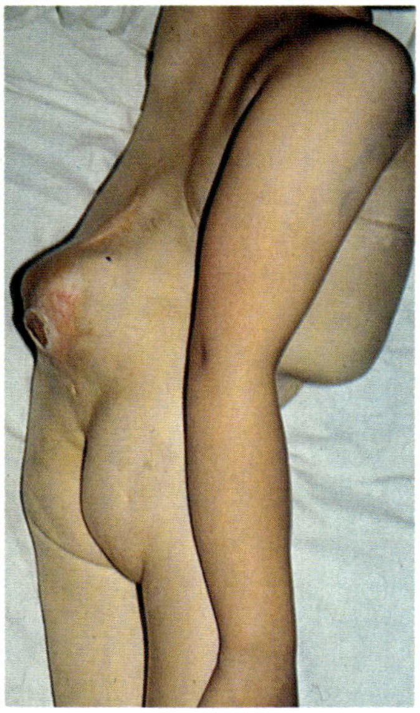

544 A more severe form of spina bifida, closed at birth, but the attenuated overlying tissue began to ulcerate converting it into an open type of spina bifida. There was complete spastic paralysis from the waist down.

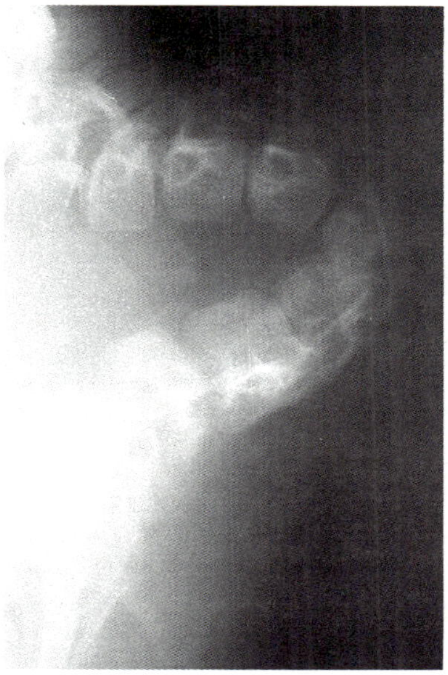

545 Radiograph showing the gross kyphosis at the site of extensive failure of fusion in the mid-lumbar segments.

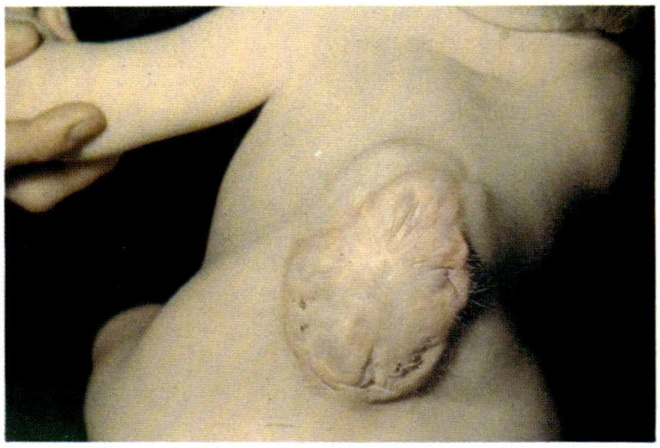

546 Open spina bifida. Elements of the meninges and surrounding fat covering the spinal cord are exposed in an older child with established kyphotic deformity and paralysis below the lesion.

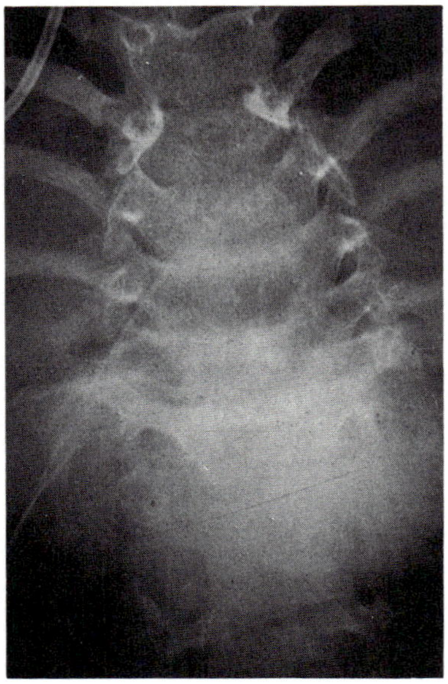

547 Radiograph showing extensive failure of fusion of the dorsilumbar segments.

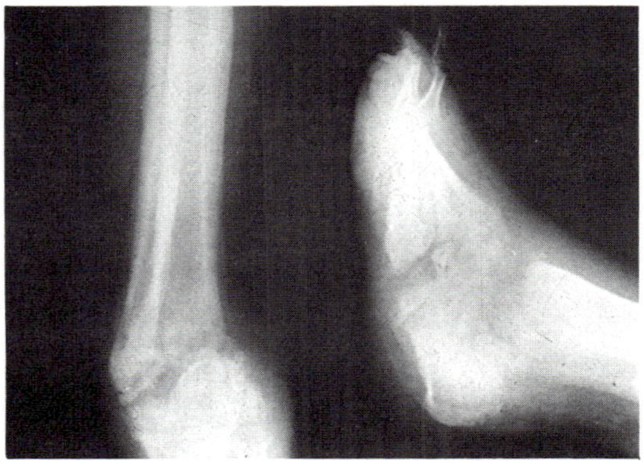

548 Neuropathic arthropathy (Charcot's joints) in the same child resulting in disorganisation of the ankle and hindfoot.

Scoliosis

Broadly speaking, scoliosis (spinal curvature) is either mobile or fixed. The mobile variety may be seen as a transient postural occurrence in adolescence, distinguished by the fact that it disappears on flexion of the spine.

Symptomatic scoliosis may occur because of inequality of leg length and consequently it disappears when the leg lengths are equalised, or when the patient sits down.

'Sciatic scoliosis' is a term applied to the lateral tilt of the spine which may accompany an acute lumbar intervertebral disc protrusion. It is caused by muscle spasm which disappears when the underlying cause has been treated. There are a variety of other less common causes of transient symptomatic scoliosis.

True structural scoliosis is always accompanied by rotation of the vertebrae so that in all cases other than some congenital curves the deformity is defined as lordoscoliotic. Varying degrees of lateral and axial vertebral body rotation result in a rib prominence on the convex side of the curve. The following are some examples of structural curvatures.

Congenital scoliosis

Owing to disturbance of foetal spinal segmental differentiation the axial skeleton may contain hemivertebrae, intervertebral bony bars, diastematomyelia, cord lesions and associated thoracic cage and rib anomalies. Other congenital visceral lesions may coexist affecting kidneys, bowel and cardiovascular system. Some types are hereditary.

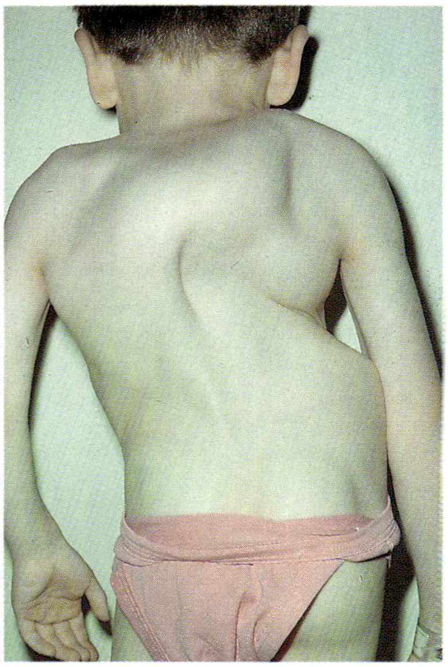

549 This boy has a sharply angled and rigid congenital curve with foreshortened trunk and thoracic cage deformities with a prominent rib hump.

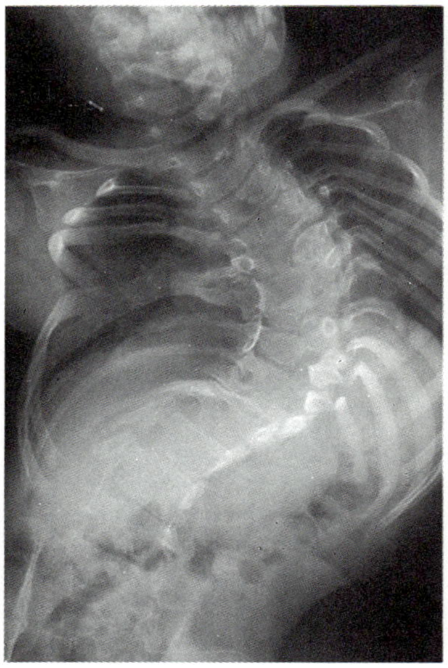

550 The postero-anterior radiograph of a child with gross scoliosis, hemivertebrae, fused ribs and posterior element defects in the lumbar area.

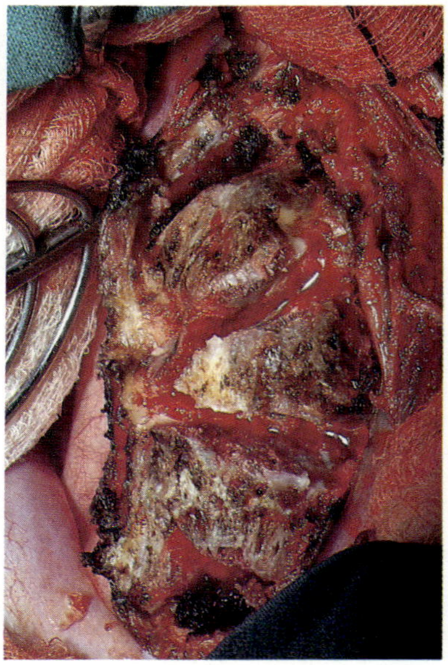

551 An operative picture of the front of the spine showing a hemivertebra prior to excision to correct the deformity.

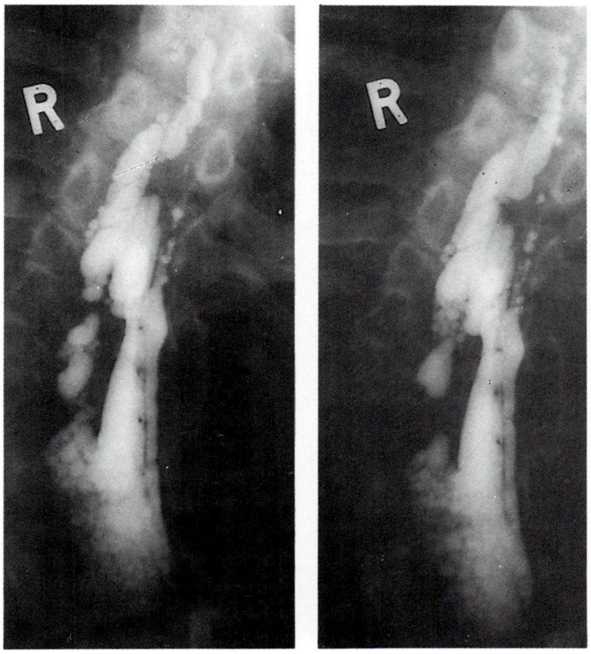

552 In a proportion of cases there are associated congenital lesions such as diastematomyelia shown here on a myelogram.

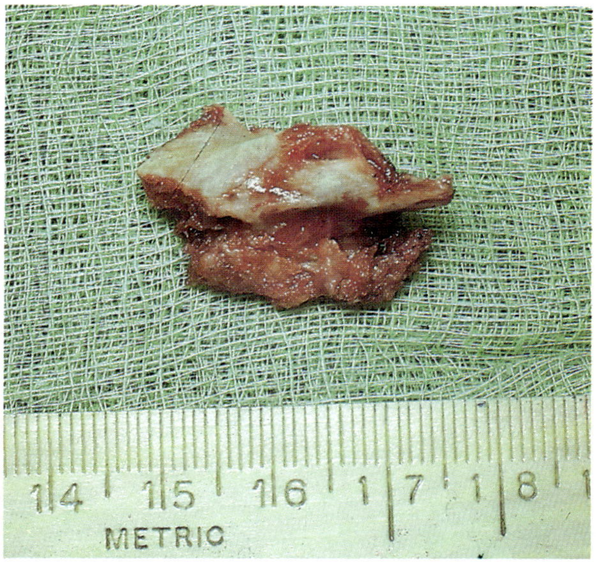

553 Diastematomyelia. A bony spur removed from the dorsal area of the vertebral canal.

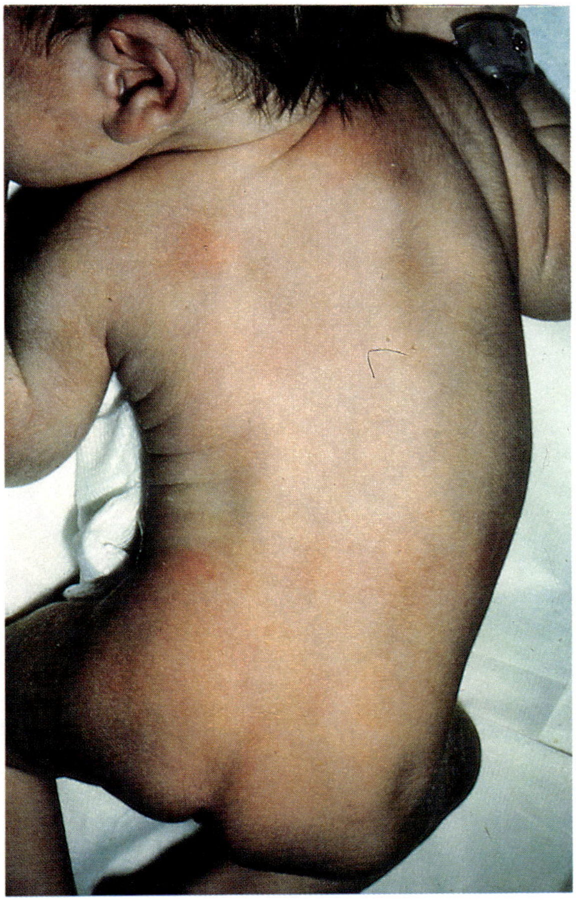

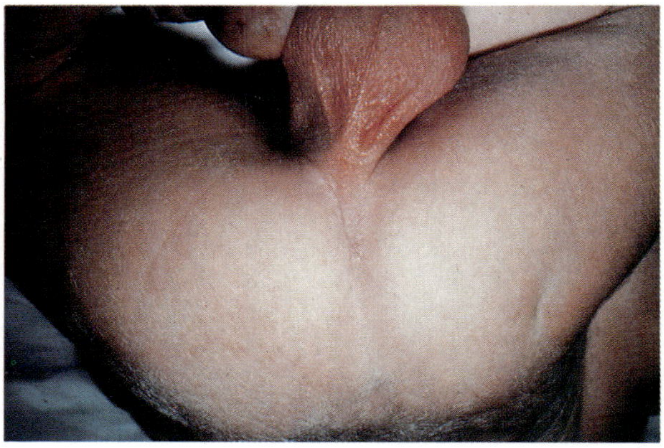

554 & 555 A baby with congenital scoliosis and an imperforate anus.

Idiopathic scoliosis

As the name implies the aetiology of these curves is still unknown. The child is symmetrical at birth, but at varying times in childhood the spine assumes a lordoscoliotic pattern. The curvatures may be of 'early onset', infantile and juvenile idiopathic forms, or 'late onset', adolescent scoliosis.

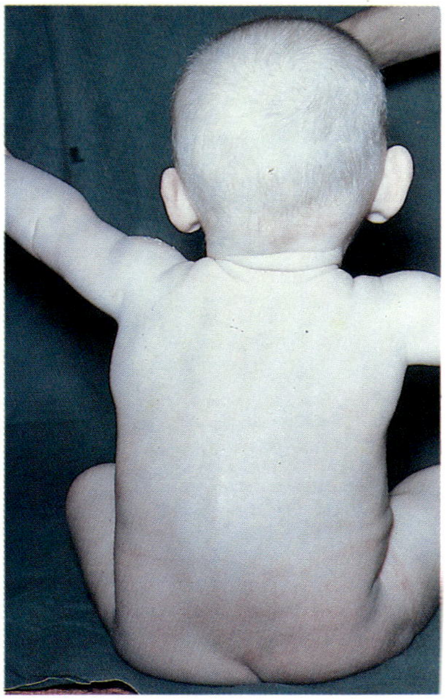

556 Infantile idiopathic scoliosis. A boy showing an early curve. A majority of these curves resolve but others progress to severe deformities frequently resulting in cardiopulmonary embarrassment.

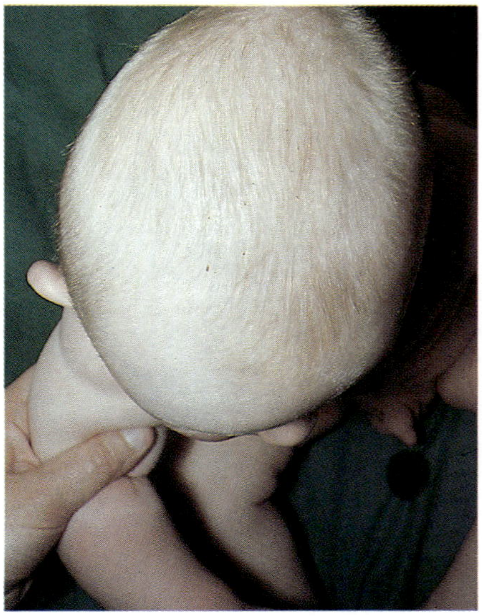

557 All infantile idiopathic scoliosis is associated initially with plagiocephaly. The same child as **556**, viewed from above shows the cephalic moulding.

A B

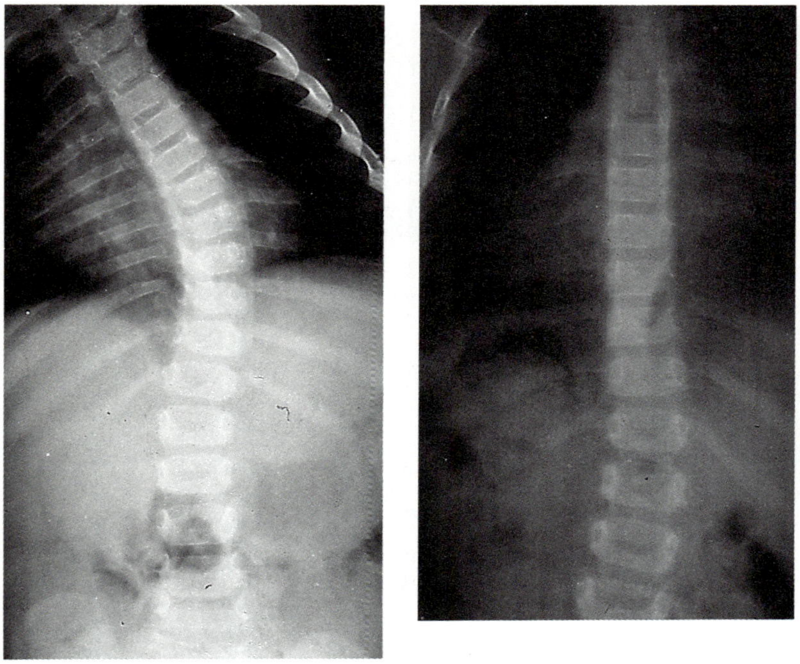

558 (A), (B) Radiographs showing an example of a spontaneously resolving infantile idiopathic scoliosis.

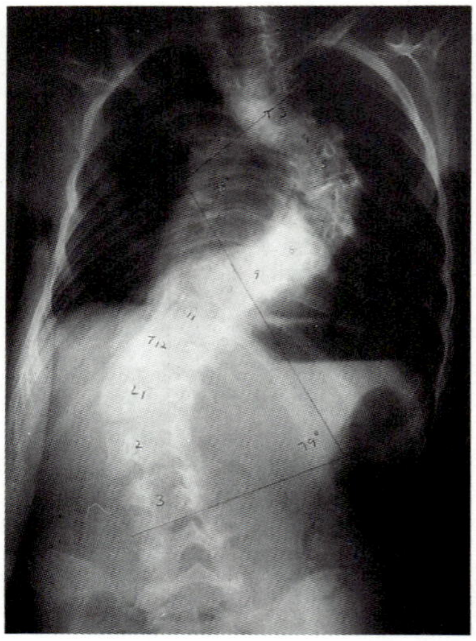

559 A severe left-sided curve in a child with progressive infantile idiopathic scoliosis.

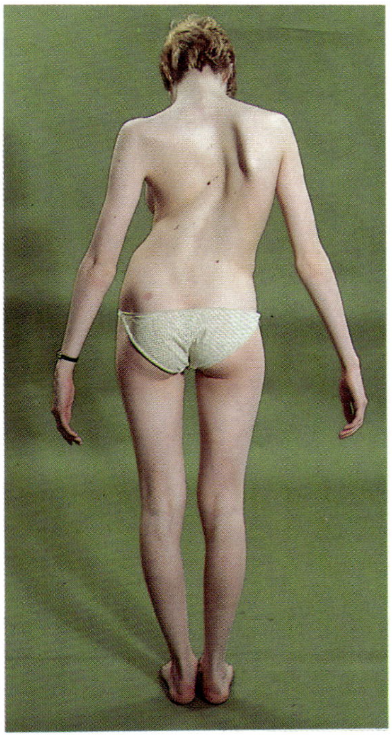

560 Adolescent idiopathic scoliosis. Some mild curves resolve but during the growth spurt many progress. A typical right-sided dorsal lordoscoliosis is seen in this adolescent girl.

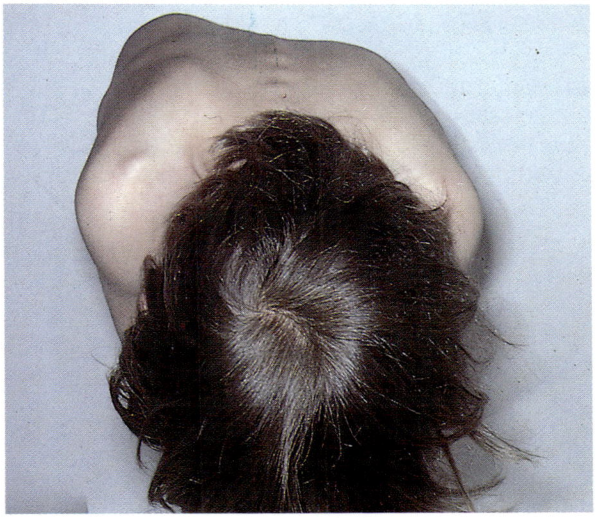

561 In the forward flexed position the skyline view of the posterior rib hump is highlighted.

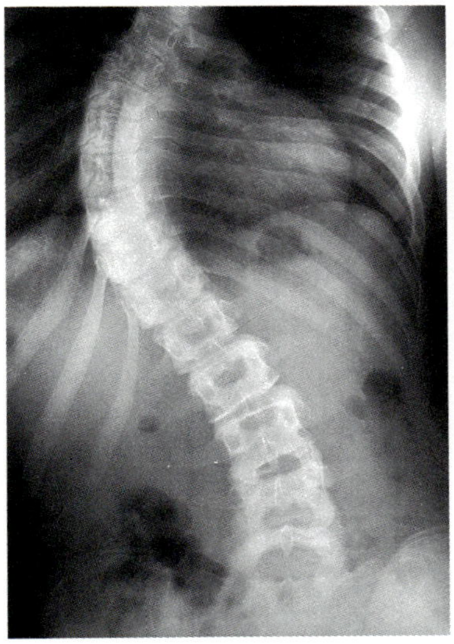

562 An AP radiograph of a typical adolescent idiopathic scoliosis.

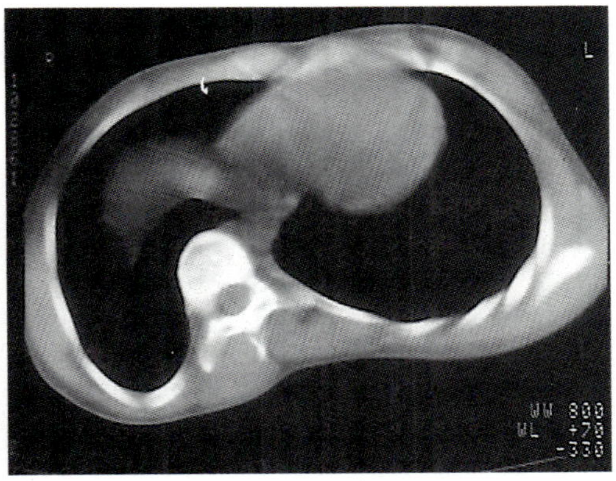

563 A CT scan of the thoracic cage in a child with scoliosis demonstrates the deformed thoracic cage and the vertebral body rotation to the convexity of the curve.

Paralytic scoliosis

Except for the congenital arch defects seen in spina bifida, radiographs of paralytic curves show otherwise normal bone and joint structure. The paralytic curves are usually long, smooth collapsing curves and may be seen in muscular dystrophy and spinal atrophy or in acquired diseases such as poliomyelitis or after spinal injury. The scoliosis arises due to trunk muscle imbalance.

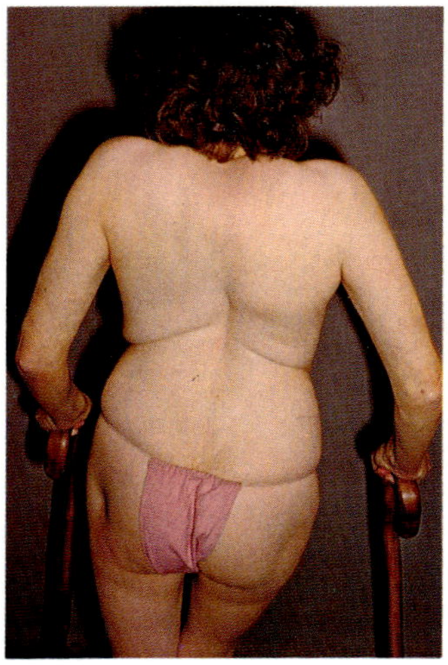

564 Spinal curvature in a patient with muscular dystrophy, still ambulant with sticks.

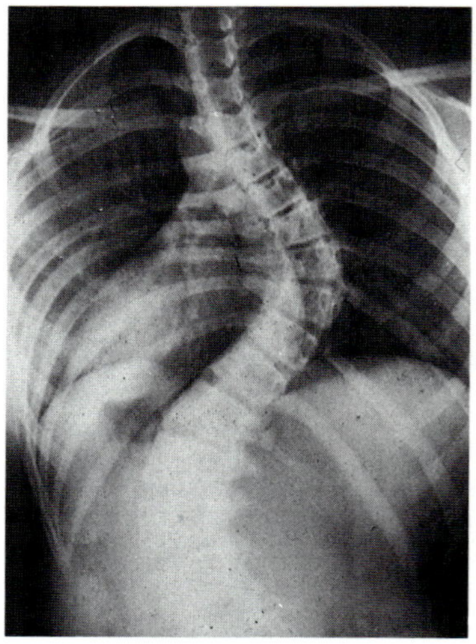

565 Radiograph of a wheel-chair bound patient with a long paralytic C-curve.

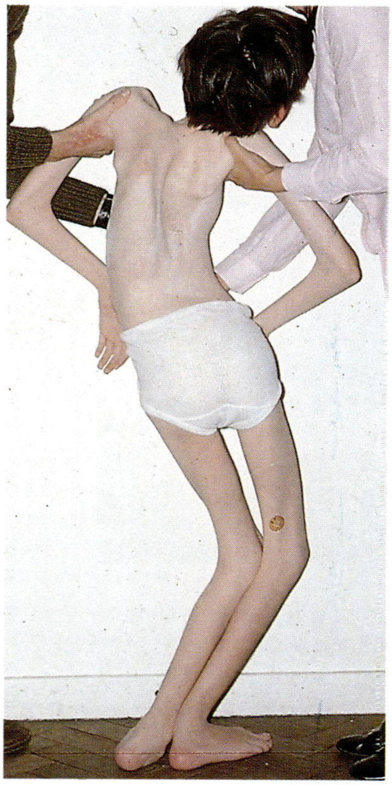

566 A boy suffering from spinal muscular atrophy with gross trunk and limb wasting and a collapsing scoliosis.

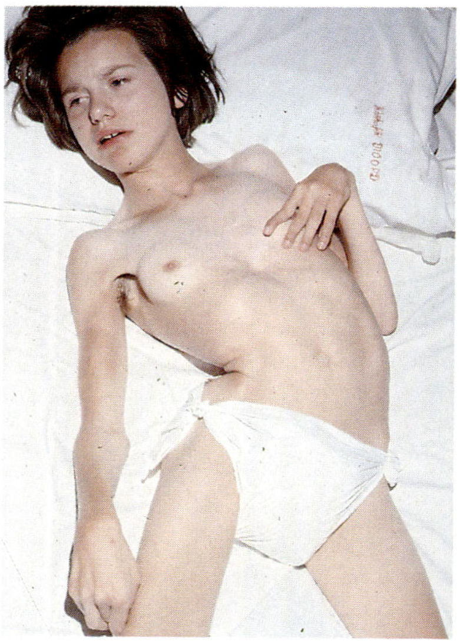

567 A girl with cerebral palsy. The facies and limb posture are typical. She also exhibits a marked lumbar lordoscoliotic curve with pelvic tilt.

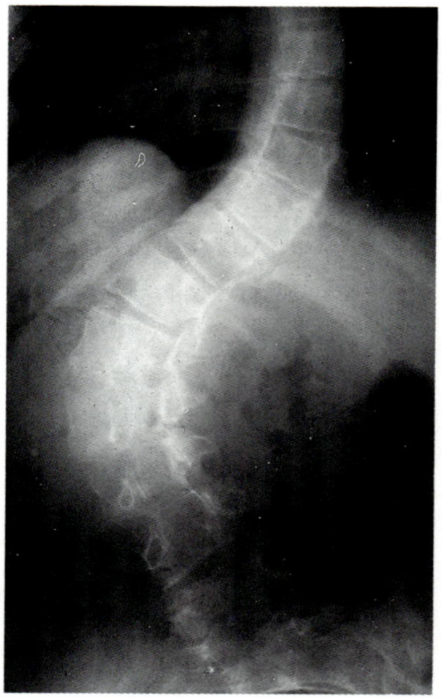

568 Radiograph of a patient with a paralytic lumbar scoliosis with gross vertebral rotation.

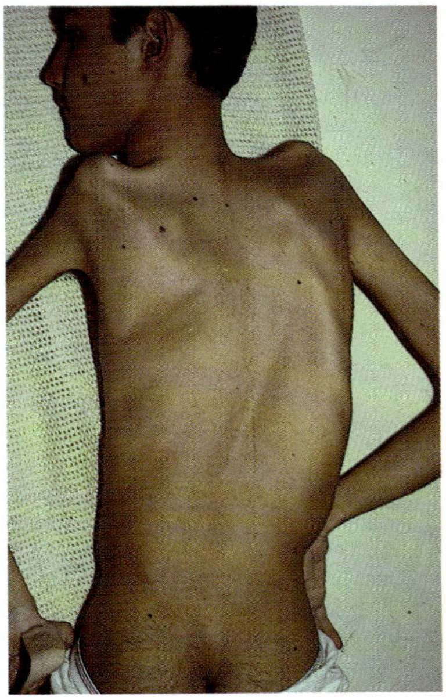

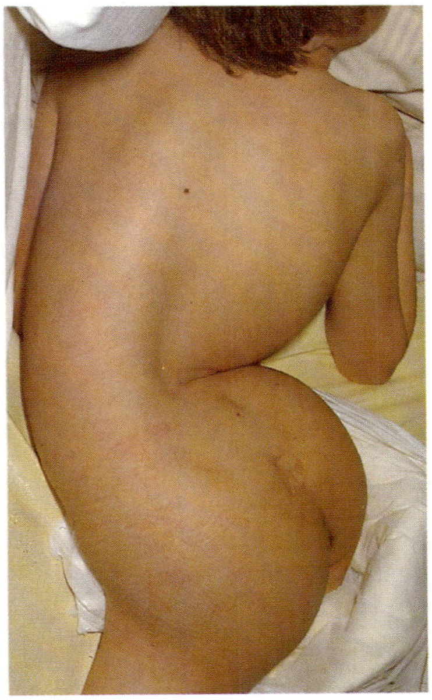

569 A long C curvature in a boy with post poliomyelitis weakness.

570 This child suffered a traumatic paraplegia at the dorsilumbar level whilst still growing. The severe pelvic tilt and lumbar scoliosis is evident.

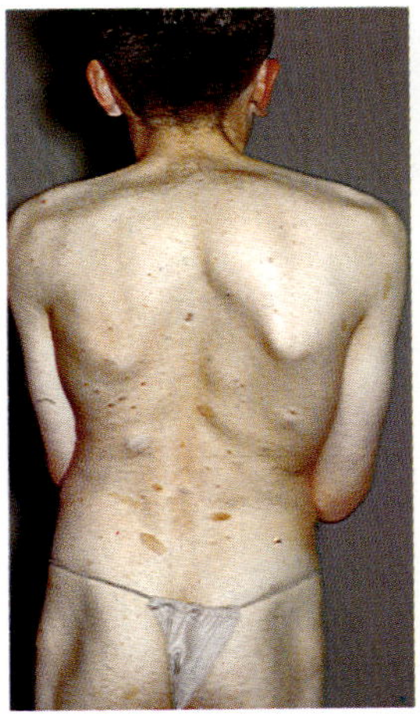

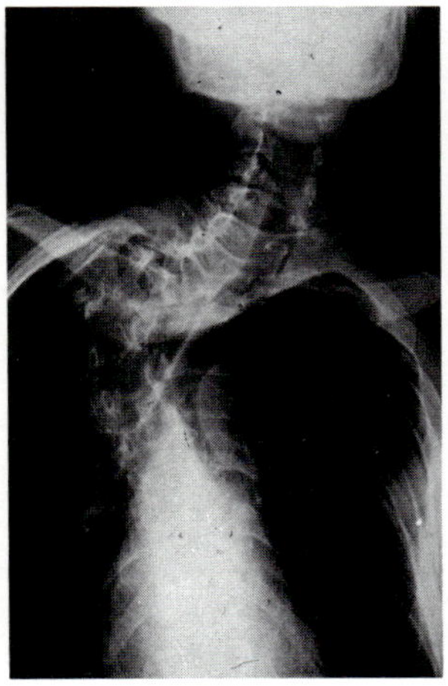

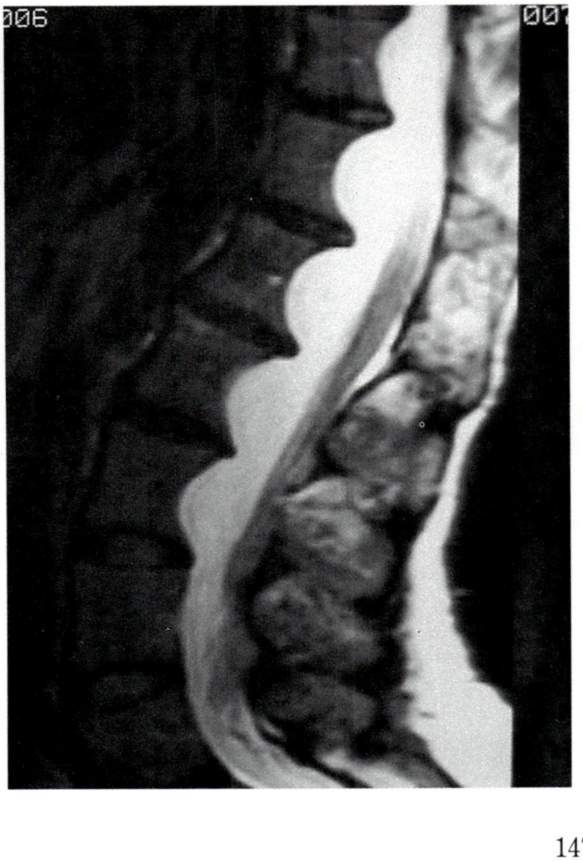

571–573 Neurofibromatosis. Probably one-third (15–40%) of sufferers will develop a scoliosis. Multiple neurofibromata and café-au-lait spots may be evident on the skin. The radiograph (**572**) shows a characteristic short, sharp thoracic curve. Scalloping of the posterior aspect of vertebral bodies, shown on the MRI scan (**573**), may occur with spinal neurofibromata. However, these are not the cause of the scoliosis.

The lumbosacral and sacral region

The lumbosacral area of the spine, because of the bipedal stance of humans, is subject to much stress and often manifests instability. Added to this there may coexist a variety of bony and neural tissue anomalies. Some of these problems, both congenital and acquired, are illustrated below.

Congenital skeletal anomalies

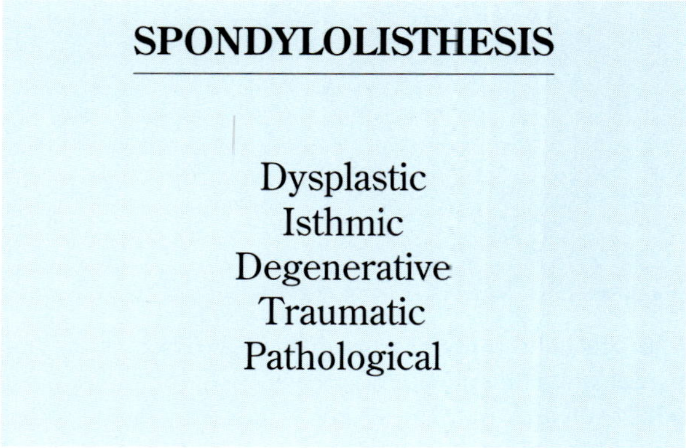

574 Spondylolisthesis is a forward shift of a vertebra upon the one below it. It is most common at the L4/5 and L5/S1 levels. The posterior facet joints either owing to congenital insufficiency, single or repeated stresses or degenerative changes fail to provide the normal locking mechanism that prevents the vertebrae from slipping forward.

The classification of the types of this condition is depicted in the figure. The only truly congenital variety is the dysplastic type which manifests itself in childhood.

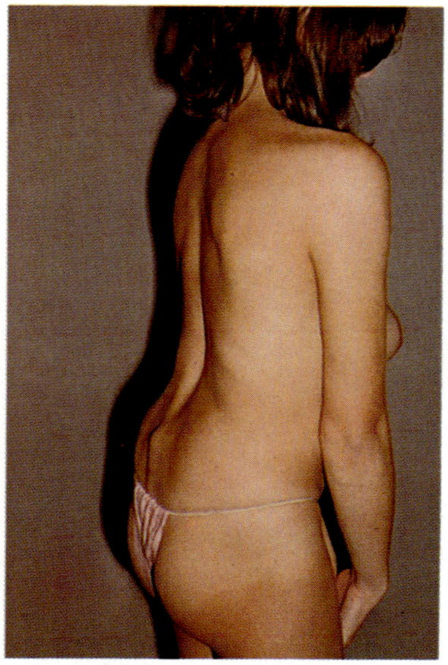

575 There is a prominence of the L5 spinous process and an increase in the lumbar lordosis above it. The sacrum below is vertical.

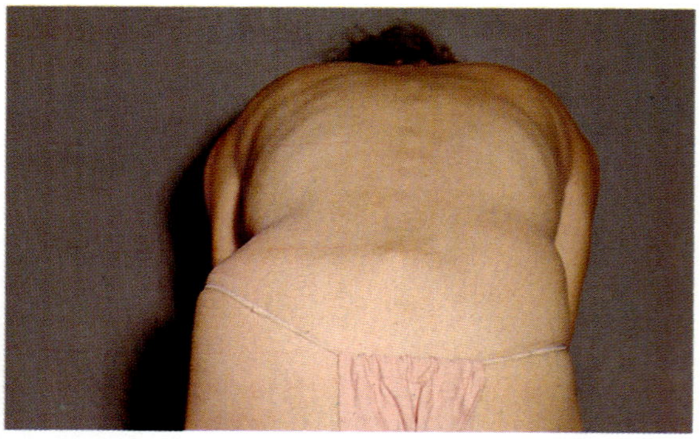

576 On forward flexion the prominent spinous process is clearly seen. It has, as it were, been left behind by the forward slide of the vertebral body.

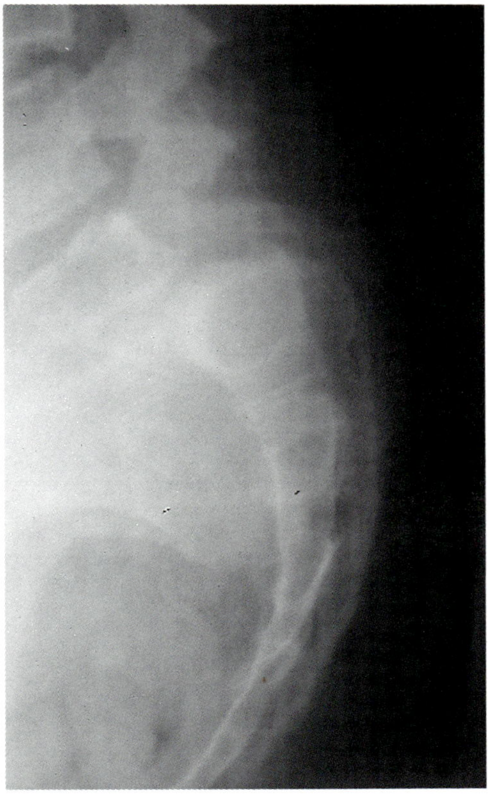

577 A lateral radiograph of an established dysplastic type of 5th lumbar slip with a vertical sacrum.

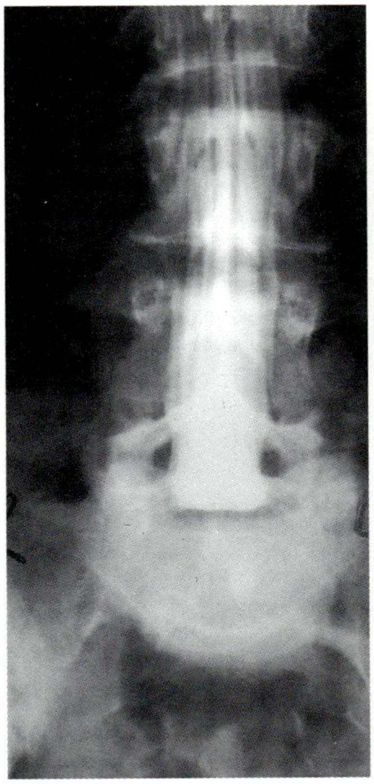

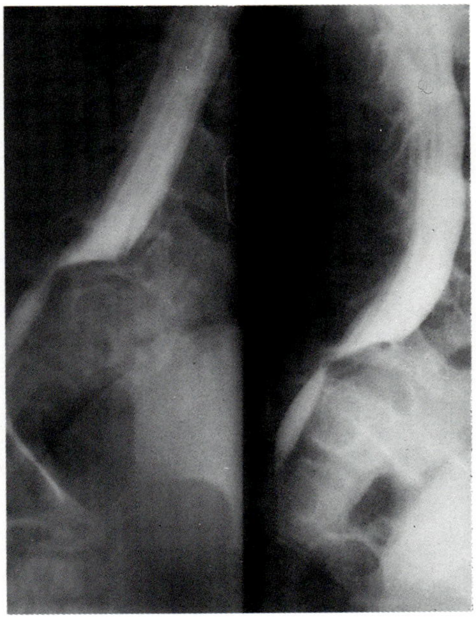

578 & **579** A myelogram showing the 'wasp waist' constriction of the spinal canal at the level of the slip.

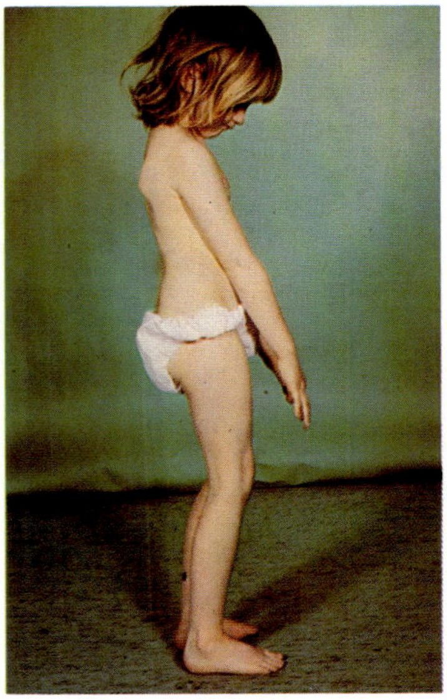

580 In an acute phase the patient is unable to flex the lumbar spine and therefore cannot touch her toes.

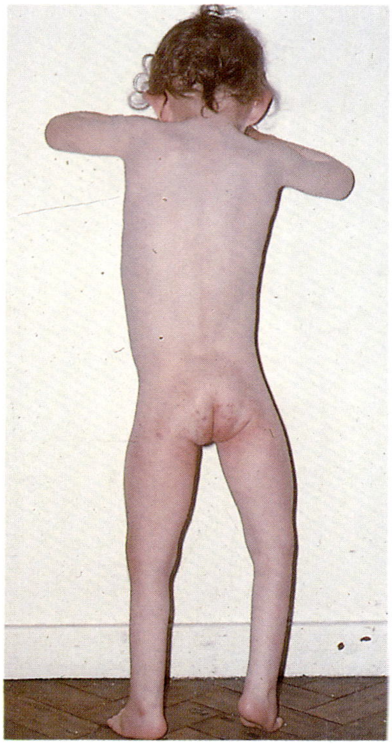

581 Sacral agenesis. This is a rare condition but important to recognise. Note the atrophic buttocks, high natal cleft and a degree of leg wasting and pes cavus.

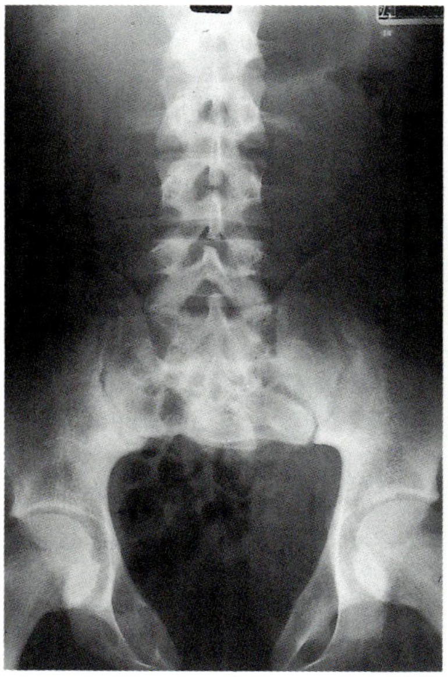

582 Radiograph showing absence of the sacrum below the first segment.

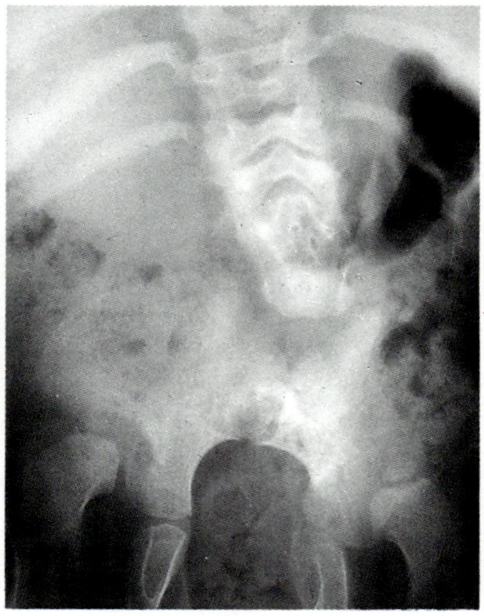

583 Total absence of the sacrum with a Robert pelvis. The patient had an arthrogrypotic appearance of both lower limbs.

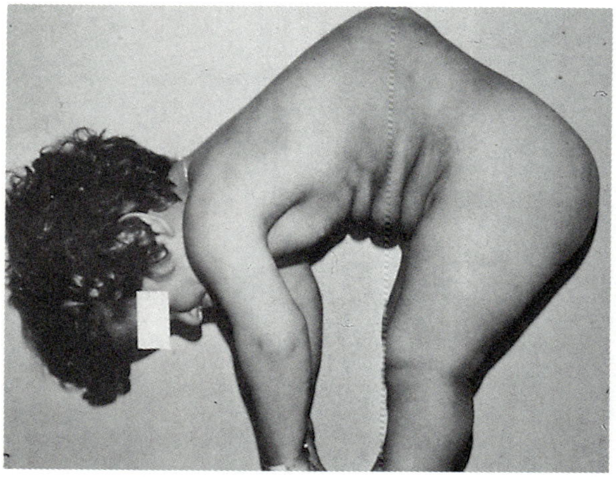

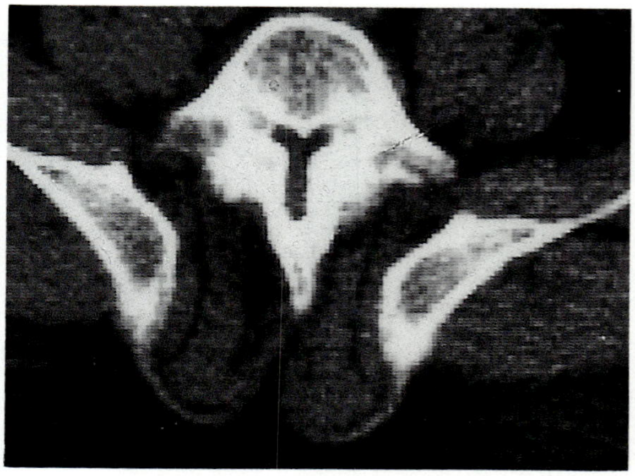

584 & **585** Achondroplastics have a tendency to develop severe lumbosacral spinal stenosis in later years. The CT scan shows a narrow trefoil spinal canal.

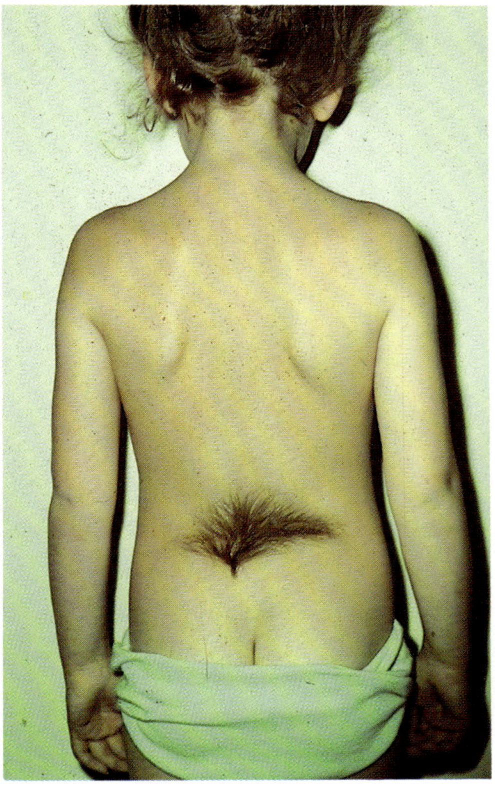

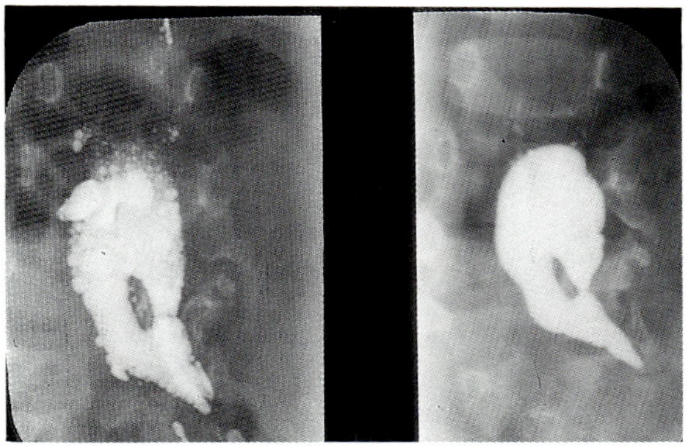

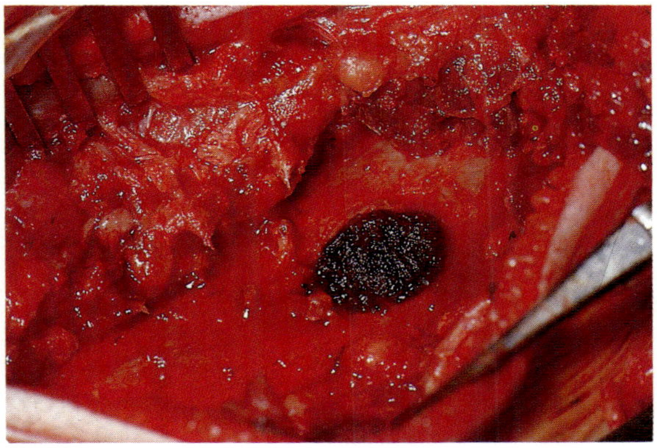

586–588 Diastematomyelia. A 'mare's tail' blemish at the lumbosacral junction. The underlying bony bar in the spinal canal is shown on the myelogram and at operation. The child had minor claw feet and suffered from enuresis.

Congenital neural anomalies

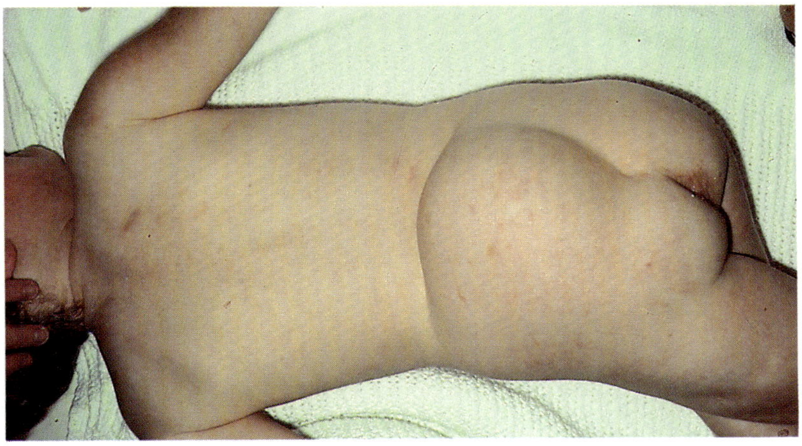

589 A child with a large, unilateral meningo-lipomatous mass but neurologically intact. A dangerous condition to treat surgically.

590

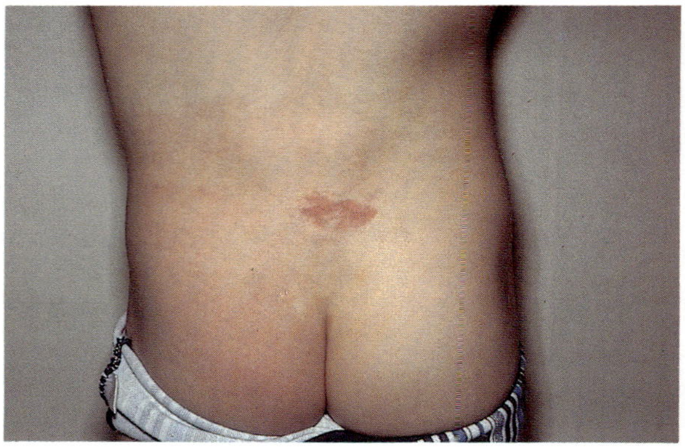

591

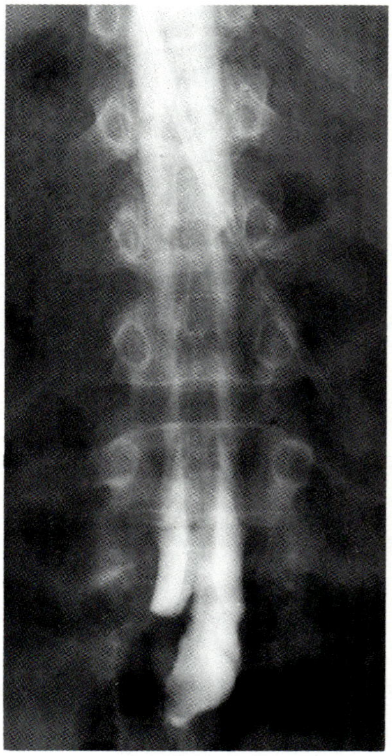

592

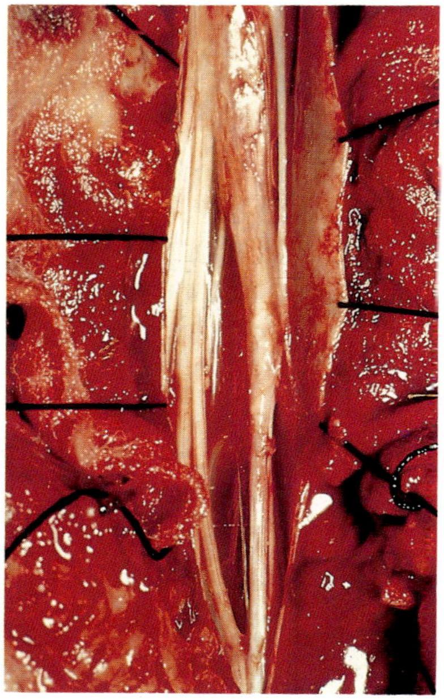

590–592 A child with a small vascular naevus in the lumbosacral skin but associated with tethering of the spinal cord and cauda equina, as shown in the radiculogram and operative picture.

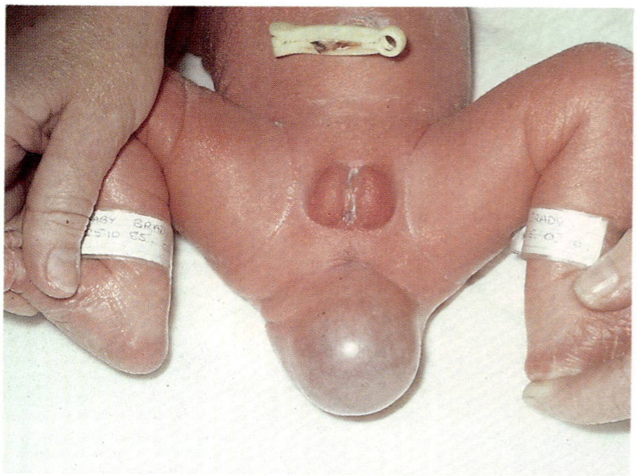

593 A baby with a large sacral meningocoele who was neurologically intact. Such lesions should not be aspirated as infection and meningitis would supervene.

Neoplastic lesions

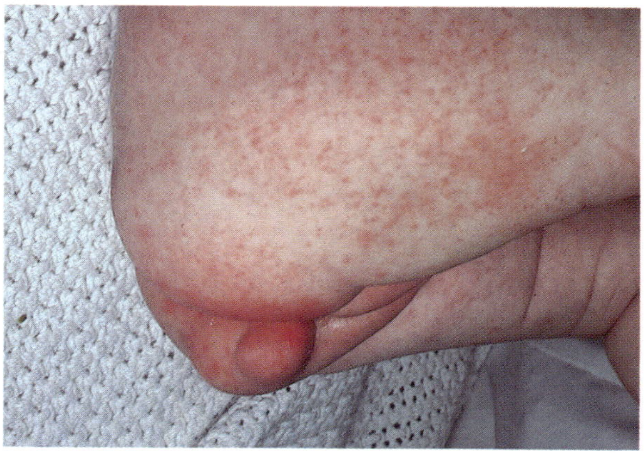

594 This baby has what appears externally to be a small sacro-coccygeal mass, but which proved to be a large malignant congenital teratoma that was ultimately fatal.

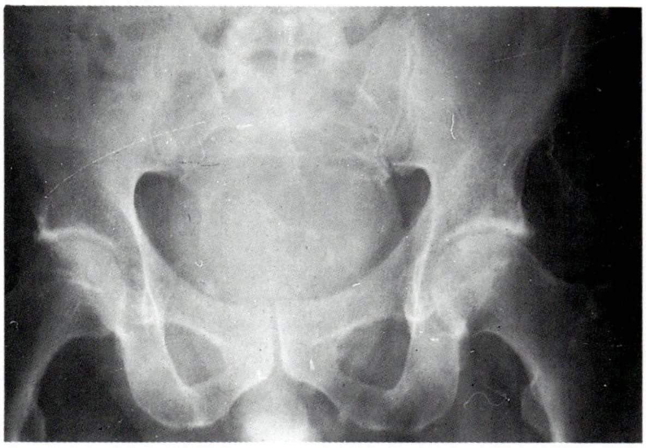

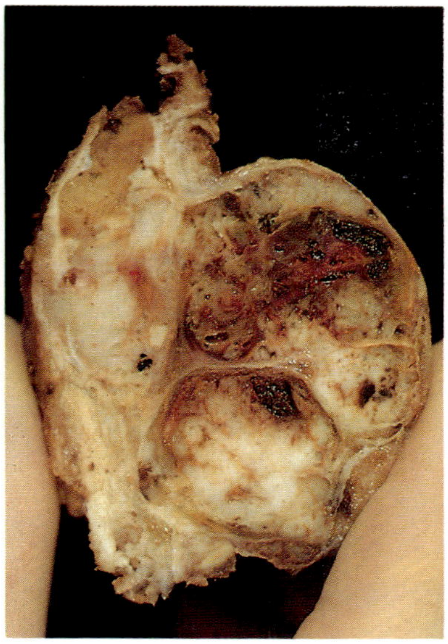

595 & **596** Chordoma. Although not strictly congenital, chordomas arise from embryonic tissues. Radiologically, a large sacral mass is seen. Although nothing is visible externally a rectal examination alerts the clinician.

Degenerative lesions and instability: Lumbar intervertebral disc protrusion

Although an intervertebral disc may protrude in any direction and at any level of the spine, by far the commonest site giving rise to symptoms is in the lower lumbar region. The syndrome of 'lumbago–sciatica' develops.

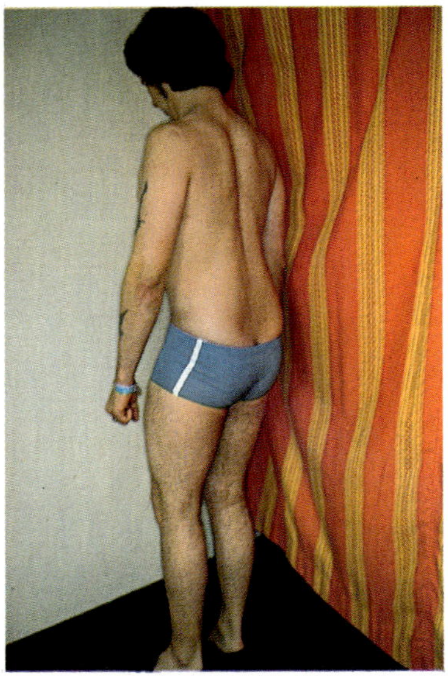

597 Obliteration of normal lumbar lordosis and the patient stands leaning forwards.

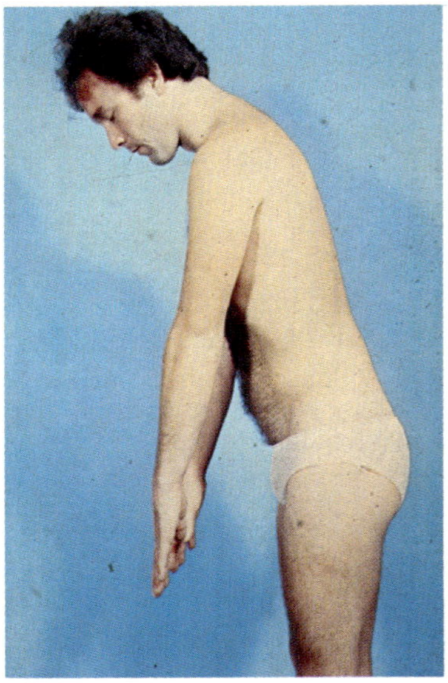

598 Restriction of forward flexion. On attempting to touch his toes the lumbar spine hardly flexes at all and the movement is grossly restricted.

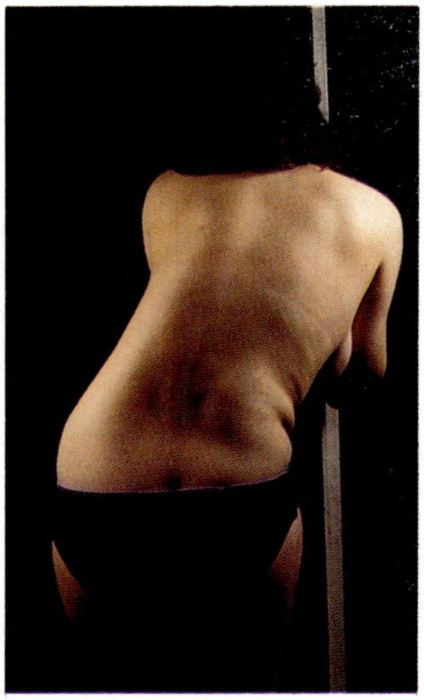

599 'Sciatic scoliosis': when the patient bends forwards there may be a marked tilt of the body, usually away from the affected side. This patient has acute left sciatica. Note the very marked list to the right, and the absence of any vertebral rotation.

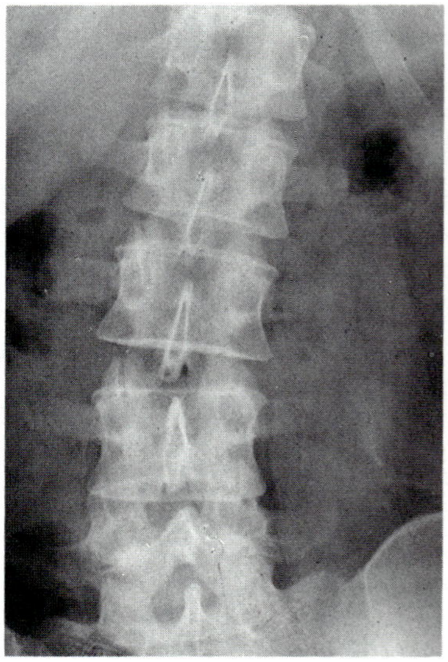

600 Radiograph shows tilting of the spine without vertebral rotation.

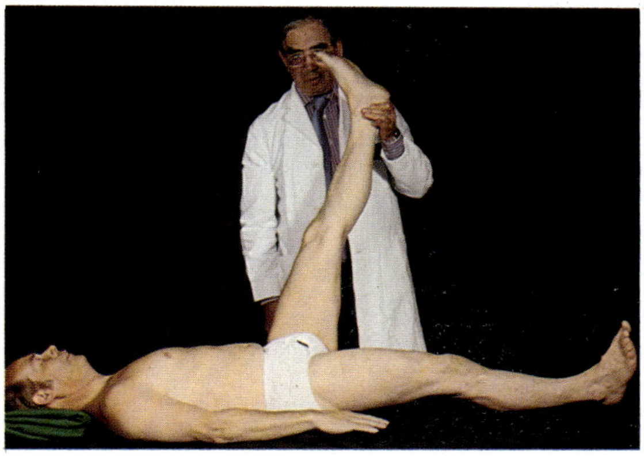

601 Straight-leg-raising test (i). The examiner raises the unaffected leg; the range is normal but at the extreme the patient may experience pain in the opposite leg.

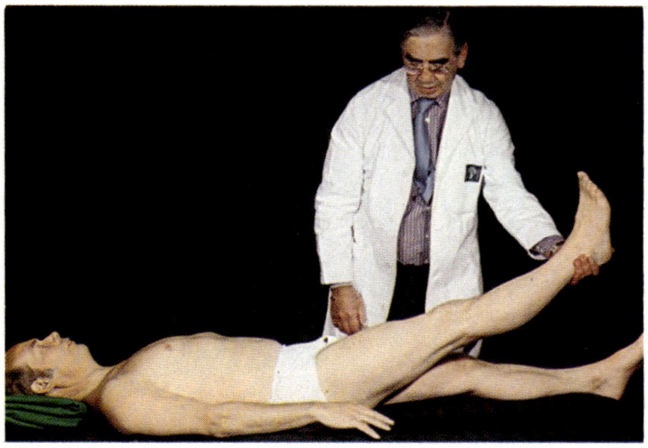

602 Straight-leg-raising test (ii). There is considerable restriction in passive straight leg raising on the affected side owing to pain and muscle spasm caused by nerve root tension.

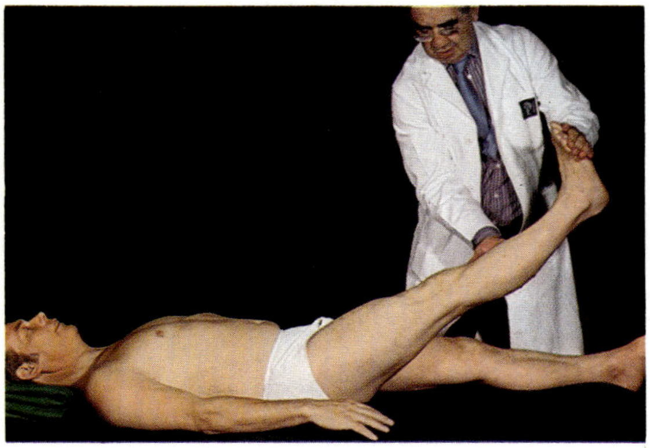

603 Straight-leg-raising test (iii). Lasegue's test: at the position of maximum straight leg raising, the ankle and foot are passively dorsiflexed, causing a marked increase of pain. A variation of this test is to rotate firmly the elevated leg internally; pain increases if positive (Troup's test).

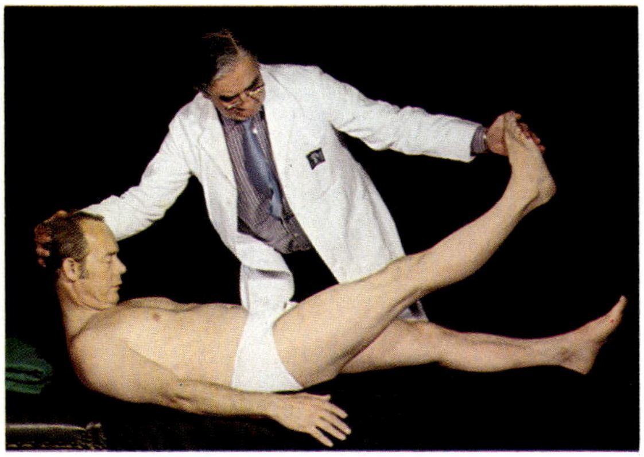

604 Straight-leg-raising test (iv). Naffziger's test: tension on the nerve root is further increased by passive flexion of neck on trunk.

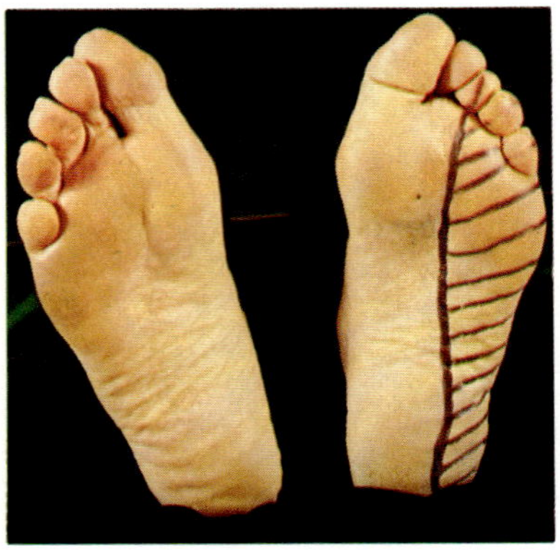

605 The area of altered sensitivity corresponds to the nerve root involved. In this patient the S1 nerve root has been compressed by a lumbosacral disc protrusion causing diminished sensitivity in the shaded area of the foot.

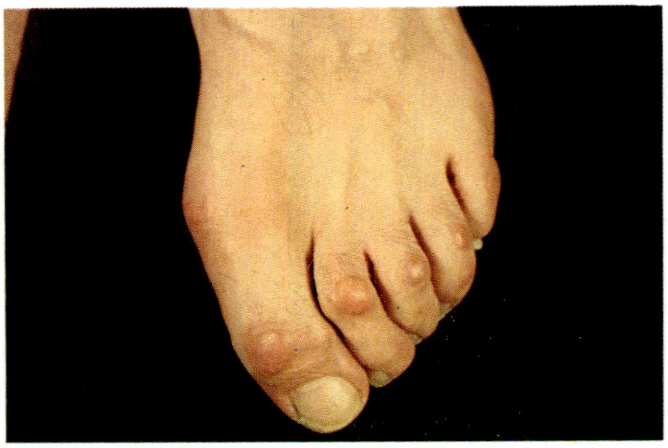

606 Severe disc protrusion 8 years previously. Weakness of the intrinsic muscles of the foot (S1) has led to clawing of the toes. Although reflex changes are frequently noted, muscle paralysis is rare.

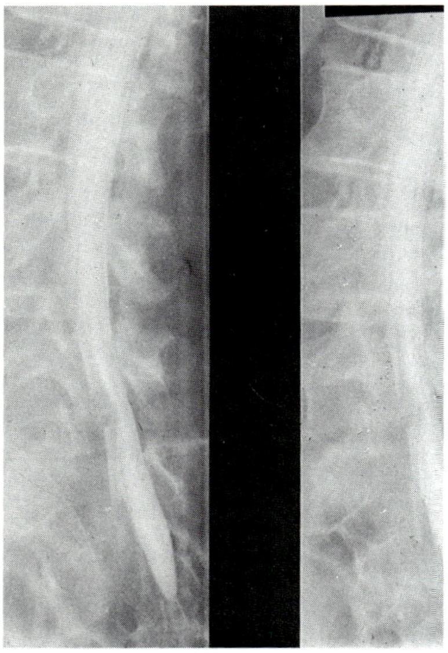

607 Radiculogram to show interruption of the flow of contrast material in the dural sheath of the L5 nerve root.

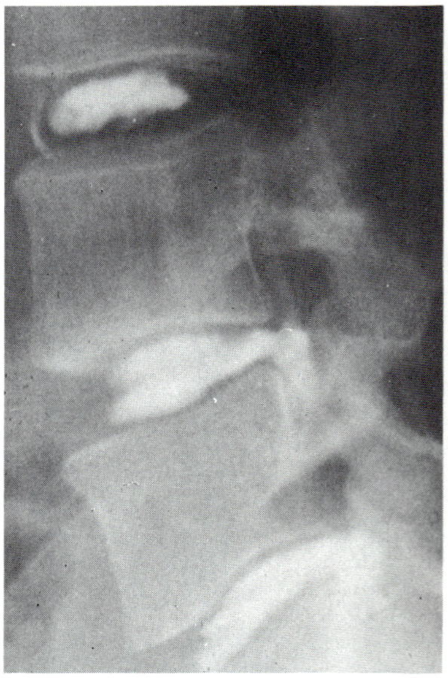

608 Discography. The nucleus pulposus of an intervertebral disc is under considerable physiological tension. It may protrude through the vertebral endplate or backwards through a ruptured annulus where it is in immediate anatomical relation with one or more spinal nerve roots.

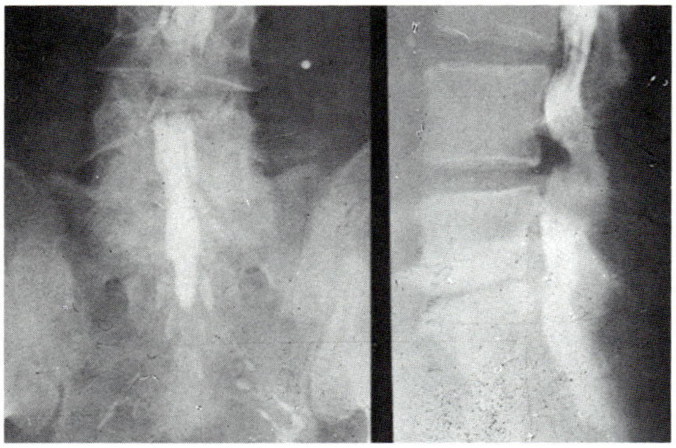

609 A massive disc protrusion of L4/5. Although the L5/S1 shows old damage, the cause of this patient's symptoms, confirmed on myelography, is a massive posterior protrusion at L4/5, causing marked interruption of flow of the contrast material.

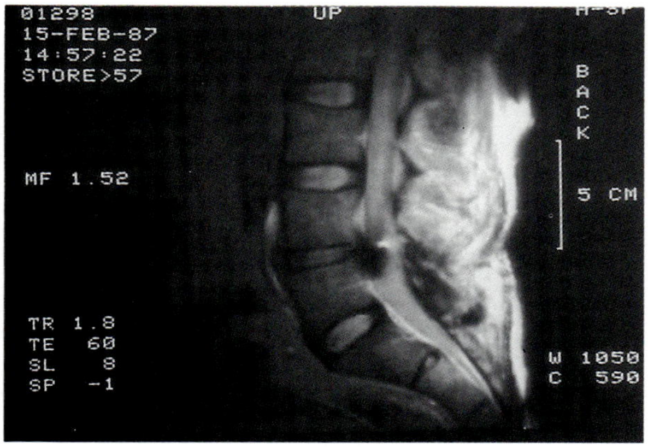

610 More recently, MRI studies reveal excellent detail in investigating disc and other tissue pathology. The degenerative and prolapsed disc material is well shown in this picture.

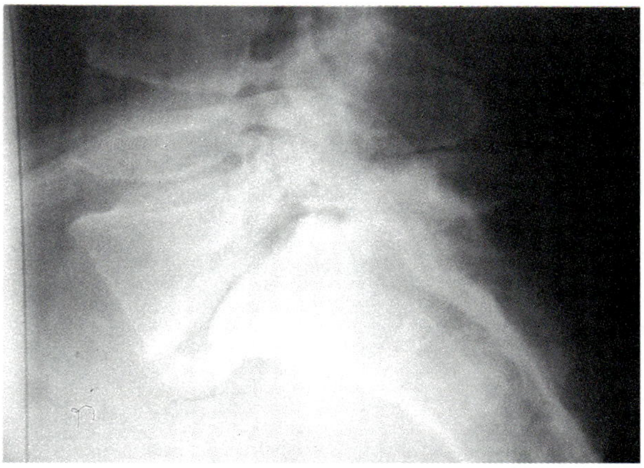

611 Instability. This can be due to disc disease with loss of disc height and secondary spondylolisthesis. This lateral radiograph shows a grade I forward slip of the 5th lumbar vertebra with extensive degenerative changes in the disc space area and facet joints.

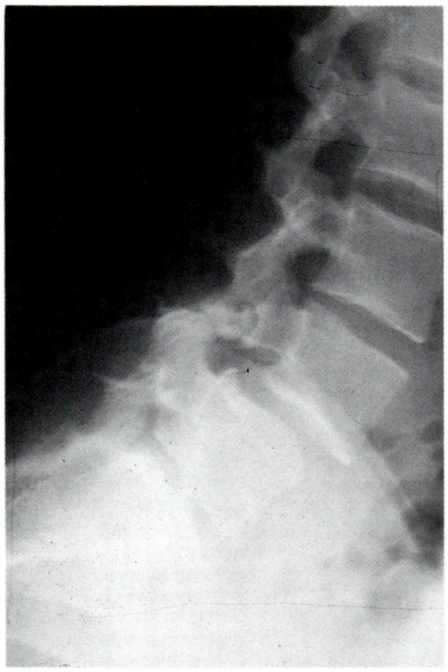

612 Another cause of instability is the isthmic type of spondylolisthesis where there is a minor defect – spondylolysis – in the pars interarticularis. Here the lesion is shown in L4 allowing slight forward slipping of L4 on L5. This lesion can be healed either with rest or surgery.

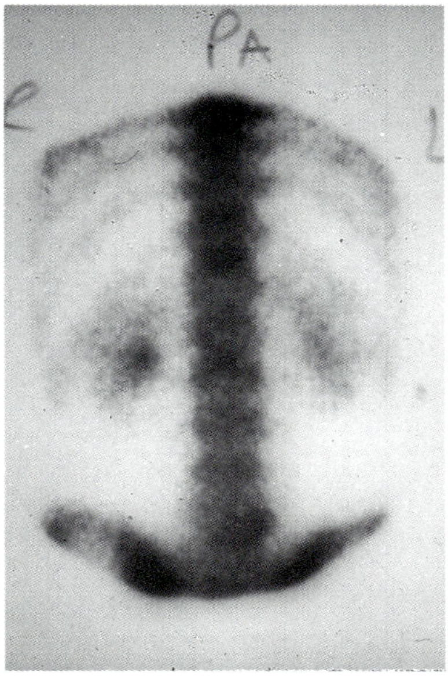

613 This radioisotope scan shows a hot spot in the left pars interarticularis of L5 indicative of possible healing of the defect.

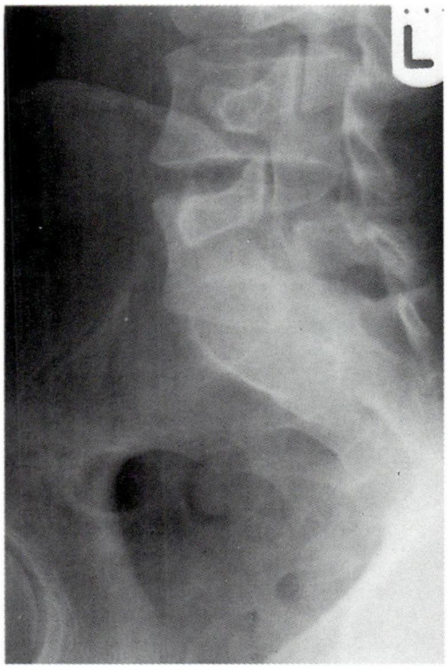

614 The spondylolytic type of spondylolisthesis is well demonstrated in oblique radiographs of the lumbar spine. The laminae and posterior facet joints imitate a series of 'scottie dogs'. The lowermost dog in this radiograph wears a collar—the spondylolytic lesion.

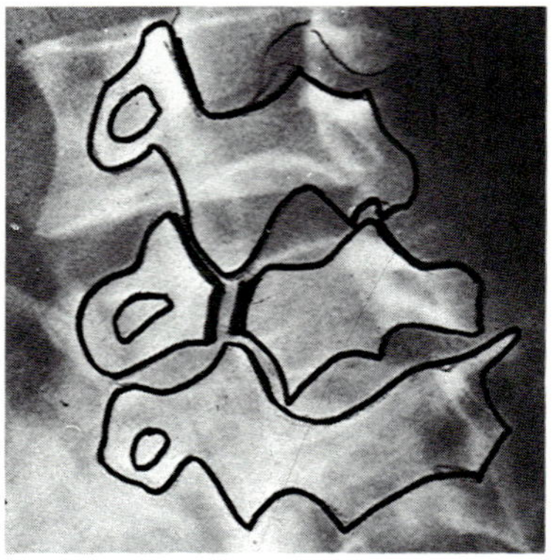

615 An outline of the 'dogs': the collar on the neck of the central dog represents a stress fracture (spondylolysis).

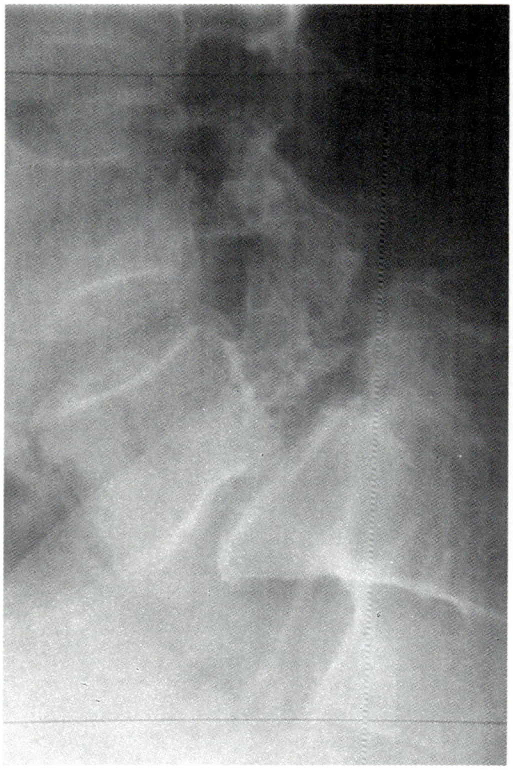

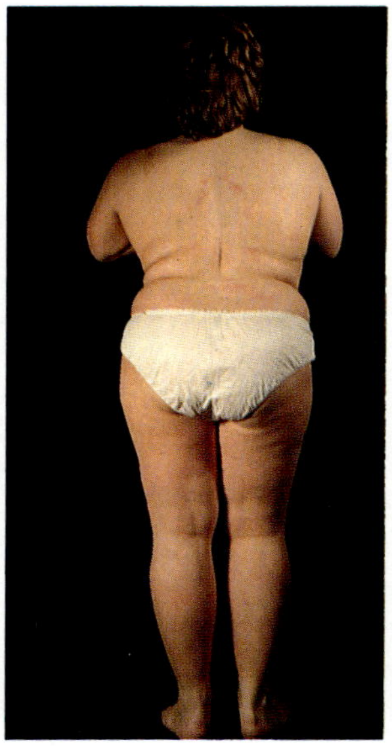

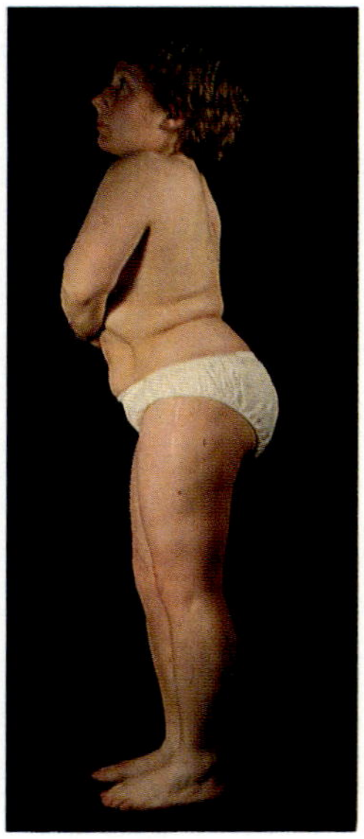

616–618 If there is an appreciable forward slip with an increased pars defect, as in this lateral radiograph, the patient may show characteristic flank skin creases.

The shoulder region

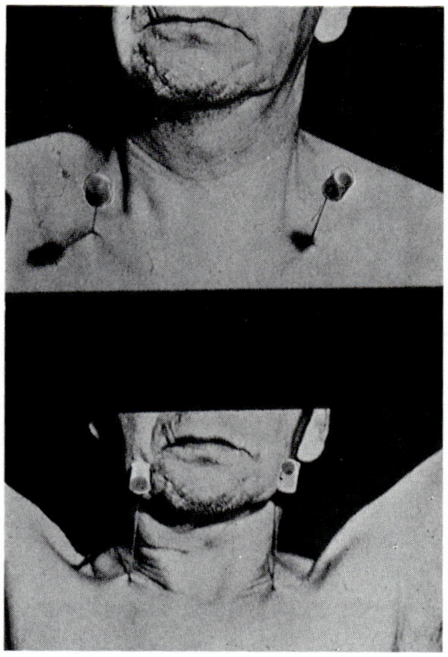

619 Axial rotation of the clavicle. Two wires have been placed into the inner ends of both clavicles; when the arms are fully abducted the wires are seen to point vertically upwards showing that during abduction the clavicles have rotated almost 90° in the coronal plane.

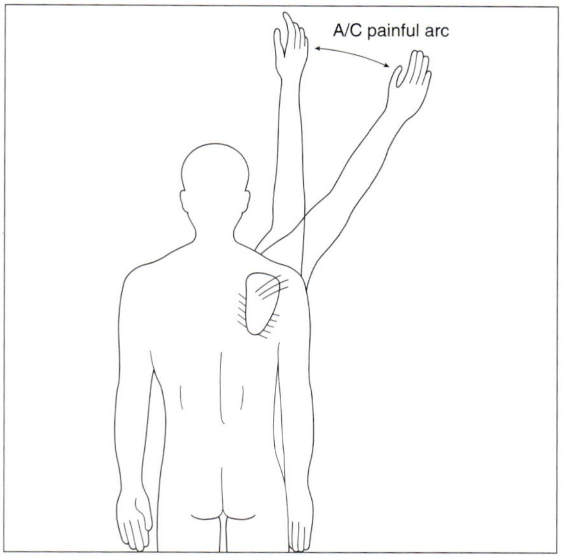

620 Acromioclavicular painful arc. Because abduction of the arm is accompanied by rotation of the clavicle the pain of acromioclavicular joint disorder is maximal at the extreme of abduction.

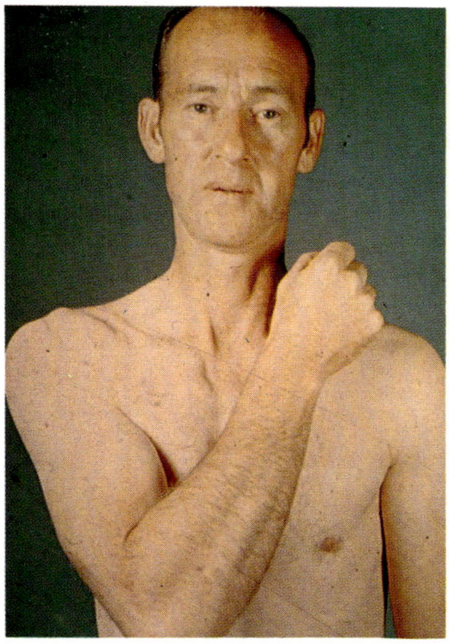

621 Occupational arthritis of the right acromioclavicular joint in a steelworker. The lump seen on top of the right shoulder is an adventitious bursa overlying an osteophyte.

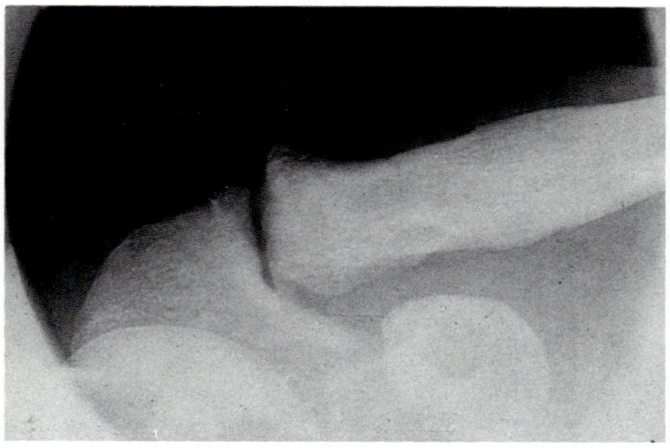

622 Typical degenerative arthritis affecting the right acromioclavicular joint with loss of joint space, sclerosis, pseudocyst formation and superior osteophytes is seen in the radiograph.

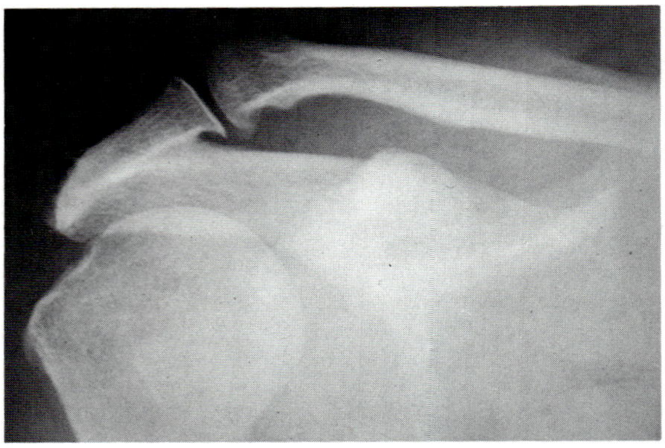

623 Severe acromioclavicular degenerative arthritis.

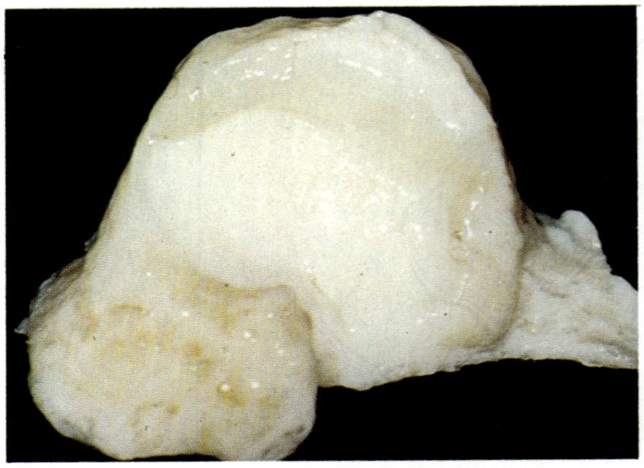

624 The intra-articular meniscus with cyst formation removed from the same patient.

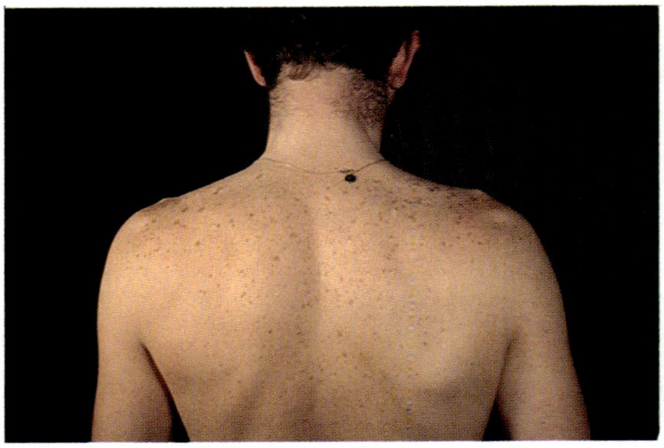

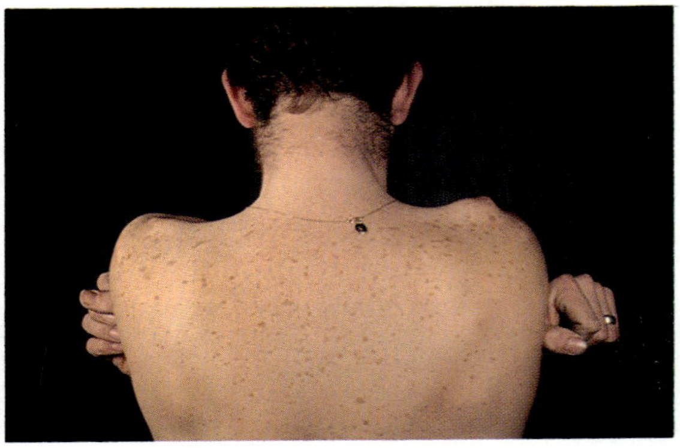

625 & **626** Subluxation of the right acromioclavicular joint due to a trivial injury long since forgotten. The prominent outer end of the clavicle is best seen from behind with the arms in full adduction.

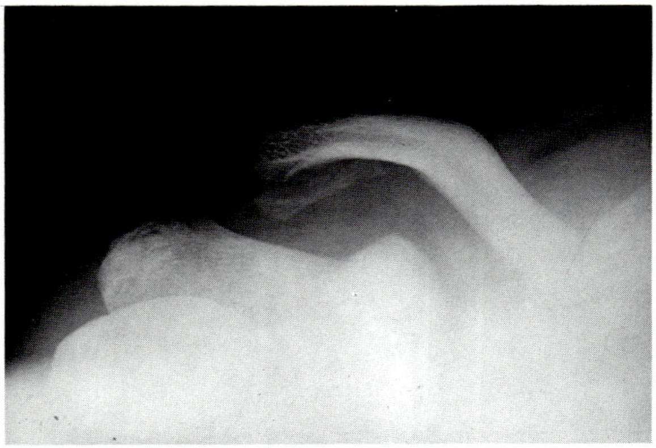

627 Radiograph of the same patient. New bone formation is seen on the undersurface of the clavicle from which the periosteum had been stripped.

Subacromial joint

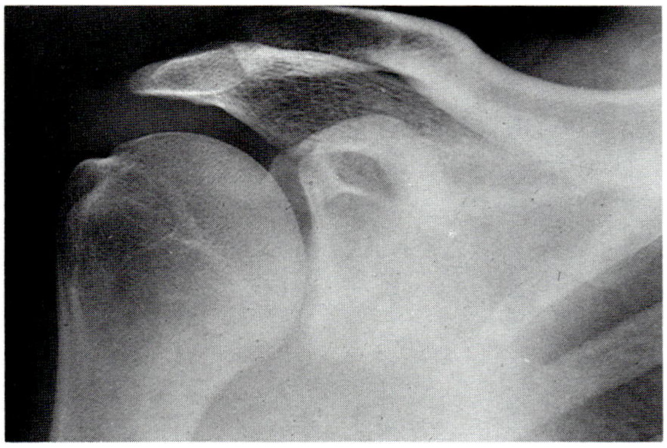

628 A normal shoulder. The anatomical area bounded above by the acromion and the coracoacromial ligament, and below by the head and tuberosities of the humerus, has been variously designated. It is most conveniently considered as a surgical joint, called here the subacromial joint.

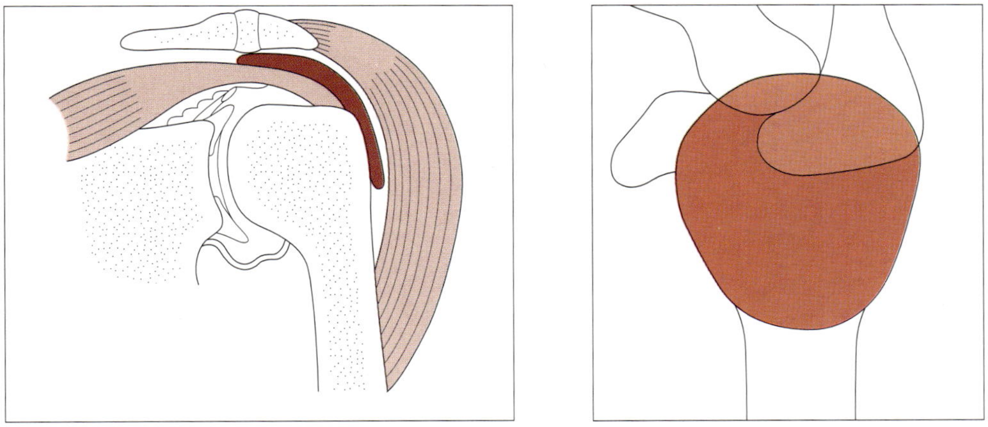

629 & **630** The joint space is formed by the subacromial bursa whose floor is centrally tethered to the tendons of the rotator muscle cuff. The extent of the bursa which serves as the synovial lining of the subacromial joint is shown.

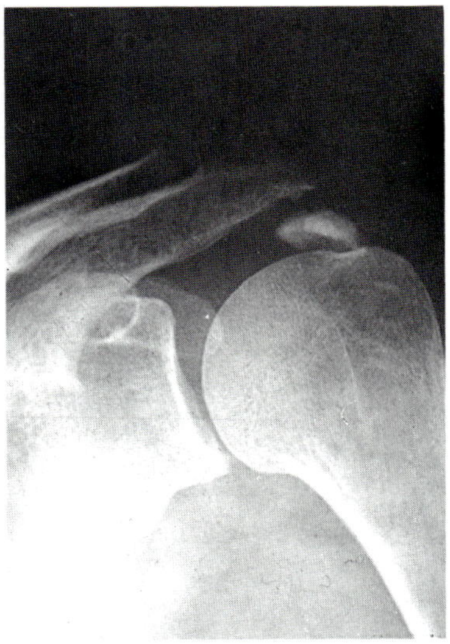

631 Acute calcific bursitis. Radiograph of a patient with intense pain in the shoulder shows a deposition of radio-opaque calcium salts. The deposit consists essentially of calcium apatite with a surrounding inflammatory reaction.

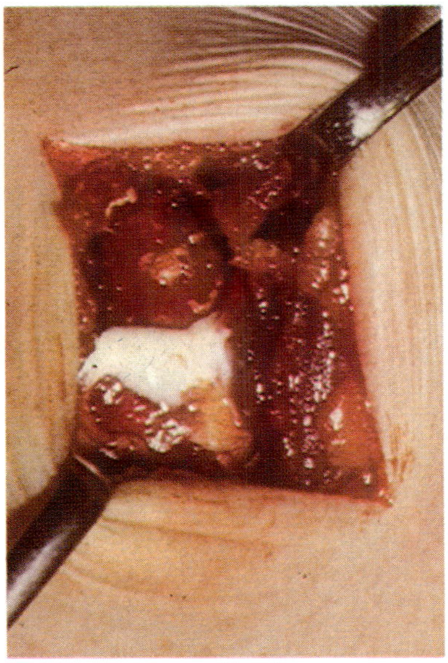

632 The consistency of the calcific deposit at operation is very variable. In the acute phase it is under considerable tension and is virtually a sterile chemical abscess.

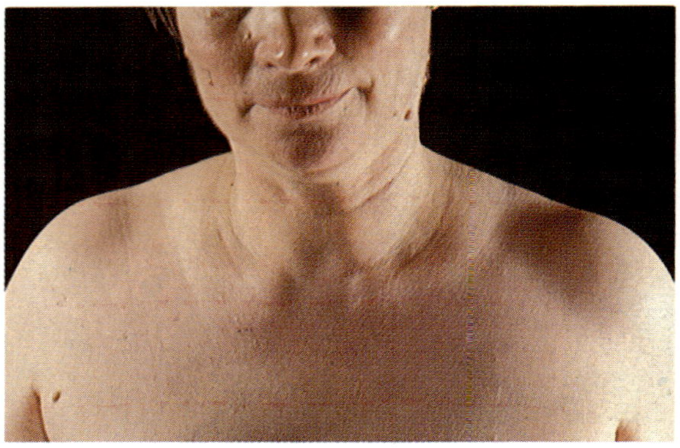

633 Chronic subacromial bursitis. The alteration of contour caused by the enlargement of the subacromial bursa on the left in a case of rheumatoid arthritis.

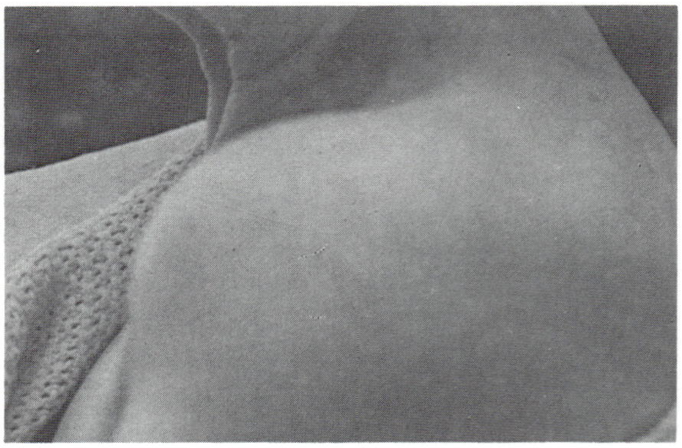

634 Subacromial bursitis highlighted from the side.

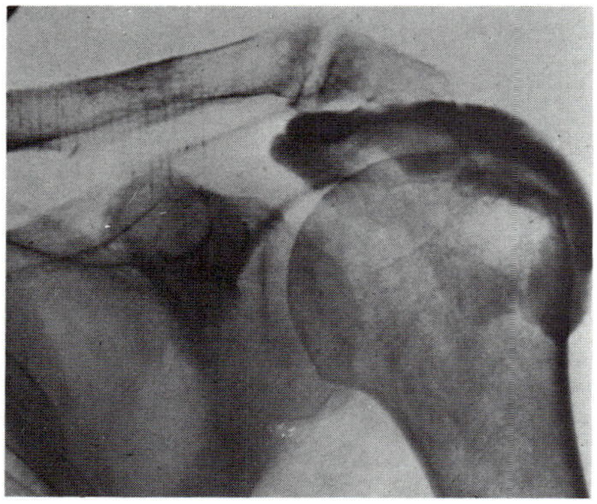

635 Contrast medium injected to produce a subacromial bursograph.

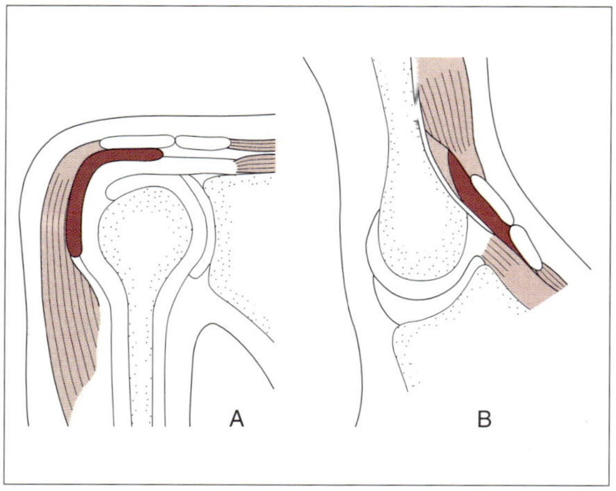

636 Note how the walls of the subacromial bursa glide with abduction of the shoulder so that points A and B come to lie opposite each other at the extremes of movement. The same gliding takes place during both abduction and rotation

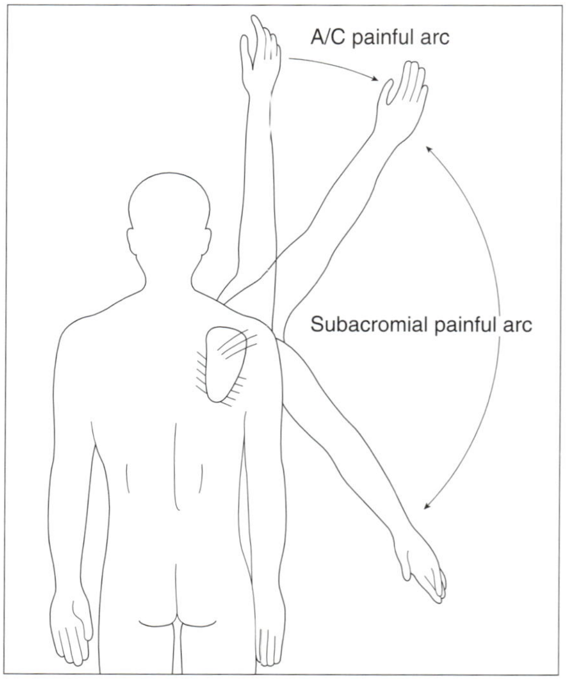

637 The subacromial painful arc. Gliding of the bursal walls and simultaneous outward rotation of the head of the humerus to achieve abduction starts at about 40° and is complete at about 120° Any inflammatory disorder of the subacromial joint therefore causes a painful arc of abduction between 40° and 120° Below and above these points the pain is less pronounced.

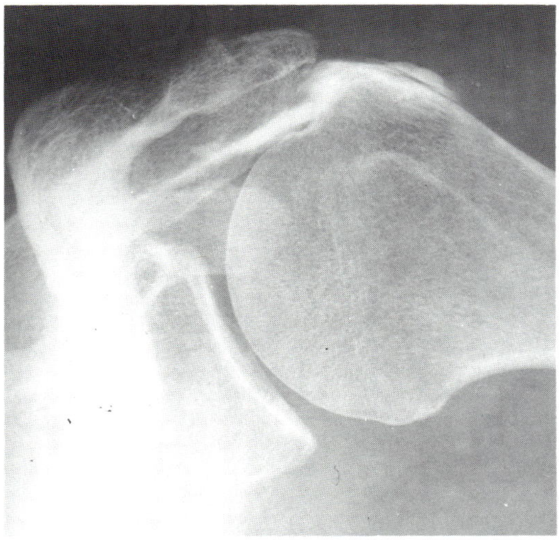

638 Before any radiographic changes are evident, soft-tissue impingement can be demonstrated by injecting contrast material. Here the supraspinatus tendon is seen kinked to a right angle by impingement of the coraco-acromial ligament. A line imagined from the tip of the coracoid to the acromion demonstrates the site of impingement.

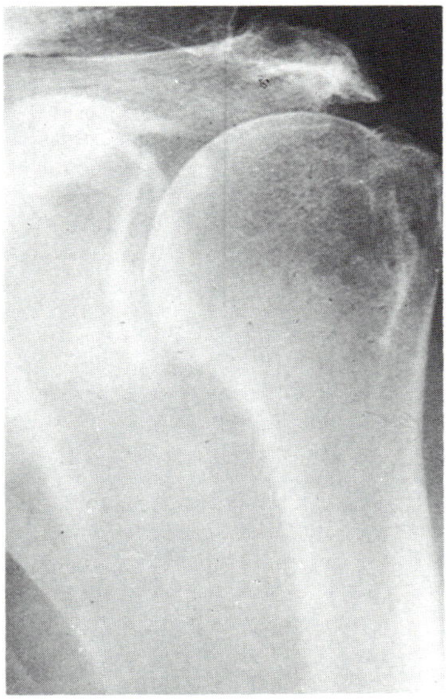

639 Intermediate stage of subacromial arthritis, illustrating that the same changes occur as in other synovial joints. There is sclerosis and osteophyte formation on either side, at the acromion and greater tuberosity.

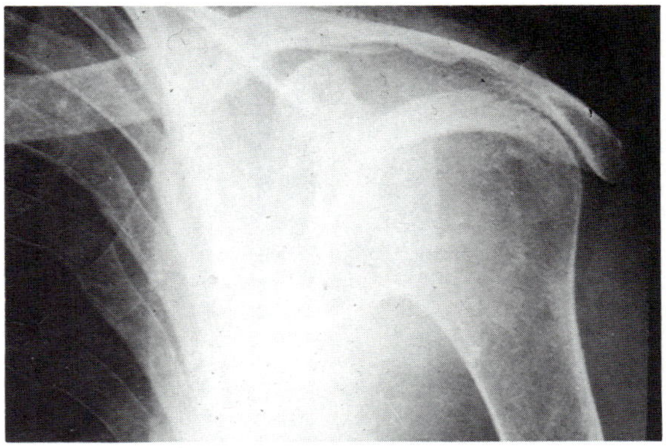

640 Subacromial degenerative arthritis in its final stage in which the intervening soft tissues give way and the atrophic tuberosity area of the humerus comes to form a secondary articulation with the undersurface of the acromion.

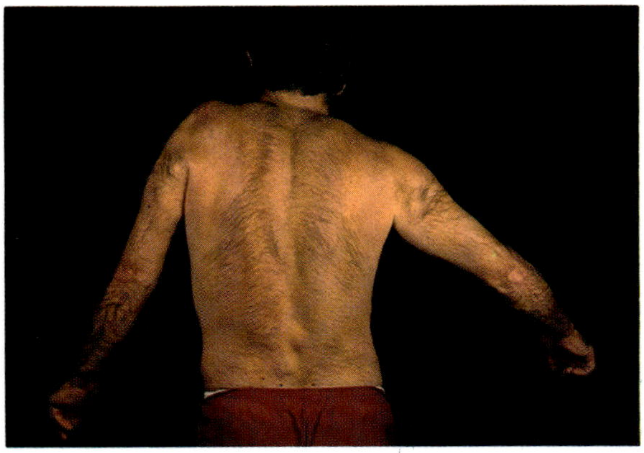

641 Rupture of the rotator cuff. The patient is unable to abduct his arm without hunching the shoulder. There is a reversal of normal scapulo-humeral rhythm. Passive movements are full.

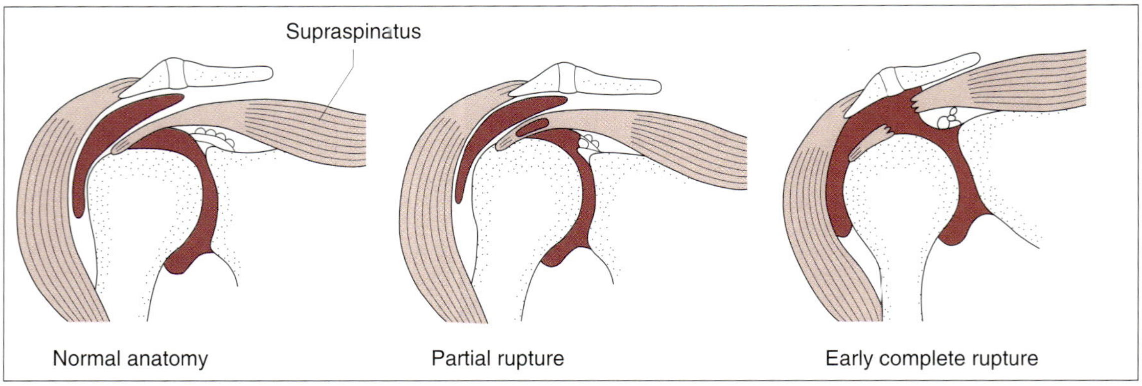

642 Varieties of rupture of the rotator cuff.

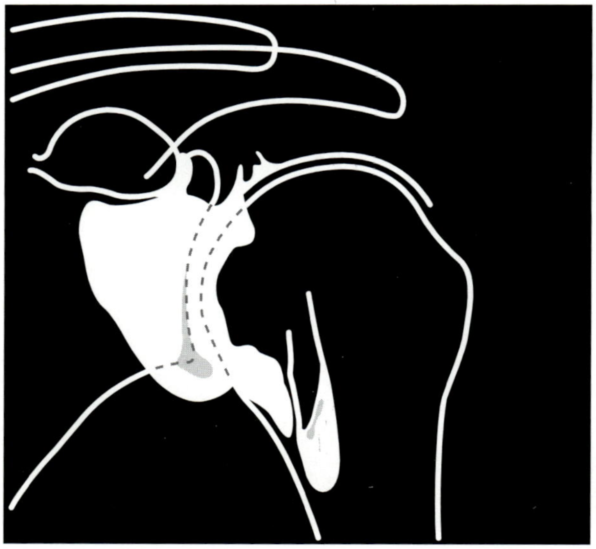

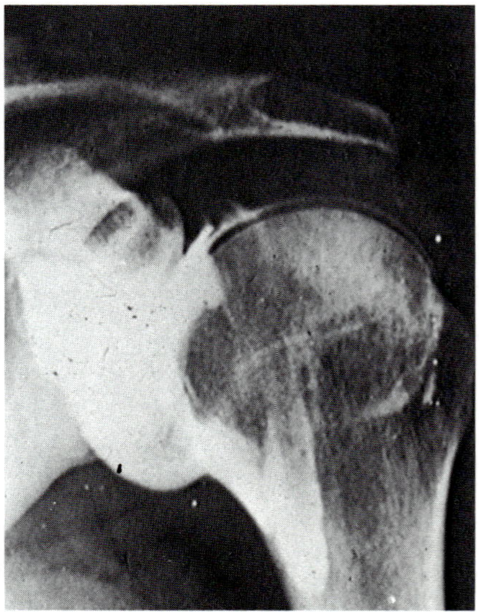

643 Normal arthrograph of the shoulder joint. Contrast material in the glenohumeral joint: it outlines the articular cartilage of the head of the humerus, the subcoracoid bursa, the inferior joint recess, and the tendon sheath of the long head of the biceps.

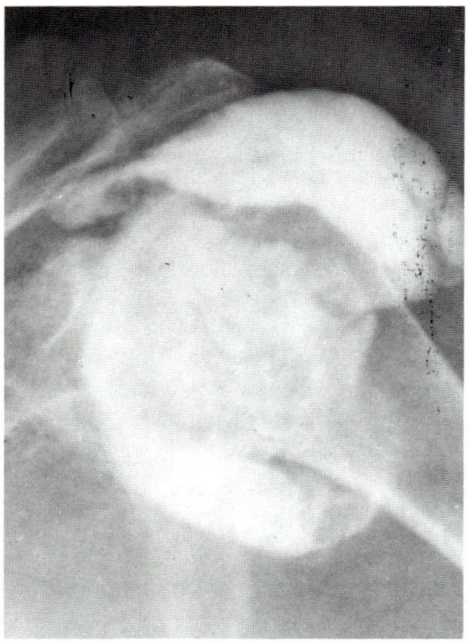

644 Total rupture of the rotator cuff. In this arthrograph of the shoulder the contrast medium escapes into the subacromial bursa, and outlines both joint and bursa.

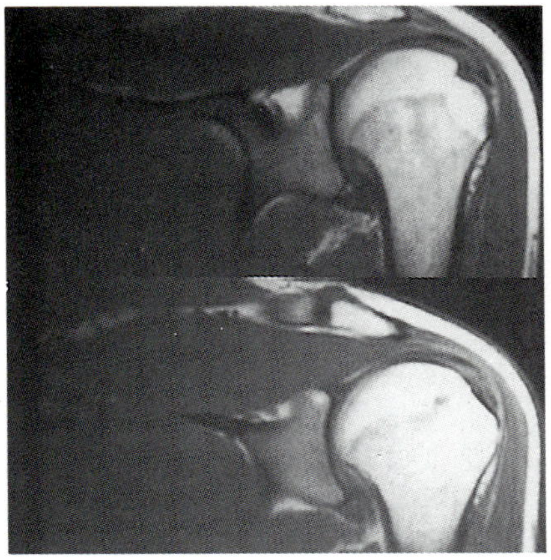

645 Normal MRI scan of the shoulder. This investigation has greatly improved the imaging of the soft tissues of the shoulder and greatly aided the diagnosis of rotator cuff pathology. Contrast enhancement of images further sharpens the diagnostic abilities

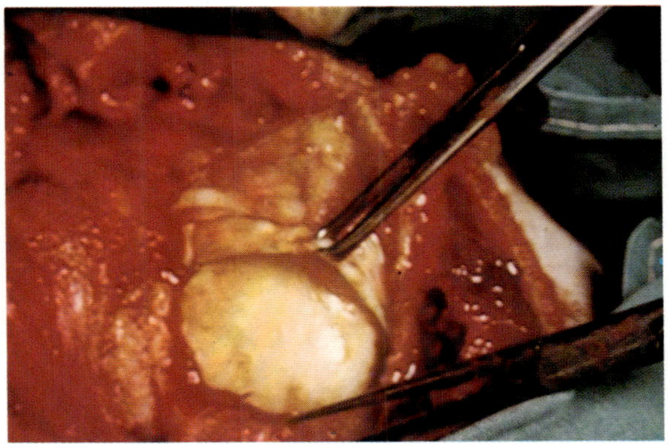

646 An acute massive rupture of the rotator cuff demonstrated at operation. The cuff has been retracted to show the underlying bare head of the humerus.

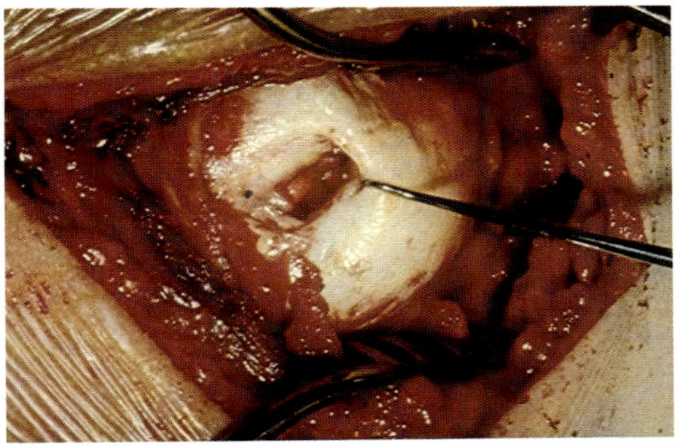

647 Chronic attrition rupture of the rotator cuff. Healing has taken place with a tough fibrous ring leaving a small defect between the subacromial bursa and the shoulder joint. Normal movements have returned but a painful arc of abduction persists.

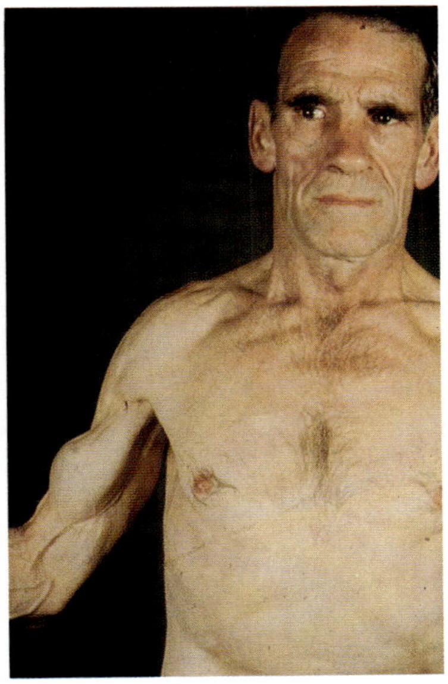

648 Rupture of the tendon of the long head of biceps. This may occur suddenly or imperceptibly without the patient's knowledge.

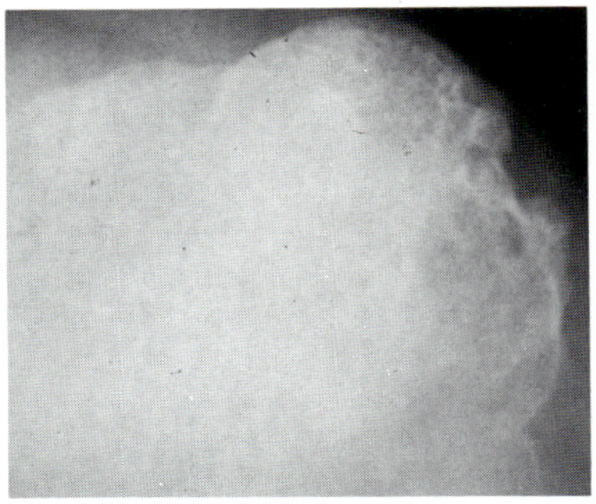

649 Radiograph of the patient's shoulder: a tangential view of the sulcus for LHB between the greater and lesser tuberosities of the humerus. Note the marked osteophyte and pseudocyst formation of degenerative joint disease.

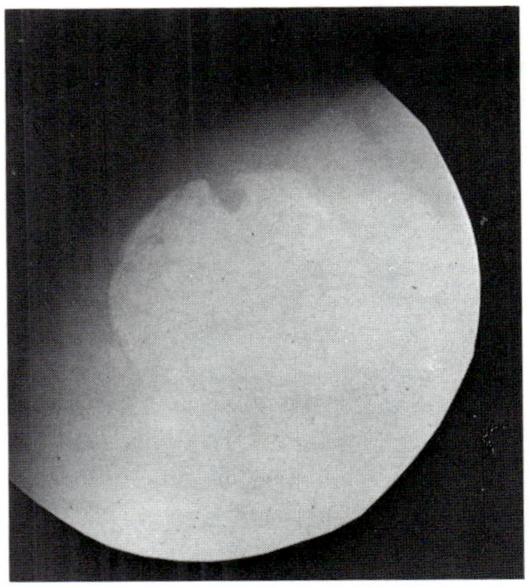

650 A normal bicipital sulcus for comparison.

Glenohumeral joint

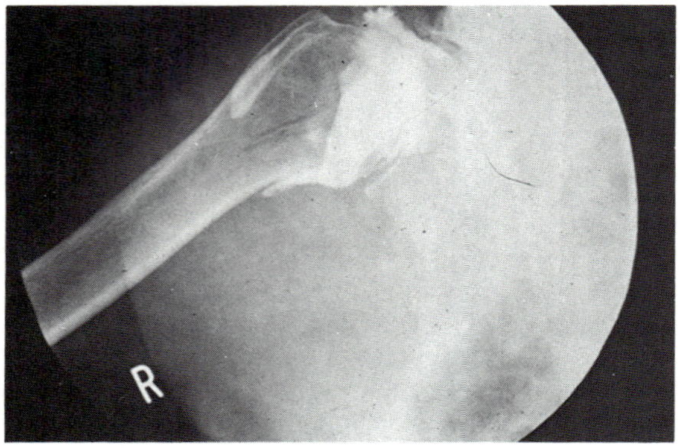

651 'The frozen shoulder'. An acutely painful and increasingly stiff shoulder is designated as a 'frozen shoulder', providing no cause can be found. An arthrograph of a 'frozen shoulder' in which there is one clear abnormality compared with the normal arthrograph, i.e. the joint space is considerably reduced, accepting only about 6–8 ml of contrast fluid compared to 25–30 ml of fluid accepted into a normal shoulder joint. Reduction of the joint space is also evidenced by the obliteration of the inferior joint recess.

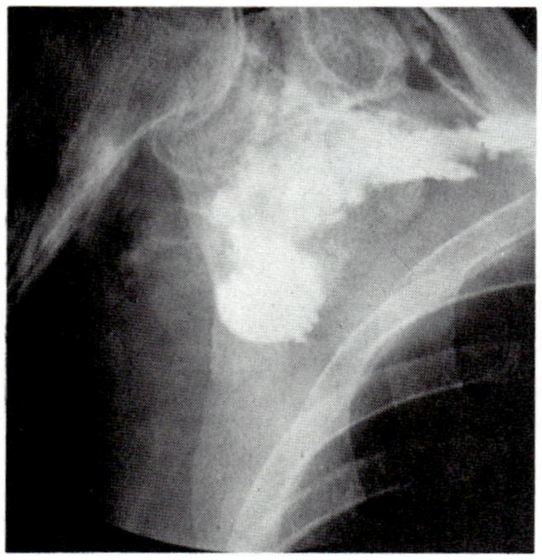

652 Radiograph of the same patient carried out immediately following manipulation of the shoulder to demonstrate how the joint capsule has been ruptured and the contrast medium flows out freely into the soft tissues in the subscapular region.

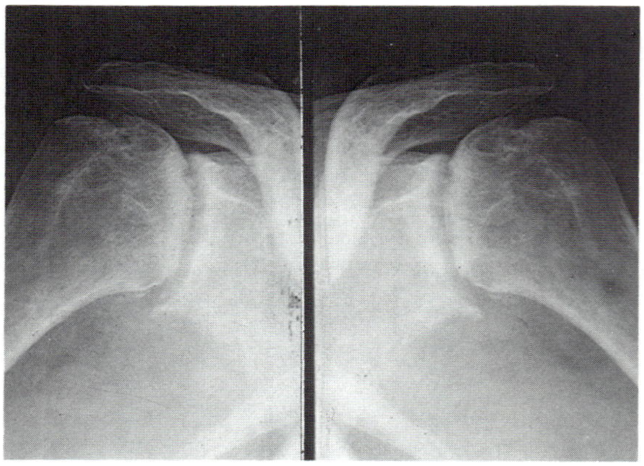

653 Rheumatoid arthritis. The glenohumeral joint is only rarely affected by any form of arthritis. Rheumatoid disease is by far the commonest cause.

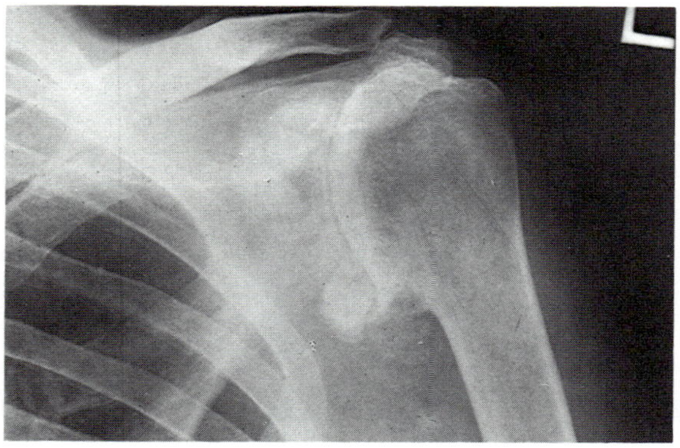

654 Synovial osteochondromatosis of the glenohumeral joint.

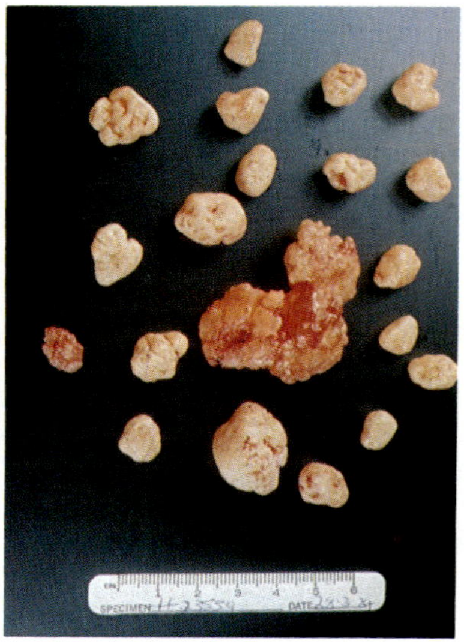

655 Multiple osteochondromata removed at operation.

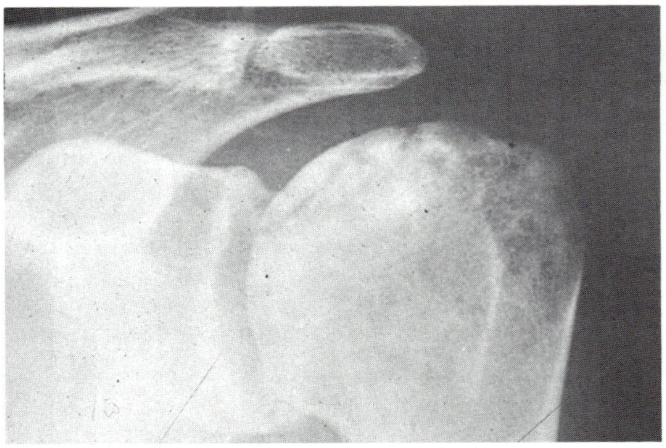

656 Caisson's disease (dysbaric osteonecrosis). The shoulder of a tunnel worker. This occupational disease is uncommon; however, when it does occur the shoulders are frequently affected. A lozenge-shaped infarct due to avascular necrosis from gas embolism, is seen on the superomedial aspect of the head of the humerus.

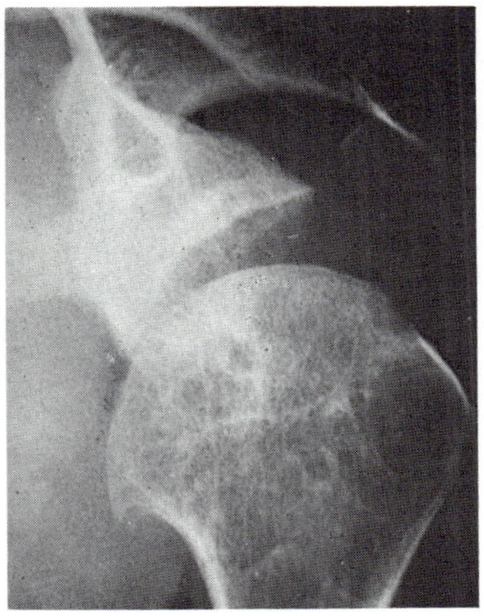

657 Haemophilic arthropathy. Shoulder of a patient suffering from another rare cause of glenohumeral arthritis.

Shoulder instability

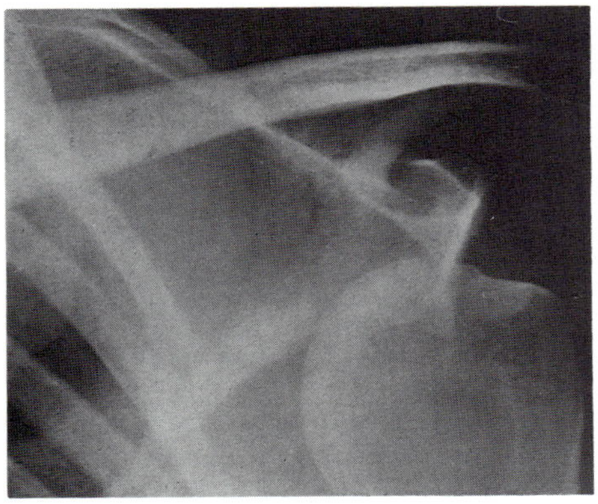

658 Recurrent anterior dislocation of the shoulder joint is a common disorder. The basic pathology consists of a detachment of the capsule from the front of the shoulder joint at the time of the original dislocation, usually combined with an impaction fracture in the posterior part of the head of the humerus.

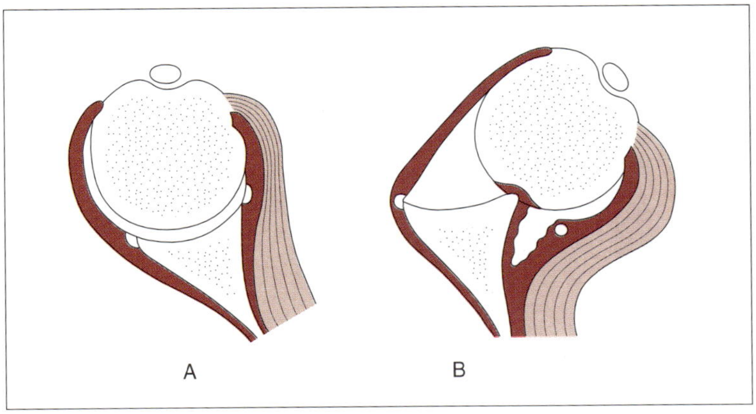

659 The diagram shows how the head of the humerus is rotated out and causes a detachment of the capsule, labrum glenoidale and periosteum from the neck of the scapula.

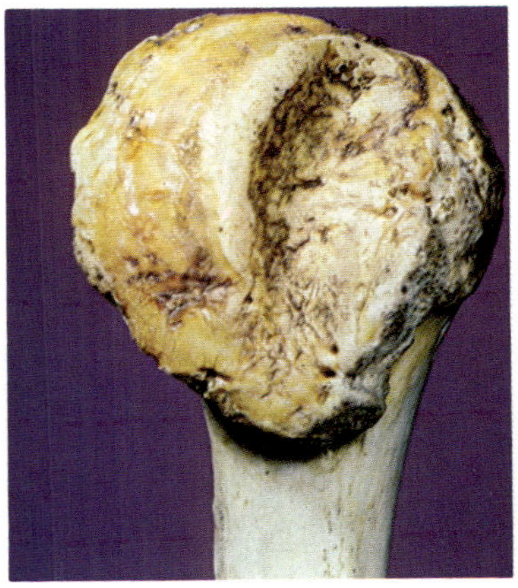

660 Hills–Sachs lesion which is probably better termed as the Broca lesion, since he was the first to describe it. Specimen of an old recurrent dislocation of the shoulder showing the impaction fracture of the posterior part of the head of the humerus.

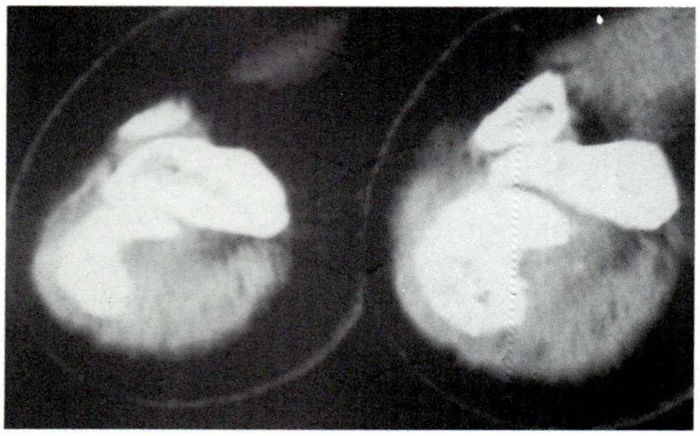

661 Broca lesion. CT scan of unstable shoulder showing large, wedge-shaped defect in the posterior aspect of the humeral head.

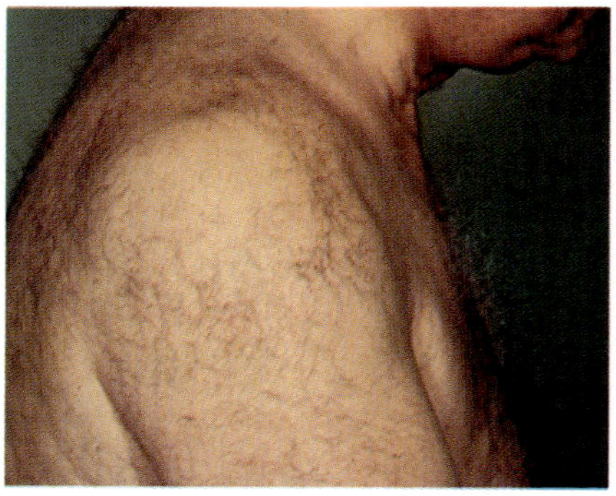

662 Posterior dislocation of the shoulder joint. The clinical appearances are very deceptive. Careful inspection reveals a bulge at the back of the shoulder, which is the head of the humerus.

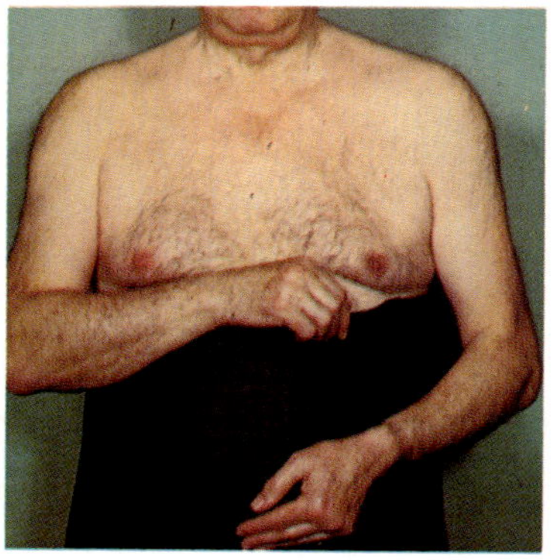

663 Fixed internal rotation of the shoulder is the single most important diagnostic sign.

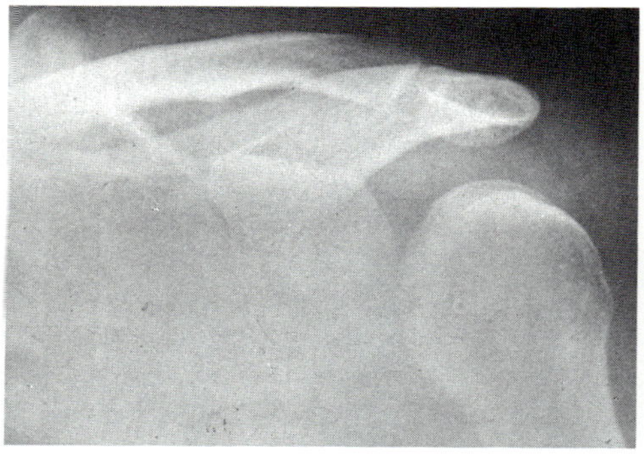

664 The standard anteroposterior radiograph can be very deceiving.

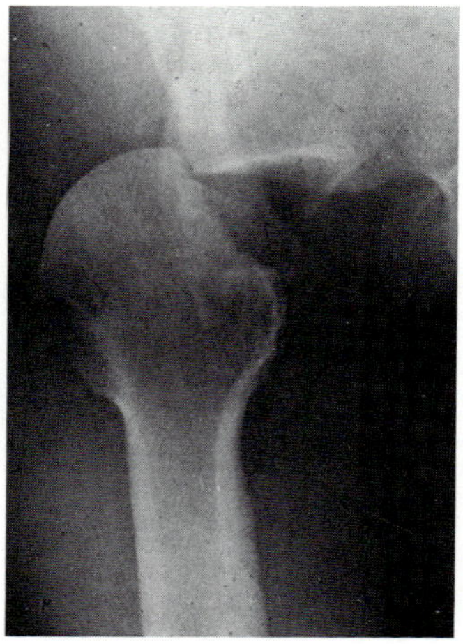

665 A lateral radiograph of the same shoulder to reveal the posterior dislocation.

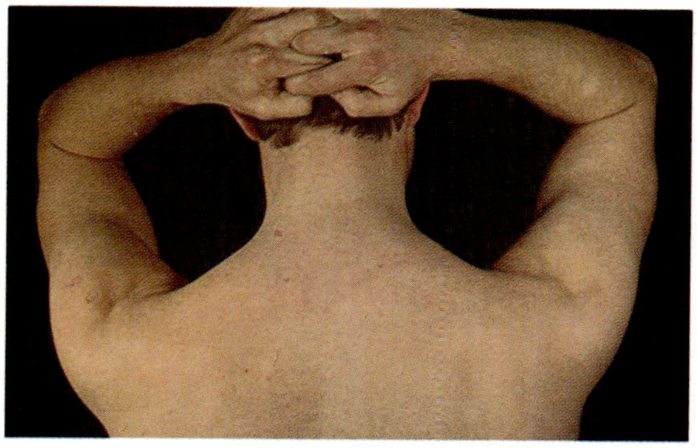

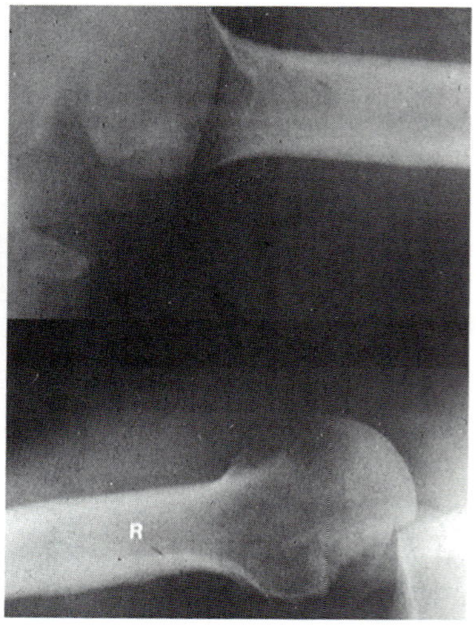

666, 667 Habitual, bilateral, posterior dislocation of shoulders.

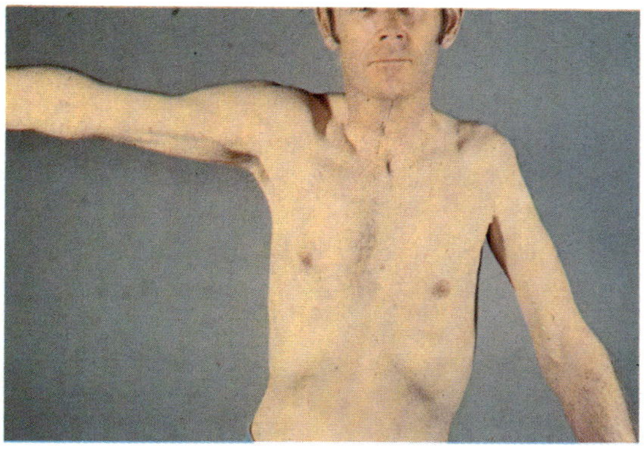

668 Neuralgic amyotrophy (Paralytic brachial neuritis or shoulder girdle paralysis). A presumed viral disease of acute onset leading to variable peripheral nerve damage. This patient has a wasted and completely paralysed deltoid muscle.

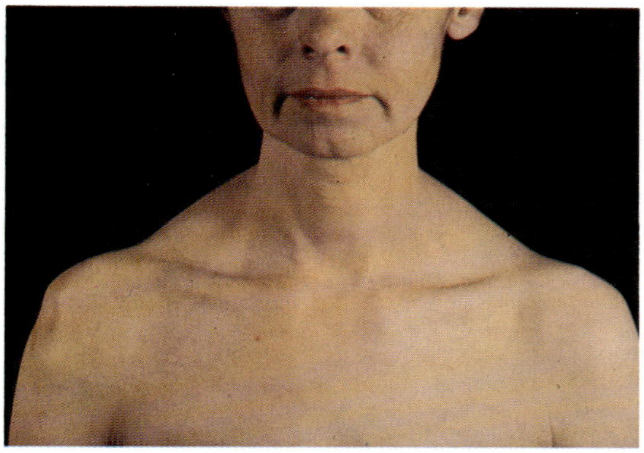

669 Deltoid paralysis following fracture dislocation of the right shoulder joint. The hollow seen on the outer aspect of the shoulder is due to downward subluxation of the head of the humerus.

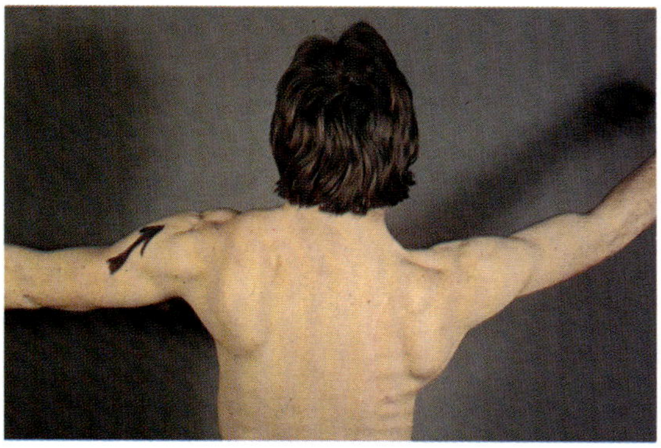

670 Facio-scapular muscular dystrophy (see also **252–254**). The muscles controlling the scapula have become gradually paralysed. On the left side the condition is untreated and the original clinical signs remain: wasting of shoulder girdle musculature, winging of the scapula, loss of range and power of abduction of the shoulder. Compare the right side on which an operation has been performed to fuse the scapula to the chest wall: improved stability of the scapula and movements of the right shoulder have been achieved.

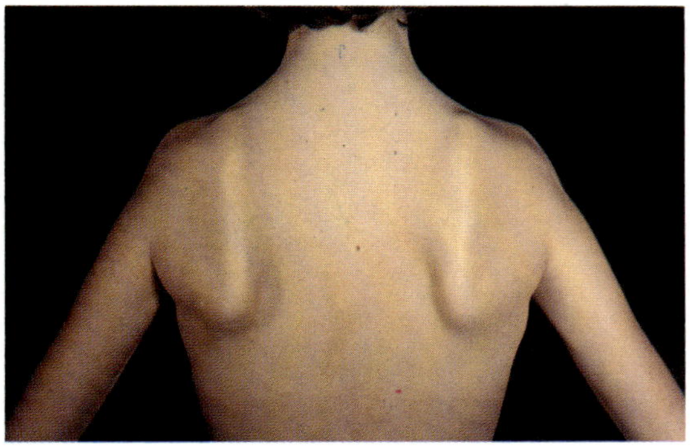

671 Contracture of deltoid caused by intramuscular injections. This patient was given a series of intramuscular injections of antibiotics, as a result of which some of the muscle was destroyed and replaced by fibrous tissue. On attempting to bring her arms to her side the shortened and tethered deltoid muscles do not allow normal adduction at the glenohumeral joints and the scapulae are forced to rotate early. The scapulae become prominent and simulate the winging of serratus anterior paralysis.

The elbow region

Deformities of the elbow

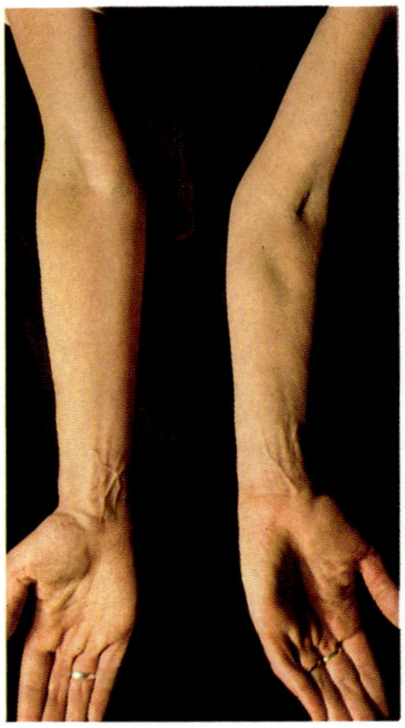

672 Cubitus valgus. This deformity is due to injury resulting in malunion or non-union of a fracture around the elbow. A more gradually developing deformity results from damage to the lower humeral growth plate. It is the classical, although not the commonest cause of tardy ulnar palsy because the ulnar nerve now has to take a longer course behind the medial epicondyle.

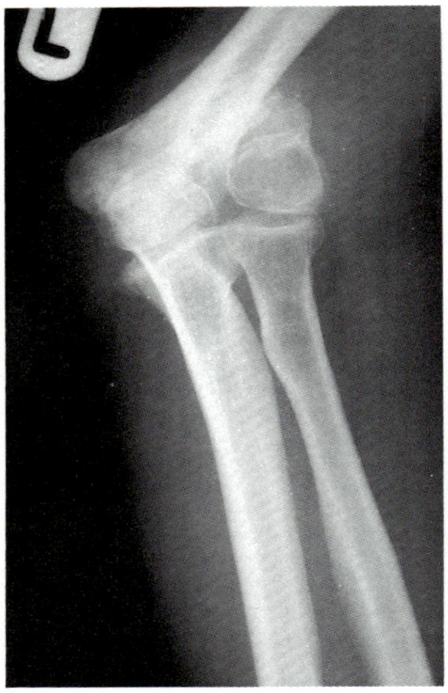

673 Cubitus valgus due to non-union of the lateral condyle of the humerus.

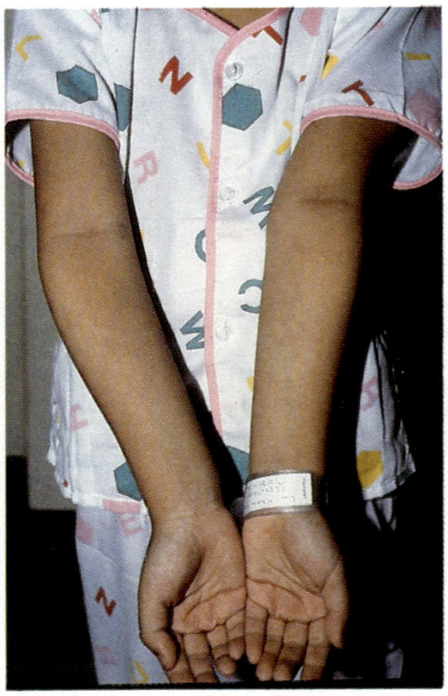

674 Cubitus varus or Gunstock deformity. This causes little functional impairment but can be extremely unsightly, requiring correction on aesthetic grounds.

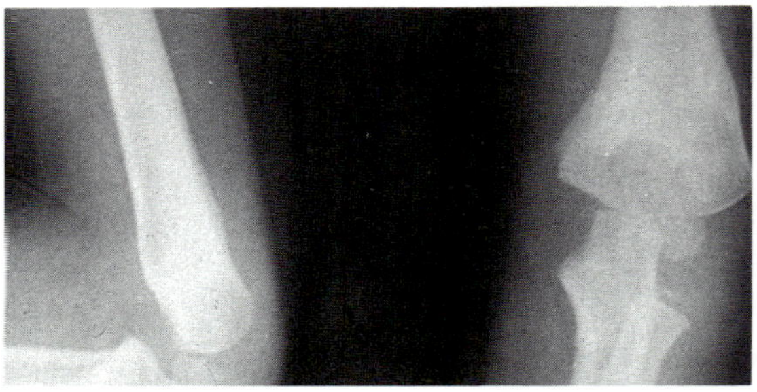

675 Radiograph shows cubitus varus due to a malunited supra-condylar fracture.

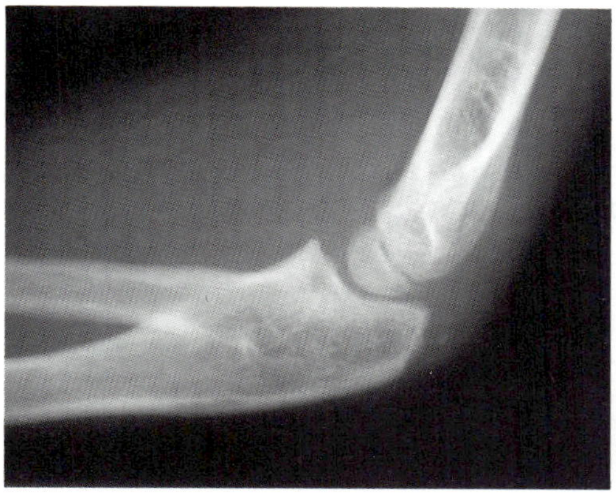

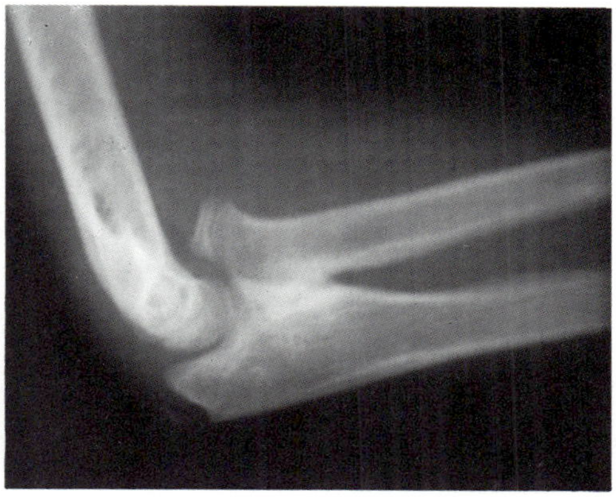

676 & **677** Congenital radio-ulnar synostosis with or without dislocation of the radial head are among the commonest congenital anomalies at the elbow. Lack of forearm rotation is only slightly inconvenient. The prominence of a dislocated radial head can be excised, particularly if it limits flexion of the elbow.

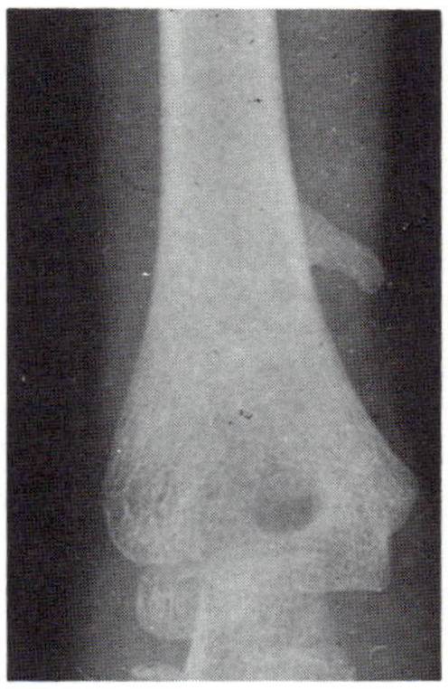

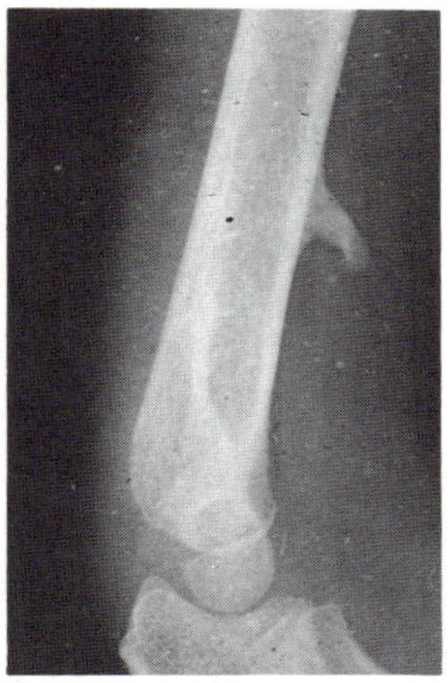

678 & **679** Supracondylar spur. This is a rare but interesting cause of neurovascular compression in the arm causing symptoms that simulate the carpal tunnel syndrome. The supracondylar process is an anatomical atavism.

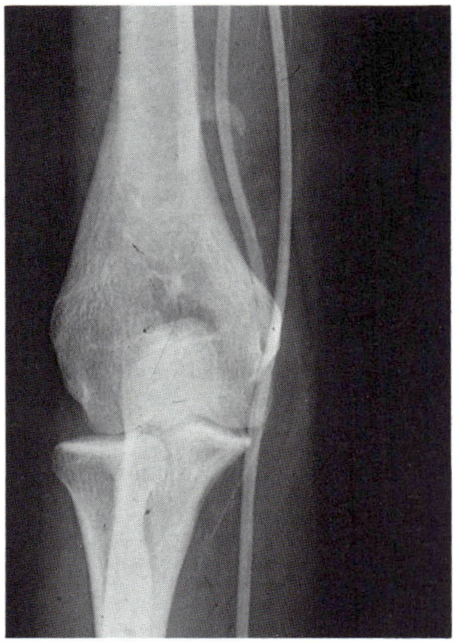

680 Brachial arteriograph showing high division of the brachial artery with impaired filling of the ulnar branch owing to compression.

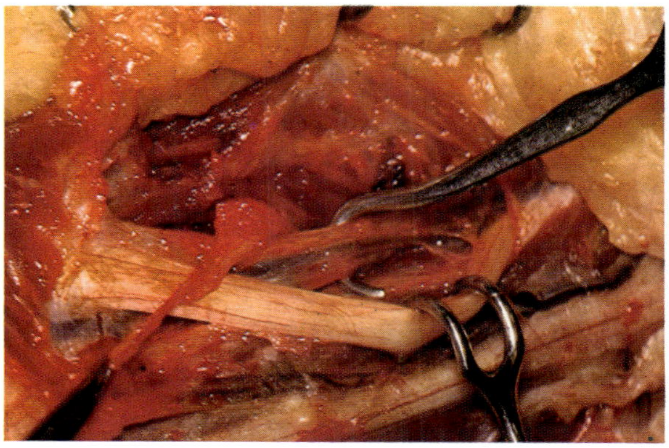

681 The area displayed at operation: from the tip of the spur the ligament of Struthers can be seen to run downwards towards the left, crossing over the median nerve and ulnar vessels.

Cubital tunnel syndrome, Tardy ulnar palsy

Compression neuropathy of the ulnar nerve can occur anywhere in the cubital tunnel from the medial intermuscular septum to the two heads of flexor carpi ulnaris. This may arise quite spontaneously or over a prolonged period of time after trauma to the elbow which results in a residual valgus deformity.

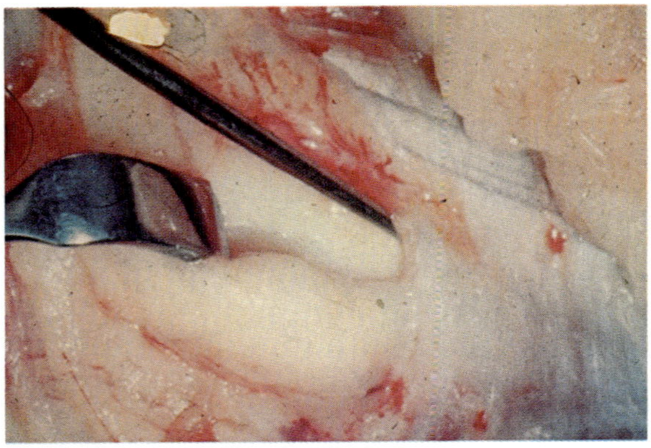

682 The ulnar nerve is seen at the distal end of the cubital tunnel passing beneath an arch of fibrous bands bridging the two heads of flexor carpi ulnaris (Osborne's bands). At the site of constriction by the bands there is an indentation of the nerve, proximal to this there is a swelling of the nerve: the neuroma. This is more accurately termed a glioma and is caused by intraneural fibrosis.

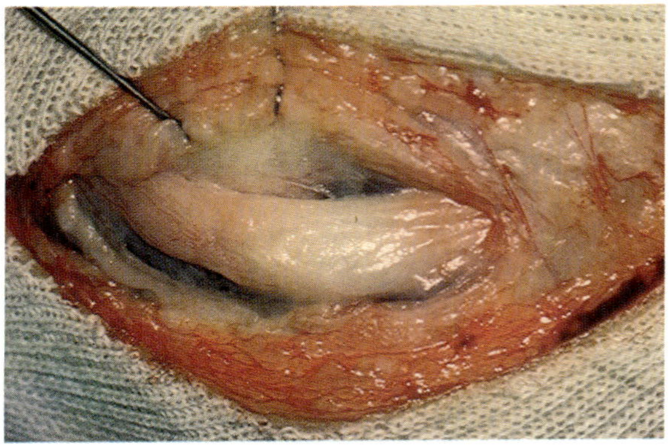

683 The ulnar tunnel has been divided and the nerve now lies free. The ischaemic area of the nerve compressed can clearly be seen.

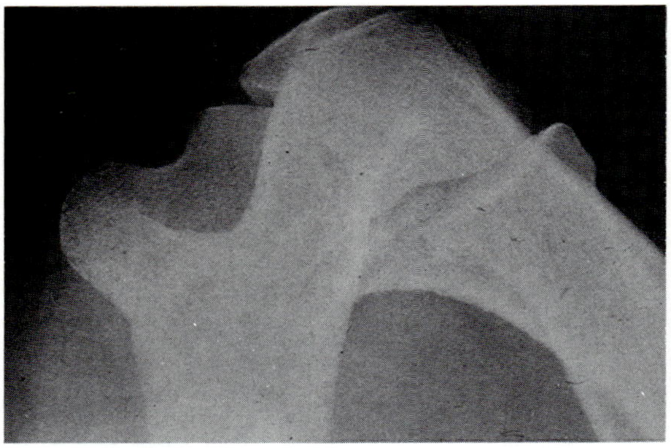

684 Tangential radiograph to show the normal ulnar groove behind the medial condyle of the humerus.

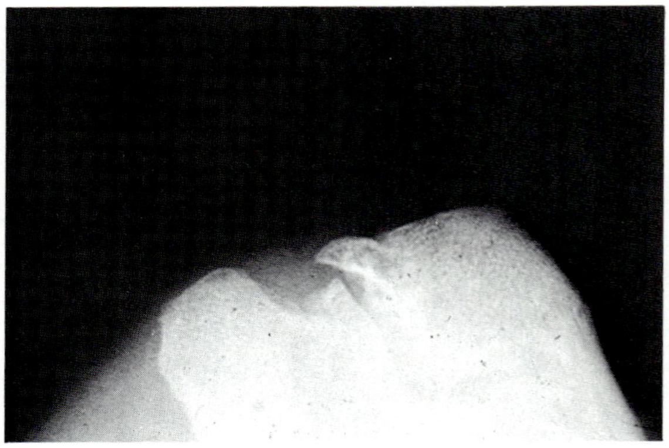

685 Radiograph of a patient suffering from tardy ulnar palsy due to encroachment on the ulnar groove by osteophytes.

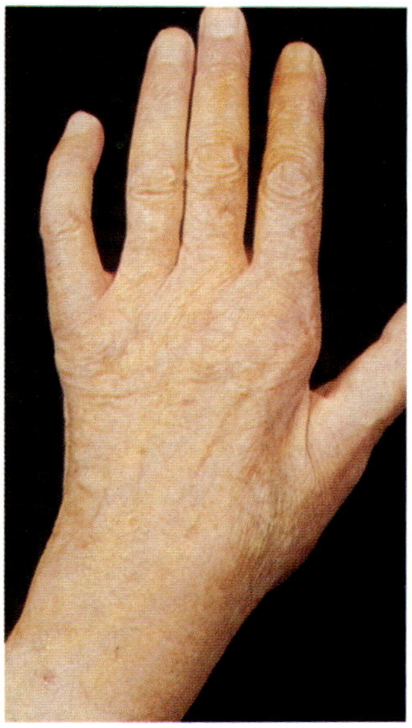

686 Intrinsic muscle wasting of the hand in a case of tardy ulnar palsy.

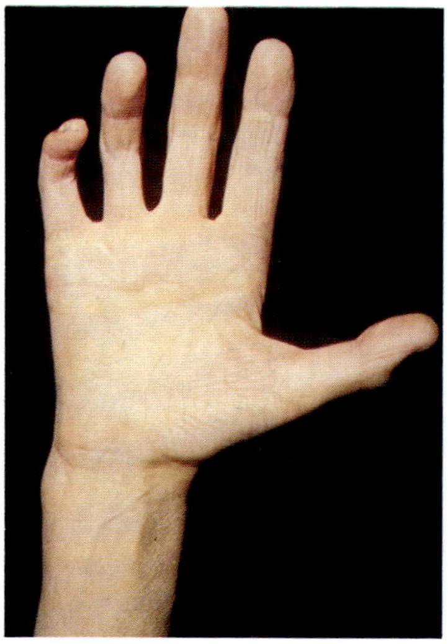

687 Ulnar claw hand due to advanced ulnar palsy by compression of the ulnar nerve at the elbow. Paradoxically, the deformity of the hand is greater when the lesion is more distal. Claw hand due to a low ulnar lesion is depicted in **818**.

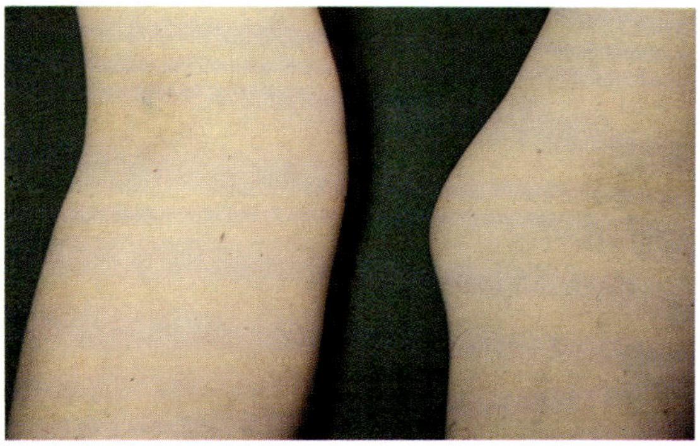

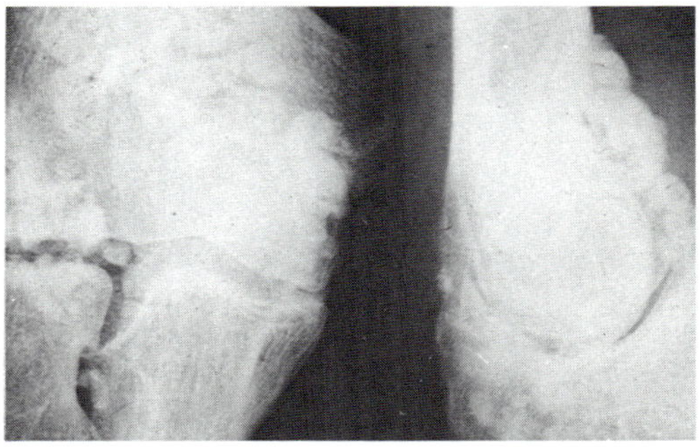

688 & **689** Synovial chondromatosis. Pronounced soft tissue swelling over the medial aspect of the left elbow. Radiographs reveal the multiple chondromata.

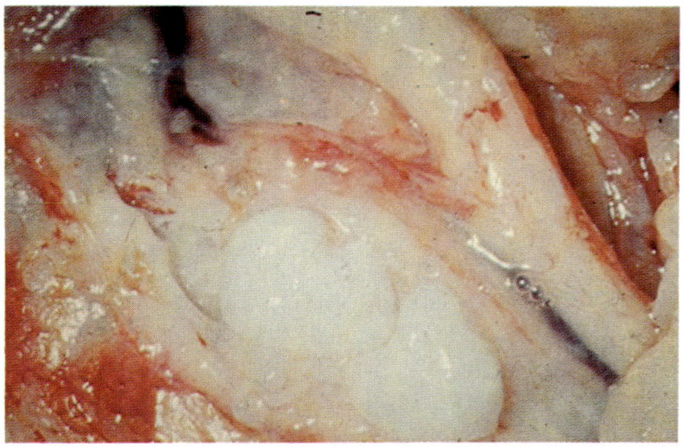

690 The chondromata escaped when the synovial membrane adjacent to the ulnar nerve was incised.

A

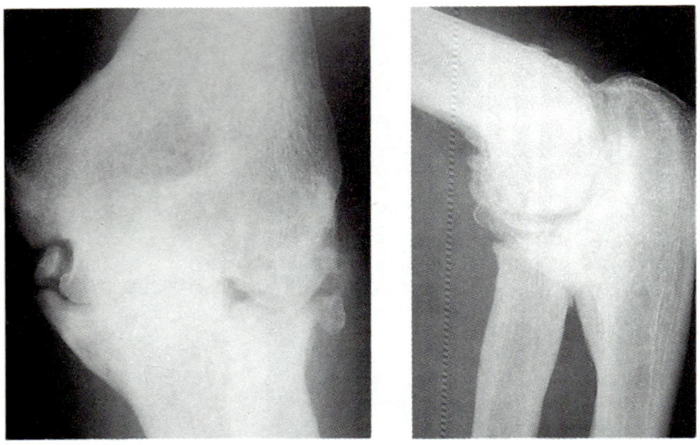

B

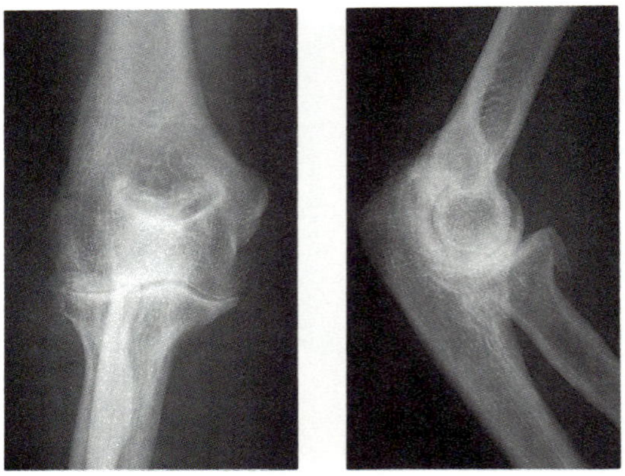

691A & **B** Osteoarthritis (OA) elbow.

692 Rheumatoid arthritis frequently involves the elbow joints. Radiographs show periarticular osteoporosis with marked loss of joint space. In later stages serious bone loss can occur.

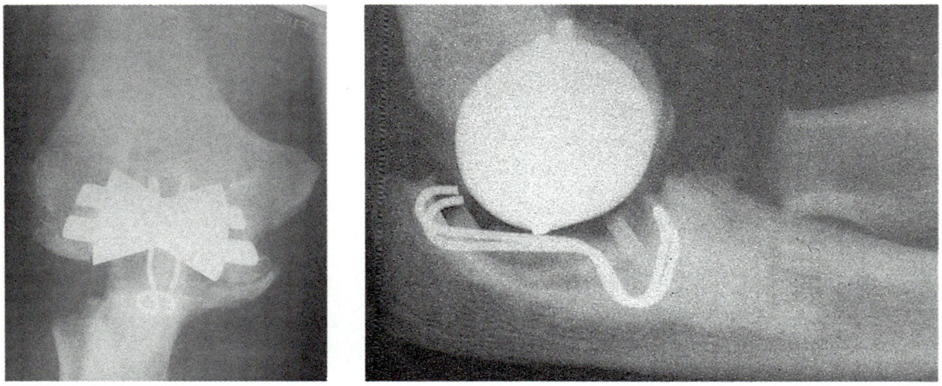

693 Rheumatoid arthritis is the majcr indication for arthroplasty of the elbow. The radiographs show one variety in use.

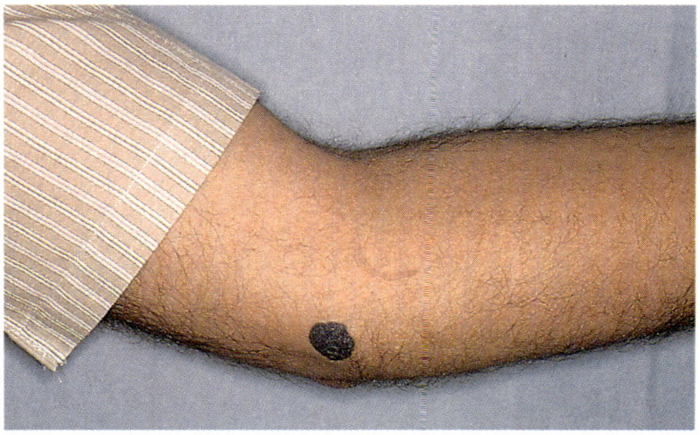

694 Golfer's elbow. Less common than lateral epicondylitis, the pain of medial epicondylitis is accurately localised to the medial epicondyle. It is caused by a sprain or tear to the fibres of the common flexor origin, usually ther flexor carpi radialis.

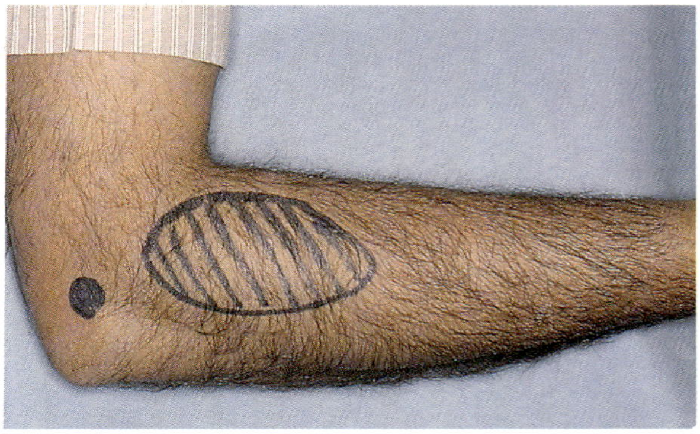

695 Tennis elbow. True lateral epicondylitis due to sprains or tears in the extensor carpi radialis brevis at the common extensor origin is a common cause of pain on the lateral aspect of the elbow. Tenderness is accurately localised to the lateral epicondyle. Discomfort from synovial fringes or annular ligament pathology is more distally and diffusely located. The less common posterior interosseus nerve entrapment produces diffuse discomfort in the muscles of the 'mobile wad of Henry' (diagonally hatched).

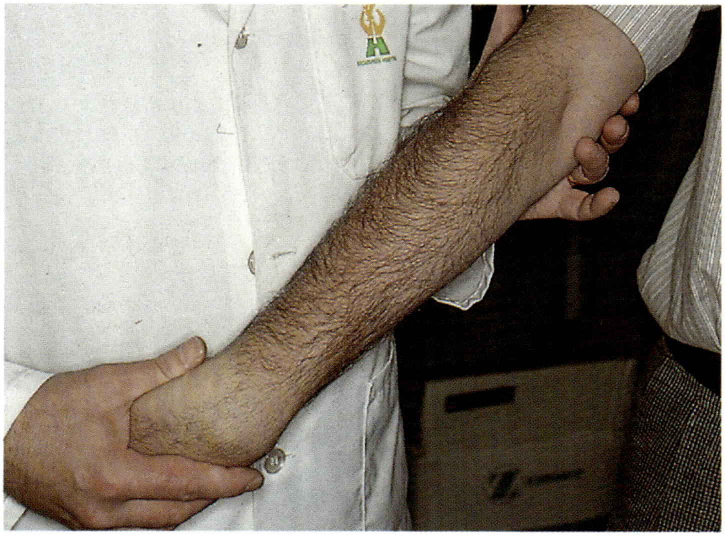

696 Mill's test. Flexion of the wrist and pronation of the forearm followed by extension of the elbow reproduces the pain of true tennis elbow.

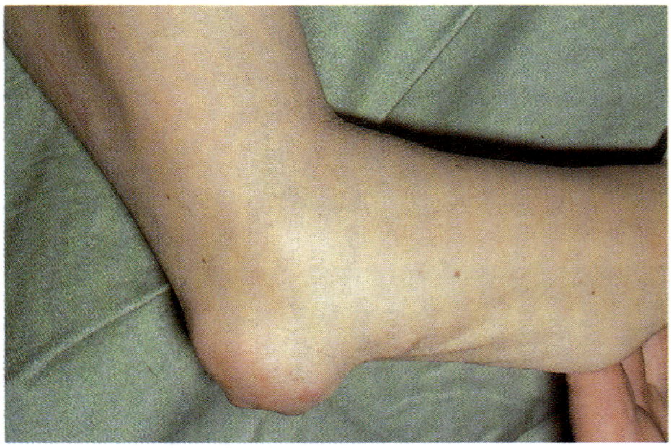

697 Olecranon bursitis. Synovial swelling with an effusion into the olecranon bursa can occur with repeated frictional trauma to the area. In this case the cause was rheumatoid arthritis.

Wrist

Careful examination of the wrist by palpation has been neglected and poorly taught in the past. As in other regions, however, a careful and systematic examination frequently reveals the cause of chronic wrist pain. All of the bones of the carpus can be individually palpated along with the sulci between them. The site of maximal tenderness is usually the site of the lesion. Stressing the intercarpal joints may produce pain or reveal abnormal mobility suggesting instability.

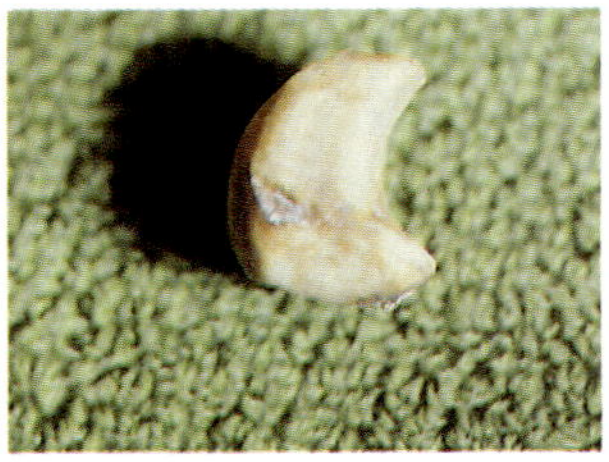

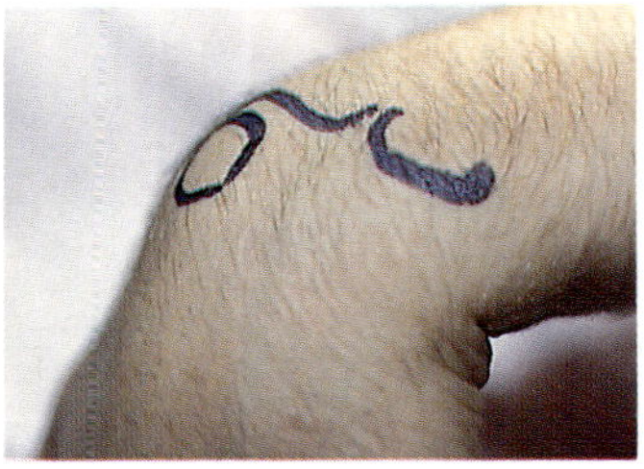

698 & **699** The 'keystone' of the carpus. The lunate forms the prominent dome shape to the palmar flexed wrist. Pain localised to the lunate occurs in fractures but is also characteristic of Kienbock's disease.

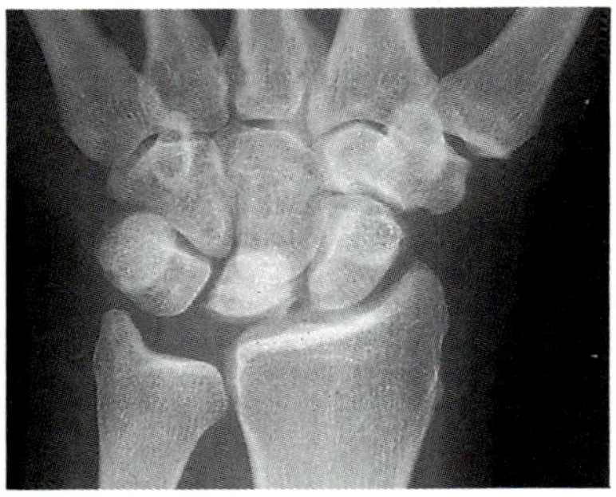

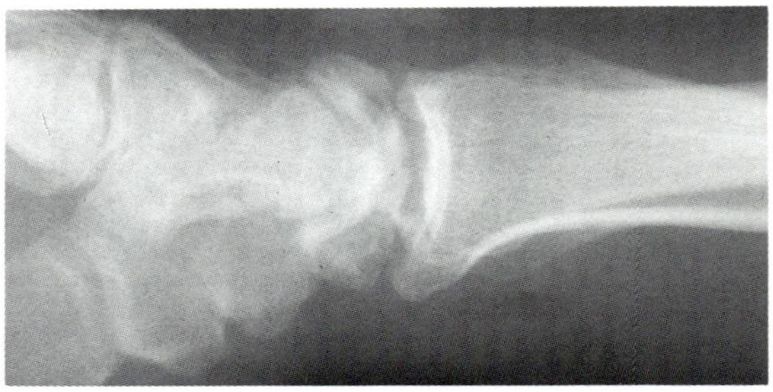

700, 701 Kienbock's disease. This disease is characterised by sclerosis and ultimate collapse of the lunate. The cause of the condition is not fully understood but is thought to be due to traumatic compromise of the blood supply to the lunate. A relative shortening of the ulna (negative ulnar variance) is a frequent association that is probably indicative of a 'susceptible' lunate.

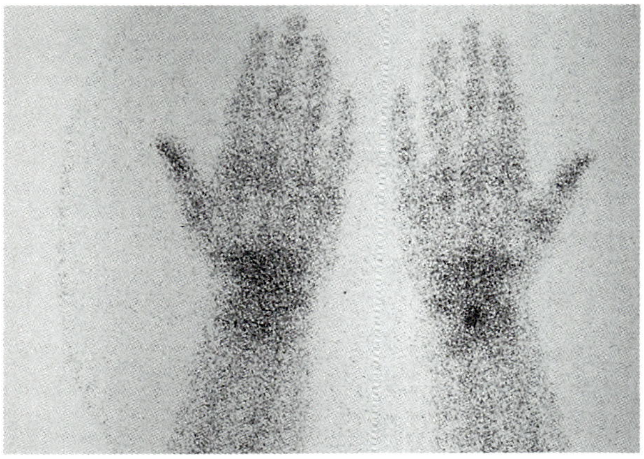

702 Kienbock's disease. In the early stages, before radiographic changes have occurred a bone scan may further indicate the diagnosis, showing an increased uptake around the lunate.

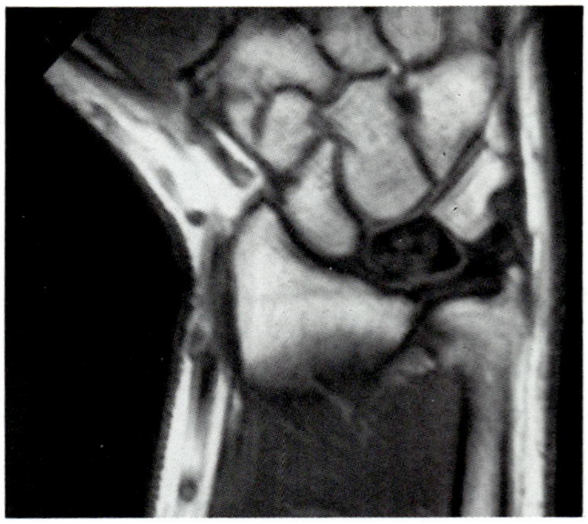

703 Kienbock's disease. More specific still for the demonstration of avascularity is an MRI scan. A diffuse diminished signal intensity is seen in this coronal (T1) weighted scan.

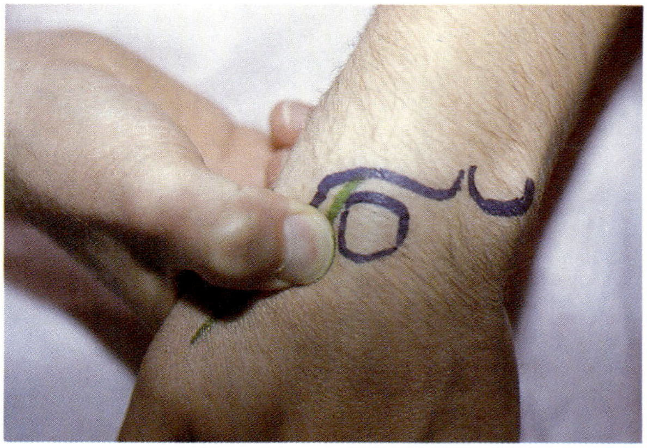

704 To the radial side of the lunate is the scapho-lunate sulcus, maximal tenderness at this site may indicate an occult dorsal scapho-lunate ganglion or a scapho-lunate instability.

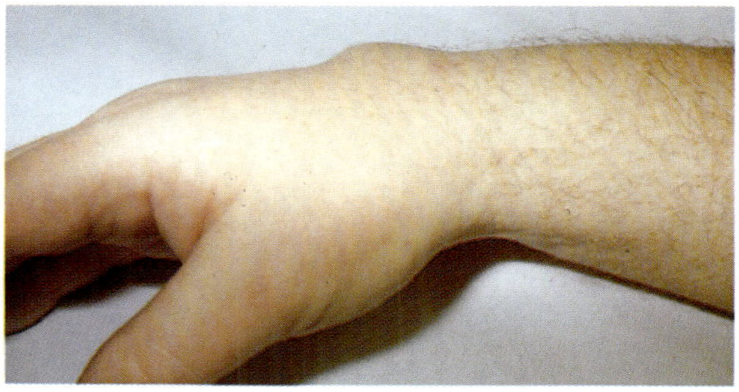

705 Ganglion. Ganglions represent 50–70% of soft tissue tumours in the hand and 60% are found in the characteristic location overlying the scapho-lunate interval. The aetiology is not clear but may be a simple synovial herniation or may be caused by mucoid degeneration of collagen.

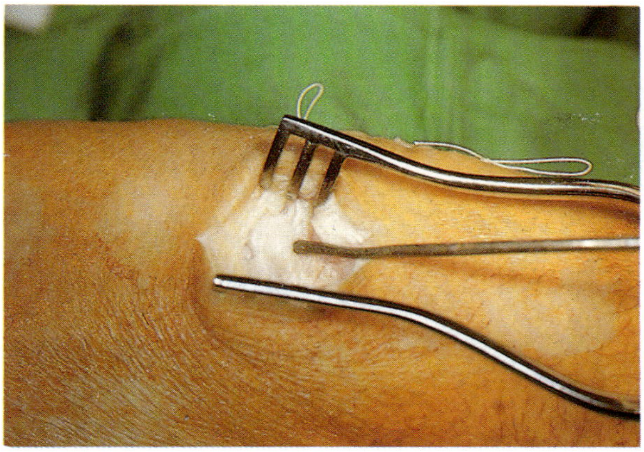

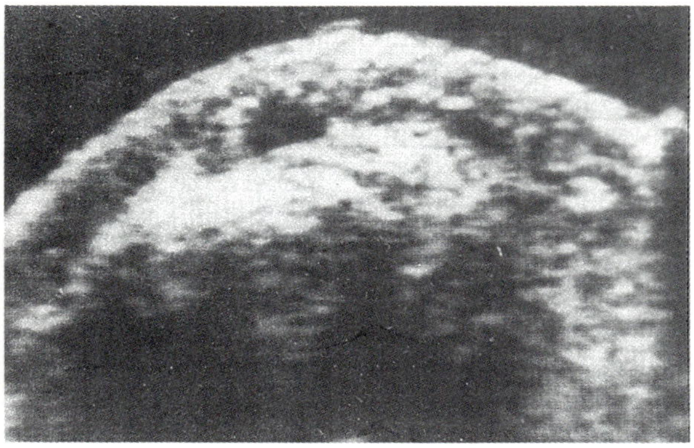

706, 707 Occult dorsal ganglion. Small intracapsular ganglia at the scapho-lunate interval are a potent cause of chronic wrist pain. With careful palpation at the scapho-lunate sulcus and comparison with the opposite side, the lesion can frequently be located. Local tenderness is disproportionate to the size of the lesion. An ultrasound scan confirms the diagnosis.

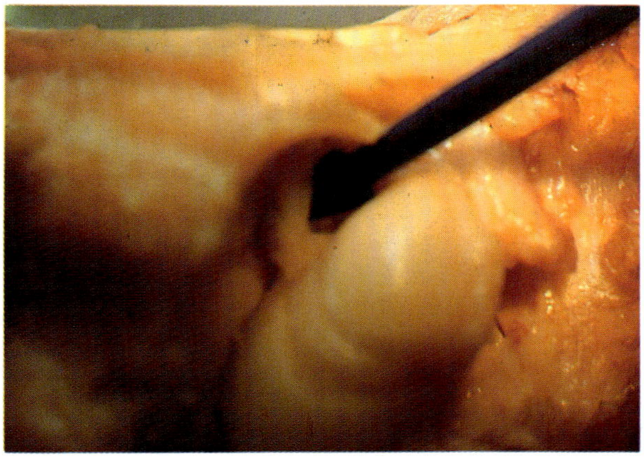

708 Scapho-lunate instability. As with all ligamentous injuries there is a spectrum of instability. Complete disruption of the intracapsular radio-scapho-lunate ligament (arrowed) and the scapho-lunate interosseous ligament results in complete scapholunate dissociation or rotatory subluxation of the scaphoid.

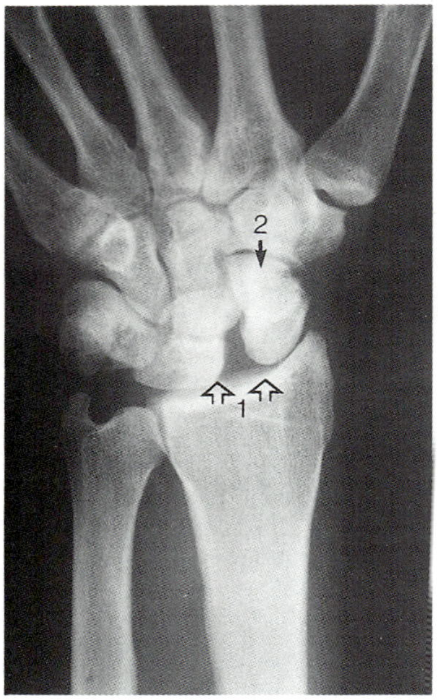

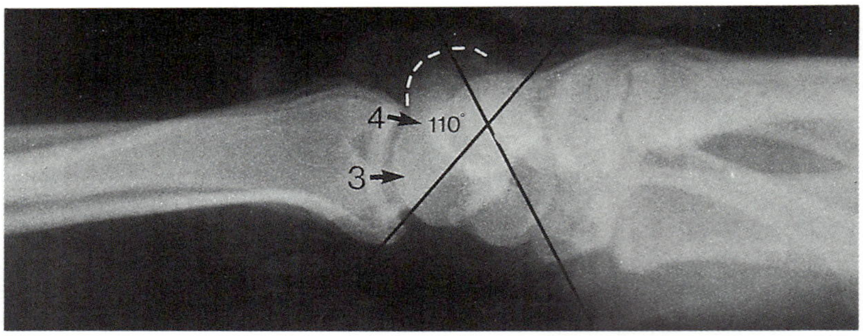

709 & **710** Scapholunate dissociation. Radiographs show a widening of the scapho-lunate interval (1). Dissociation of the scaphoid from the lunate permits the scaphoid to palmarflex, the foreshortened appearance on X-rays resulting in the 'ring' sign (2). The dissociated lunate dorsiflexes producing the DISI (dorsiflexed intercalated segment instability) deformity on lateral films (3). This divergence of the scaphoid and lunate produces an increase in the scapho-lunate angle (4), from the normal 30–60°. The subluxated proximal pole of scaphoid (outlined) may be prominently seen or palpated on the dorsum of the wrist.

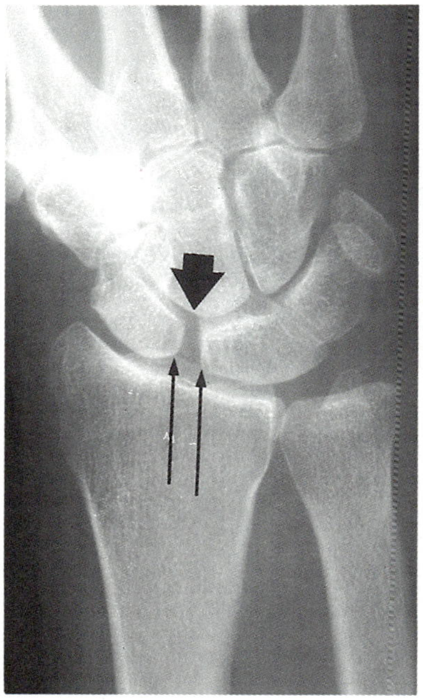

711 Scapholunate instability. Lesser degrees of instability may only be seen in the 'dynamic' situation when a compressive force across the carpus (by clenching the fist) reveals the scapho-lunate gap.

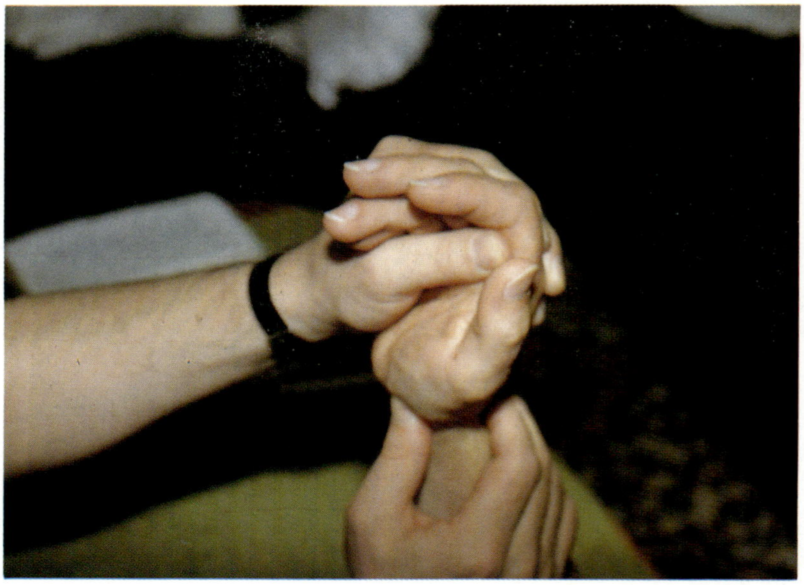

712 Watson's 'scaphoid shift' test. The thumb of the examining hand is placed over the scaphoid tubercle and the pulps of index and middle fingers over the radial joint line. With the free hand the wrist is moved from ulnar to radial deviation; pressure from the thumb over the tubercle prevents the normal scaphoid palmar flexion. In scapholunate instability the scaphoid may be felt to subluxate dorsally, lesser degrees of abnormal movement may be appreciated by comparison with the normal wrist. Pain is reproduced or a click from the joint may be felt.

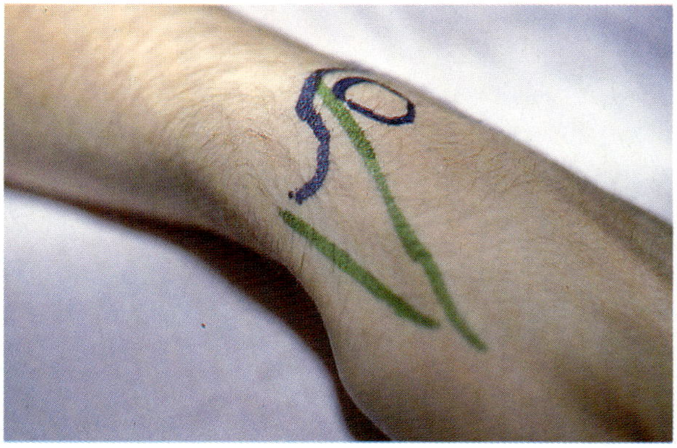

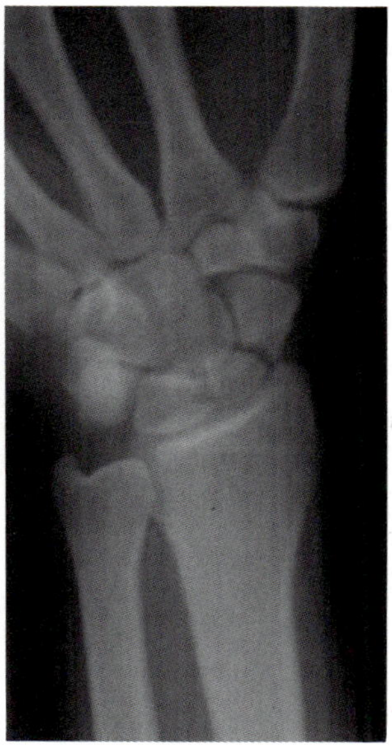

713 & **714** The anatomical snuff box. The association of pain in the snuff box with scaphoid fractures and non-unions is well known, but pain may also be felt in scapho-lunate instability and more distally in arthritis of the scaphoid–trapezium–trapezoid joint (STT joint).

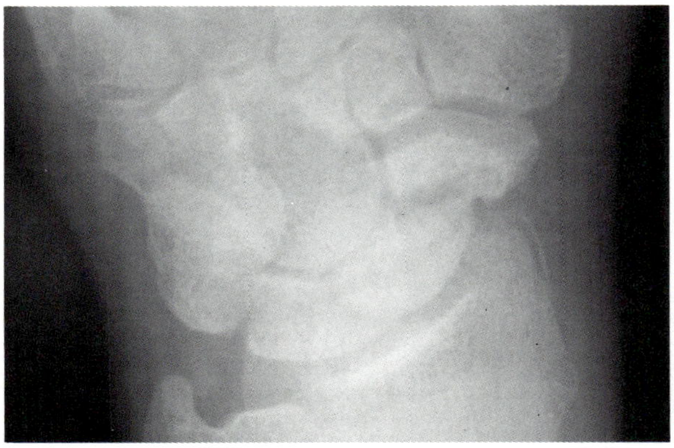

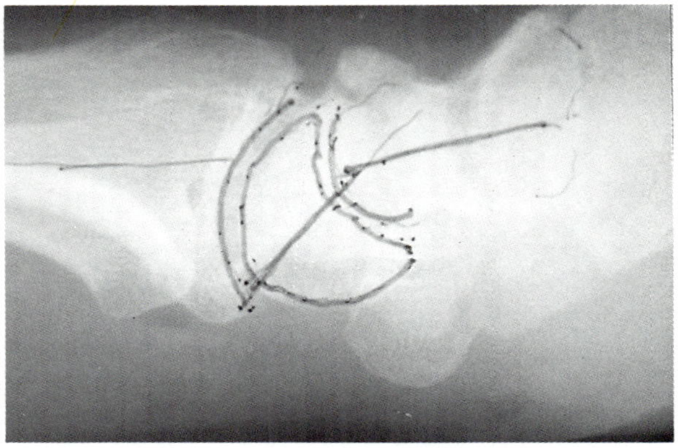

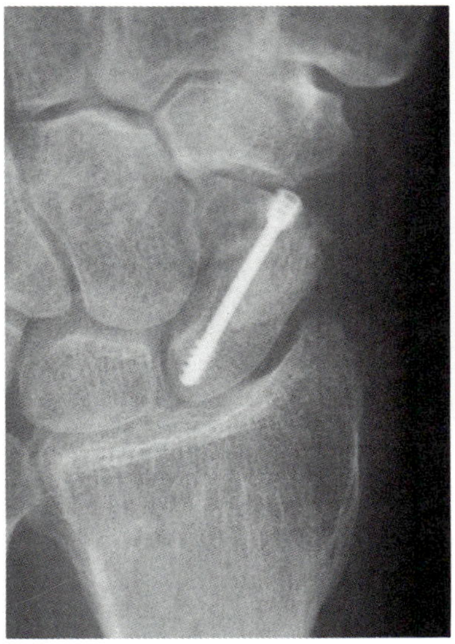

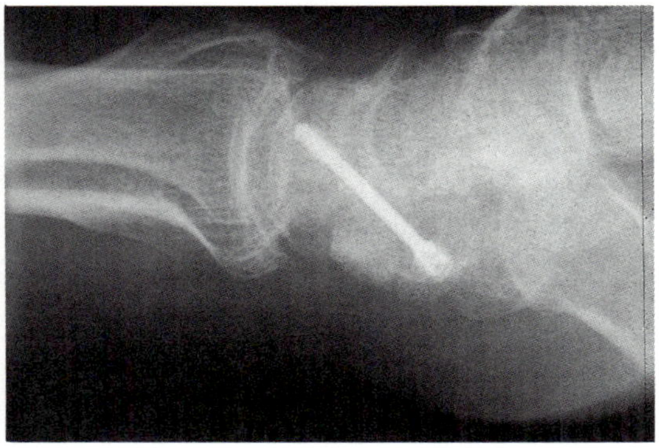

715–718 Non-union of the scaphoid. Collapse of the carpus can be appreciated on lateral radiographs and corrected by grafting with a volar wedge.

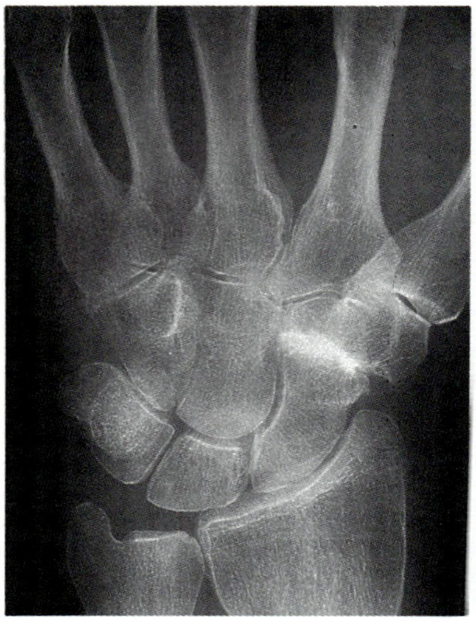

719 STT arthritis. Less common than arthritis in the basal joint of the thumb but just as debilitating.

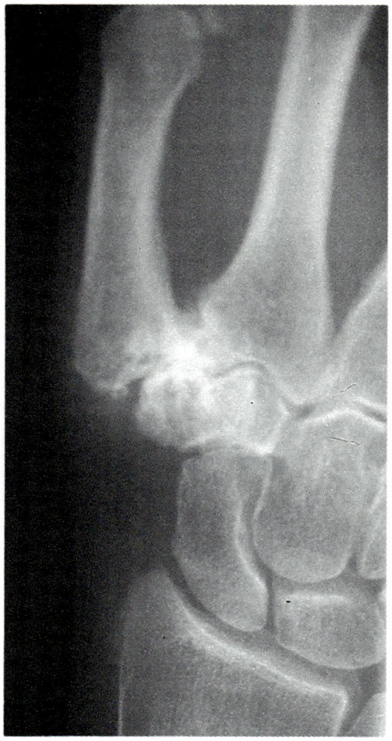

720 Trapezio-metacarpal arthritis. Basal joint arthritis of the thumb is common. Adduction of the first metacarpal is a frequent deformity in advanced cases.

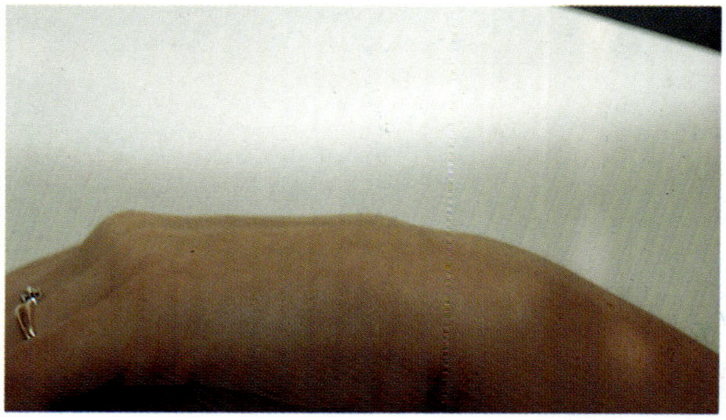

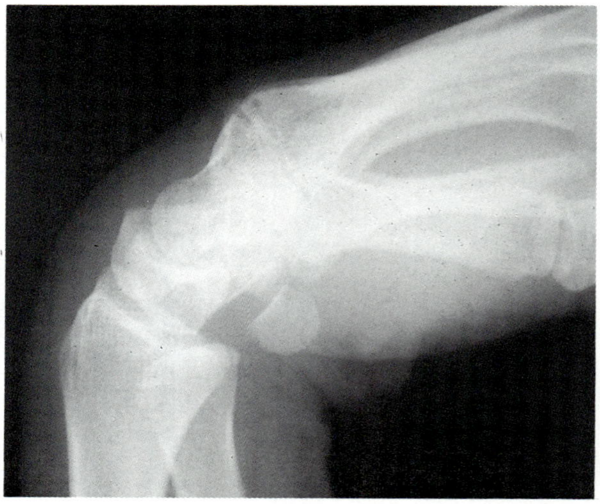

721 & **722** Carpo-metacarpal joint of index and middle fingers. Fractures and instability may occur following trauma. The commonest affliction of these articulations is the carpal boss, frequently accentuated by an overlying adventitial bursa or ganglion. Radiologically, the boss is due to dorsal osteophytes most commonly arising from the third metacarpal and capitate, although the second ray may also be involved.

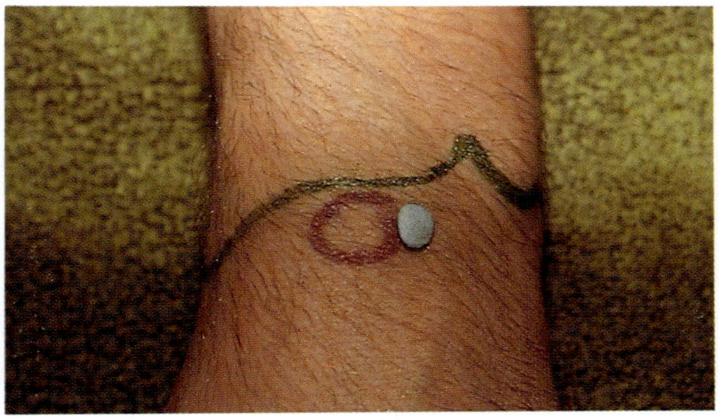

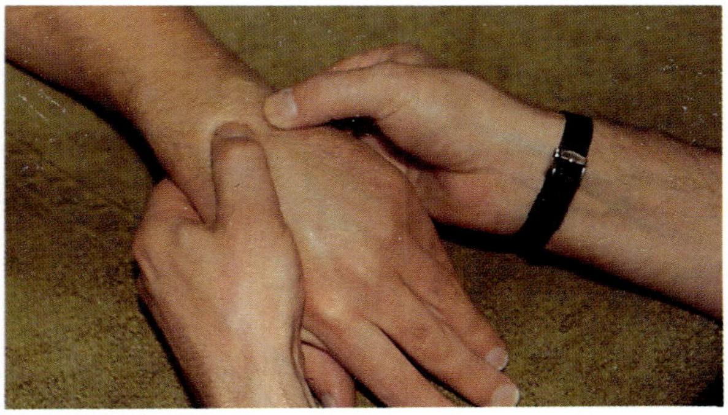

723 & **724** Triquetro-lunate sulcus and triquetral. Maximal tenderness in these sites may indicate triquetro-lunate instability or triquetral fractures. Instability may be demonstrated by triquetro-lunate ballotment. The triquetral and pisiform are grasped between finger and thumb of one hand and the lunate stabilised between finger and thumb on the other hand. Dorsal and volar mobility can be assessed comparing with the opposite side. Pain is reproduced in sprains or instability.

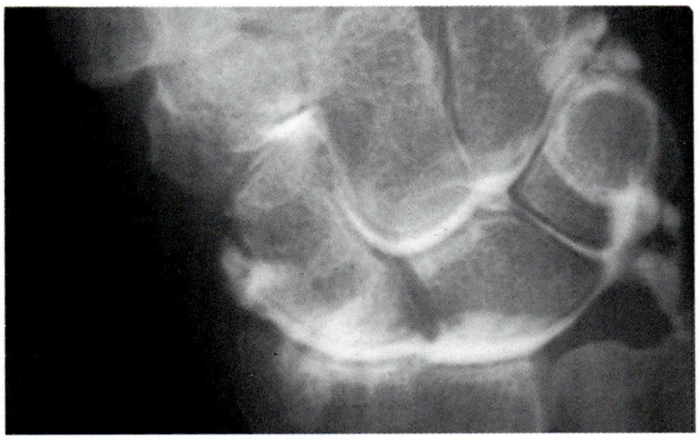

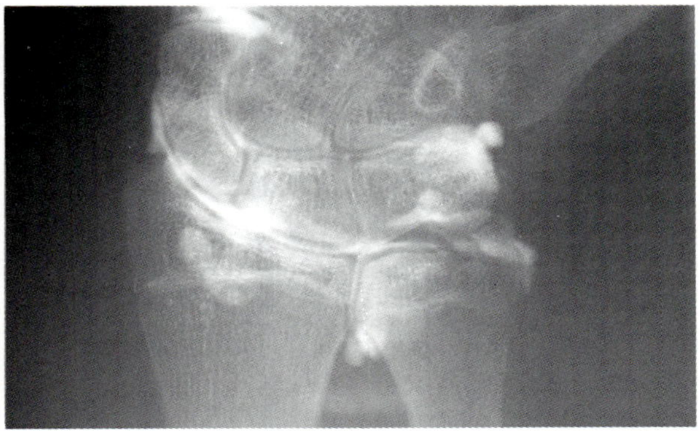

725 & **726** Arthrogram demonstrating a dye leak through triquetro-lunate interval. There is also a leak into the distal radio-ulnar joint. Triquetro-lunate instability is frequently associated with damage to the triangular fibro-cartilage complex with instability of the distal radio-ulnar joint.

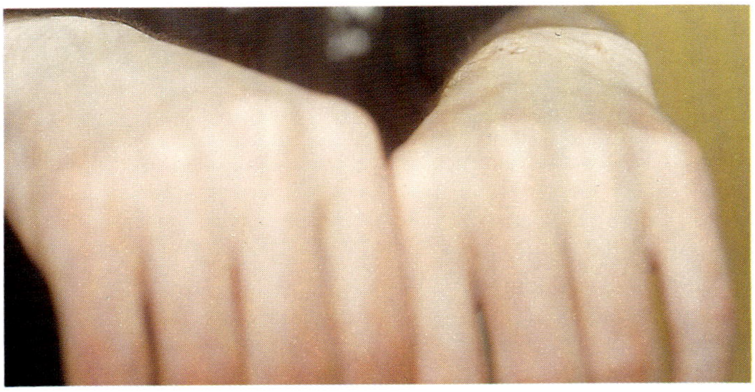

727 Dorsal instability of the distal radio-ulnar joint is most evident in pronation.

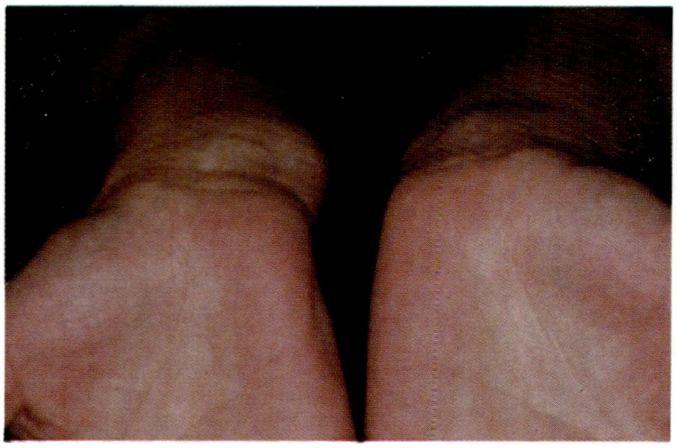

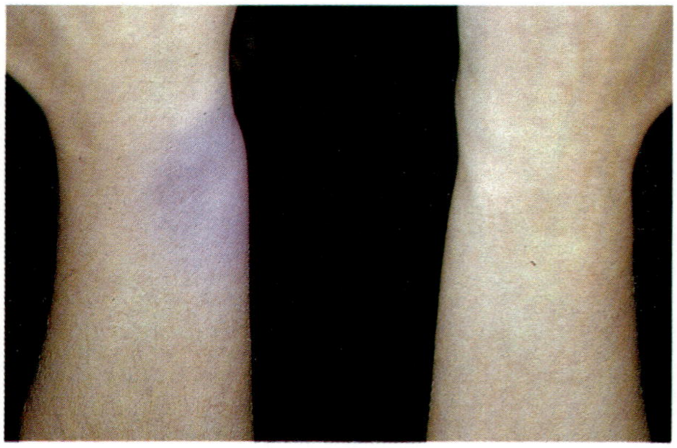

728 & **729** Volar instability of the DRUJ. The head of the ulna can be seen prominently on the volar surface of the right wrist with the arms supinated. A depression can be seen on the dorsal aspect of the wrist, again with the forearms supinated.

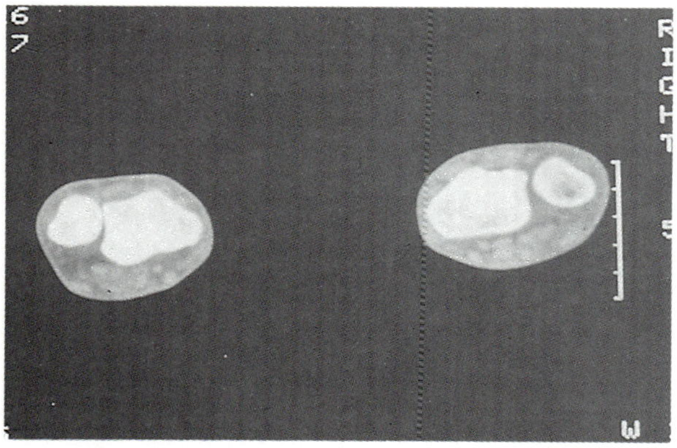

730 CT remains the most reliable investigation for DRUJ instability. This examination reveals a dorsal subluxation on the right.

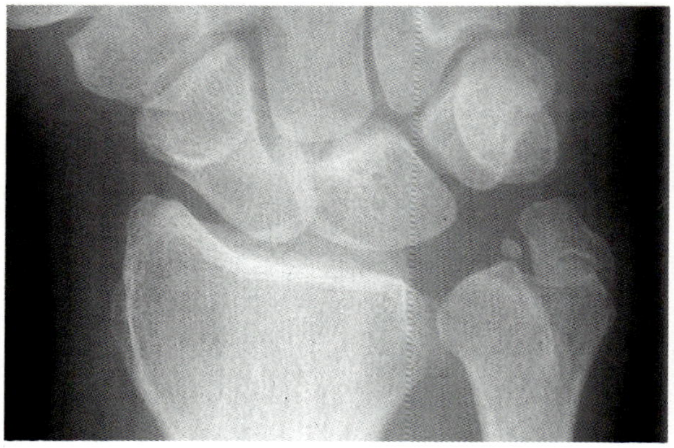

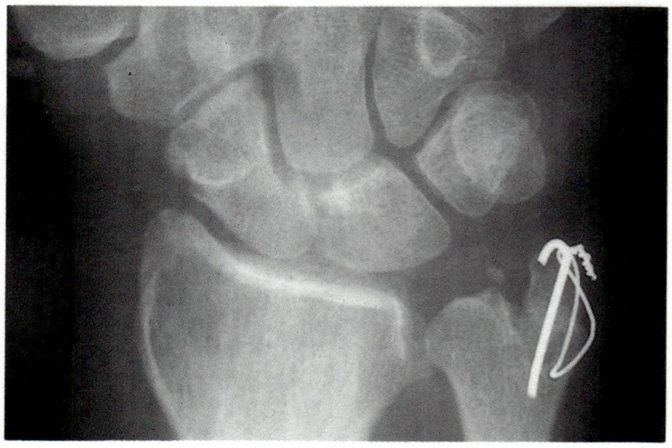

731 & **732** Non-union of a large ulnar styloid fragment is a common cause of instability. Failure to recognise DRUJ instability and removal of the styloid fragment, assuming the non-union to be the cause of symptoms, frequently leads to worsening of the instability and symptoms. Reattachment of the styloid solves the problem.

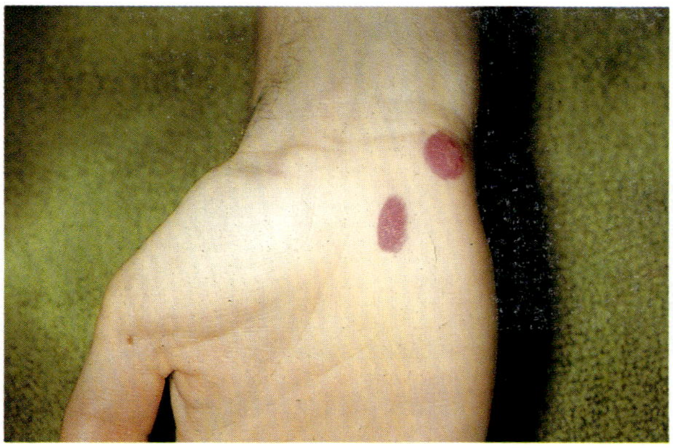

733 Pisiform and hook of hamate. Pain in these sites may indicate fractures or piso-triquetral arthritis.

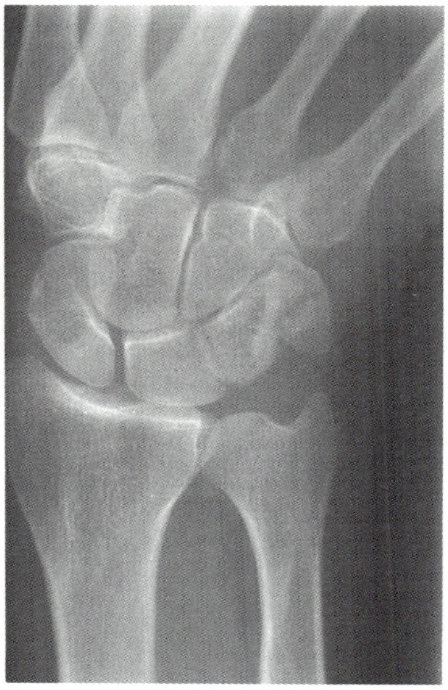

734 A fracture of the pisiform.

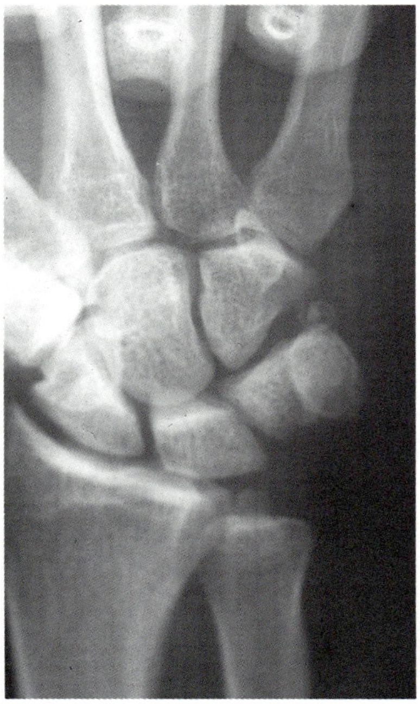

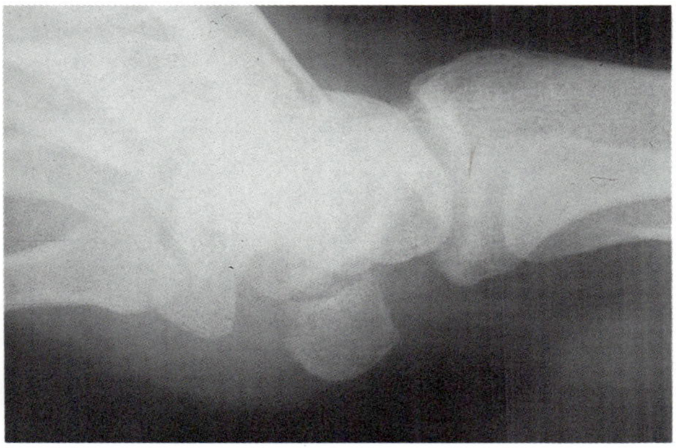

735 & **736** Crepitus and pain on moving the piso-triquetral joint confirms the diagnosis. In this case a loose body was present in the degenerative joint.

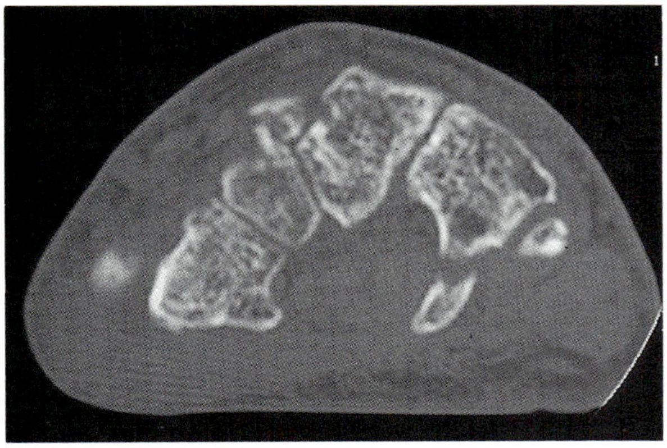

737 Pain from a hook of hamate non-union is frequently complained of on the dorso-ulnar aspect of the hand. Tenderness is elicited directly over the hook. A carpal tunnel view or CT scan will confirm the diagnosis. Removal of the hook is the treatment of choice.

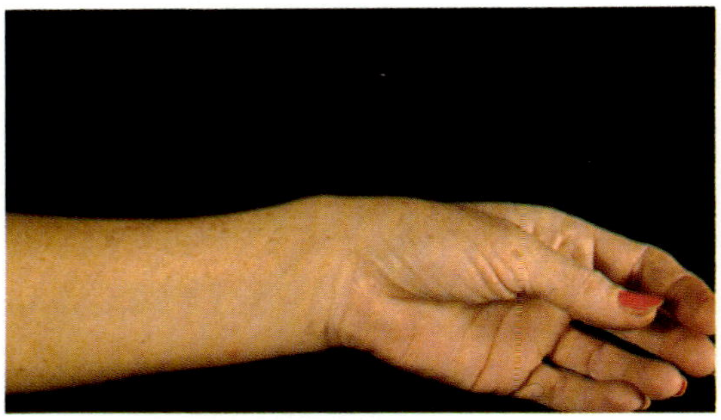

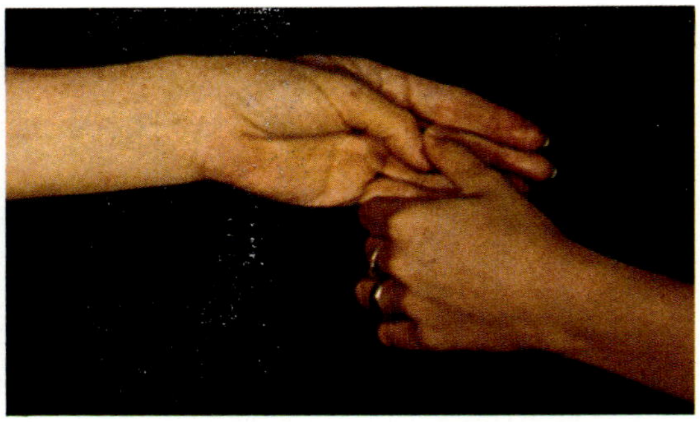

738 De Quervain's disease. Stenosing tenovaginitis of the first extensor compartment containing the long thumb tendons is a common condition causing pain on the radial side of the lower forearm extending into the thumb ray. The swelling is seen in profile on the radial aspect of the wrist. The condition needs to be differentiated from a number of other conditions producing similar symptoms (see Table 3).

739 Finkelstein's Test. Passive adduction of the thumb sharply aggravates the pain in DeQuervain's disease. It is not, however, specific for the condition, being positive in the much less common superficial radial nerve entrapment (Wartenberg's syndrome).

Table 3. Differential diagnosis of De Quervain's disease

Condition		
Intersection syndrome	—	Stenosing tenovaginitis of second extensor compartment
Wartenberg's syndrome	—	Superficial radial nerve entrapment
STT joint disease	—	Arthritis or instability
Trapeziometacarpal joint disease	—	Arthritis or instability
Scaphoid non-union		

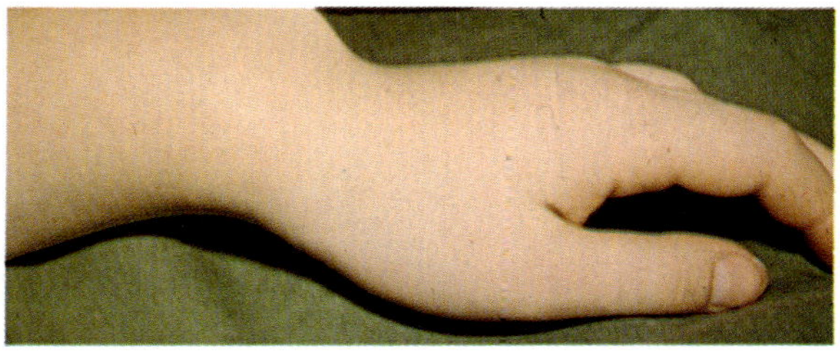

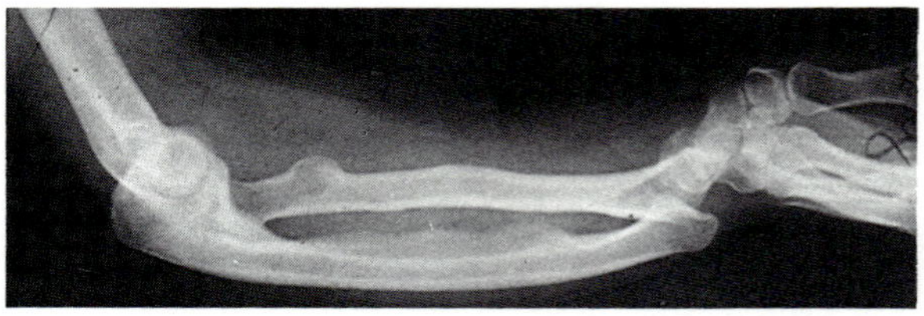

740 & **741** Madelung's deformity of the wrist.

Hand

Congenital anomalies

Classification:
- Failure of formation: Transverse deficiencies; Longitudinal deficiencies.
- Failure of differentiation.
- Duplication.
- Overgrowth.
- Undergrowth.
- Congenital constriction band syndrome.
- Generalised skeletal abnormalities.

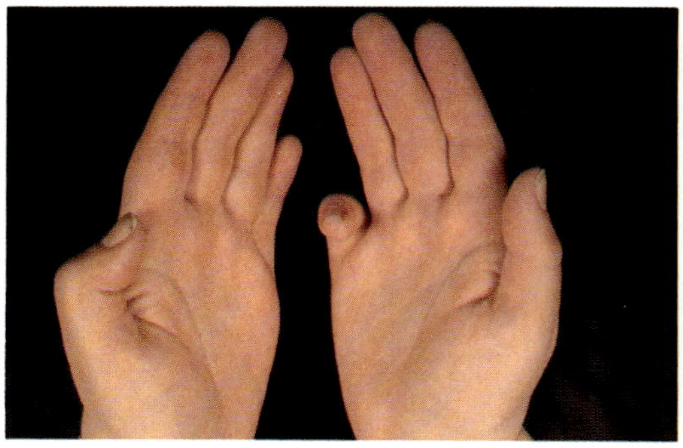

742 Camptodactyly. Distinguished from other finger contactures by its presence from birth, and the fact that it is always the proximal interphalangeal joint of the little finger alone that is affected.

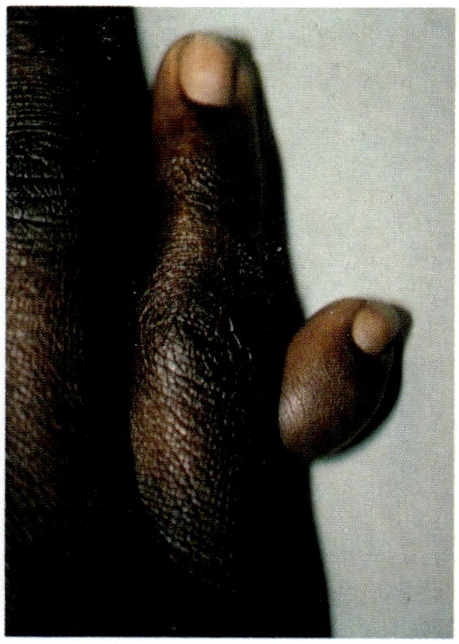

743 Supernumerary digit.

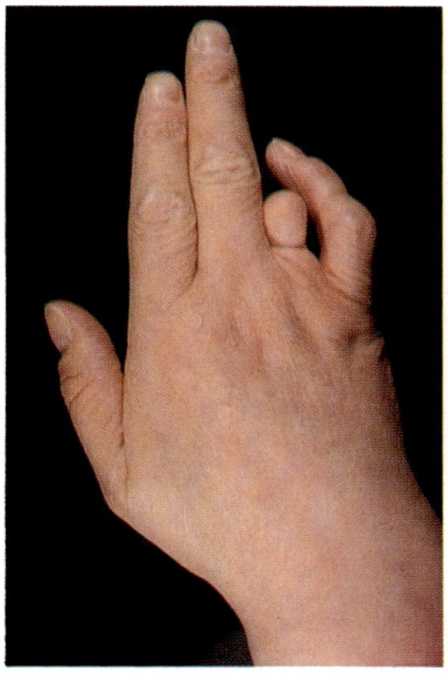

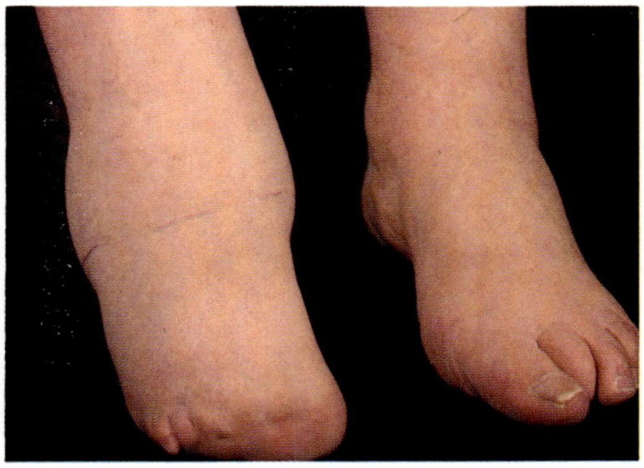

744 & **745** Congenital amputation of the fingers and toes. Its occurrence in both hand and foot of the same patient show it to be a developmental disorder rather than due to intrauterine constriction.

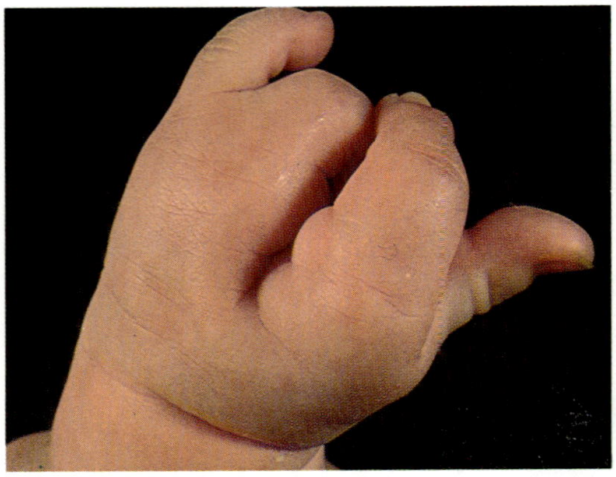

746 Congenital central ray deficiency.

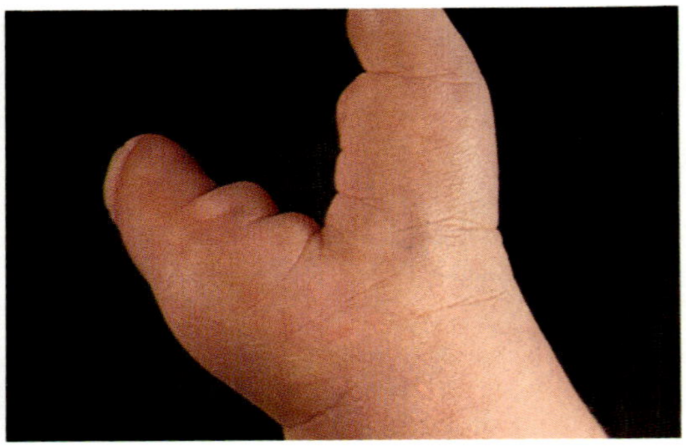

747 There is often very good movement of the hand with good function.

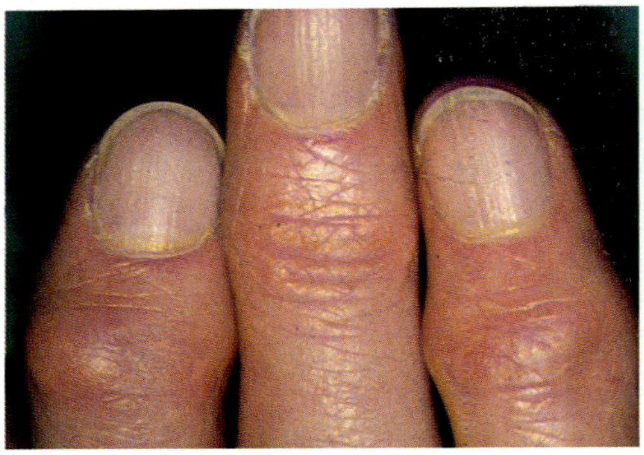

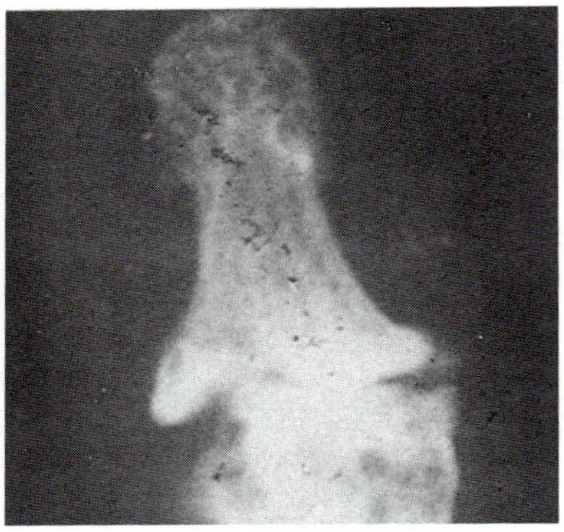

748 & **749** Osteoarthritis of the hand typically affects the distal interphalangeal joints. Heberden's nodes being due to the underlying marginal osteophytes.

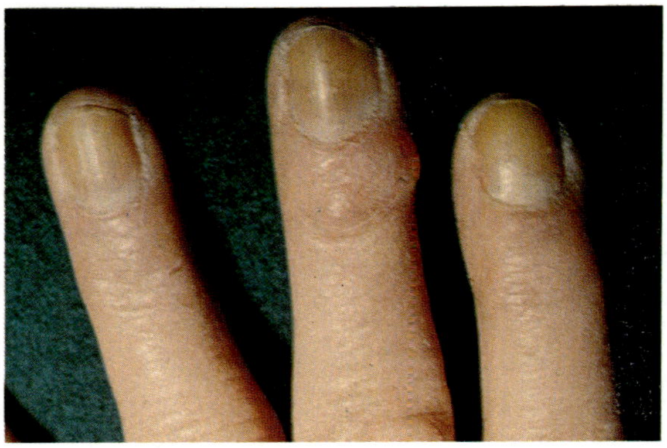

750 Mucous cysts on the dorsal aspect of the distal interphalangeal joints are common in osteoarthritis. Because of the thin overlying skin they occasionally spontaneously discharge their mucinous contents. They are, however, only ganglia of the distal interphalangeal joint. Recurrence after removal is common unless the communication with the joint is traced and excised along with a debridement of the associated marginal osteophytes.

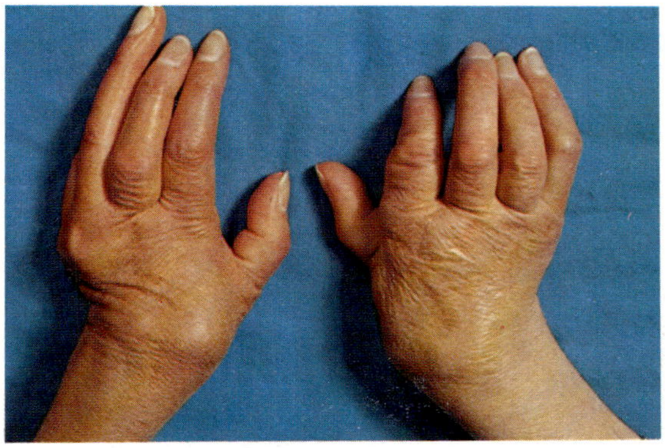

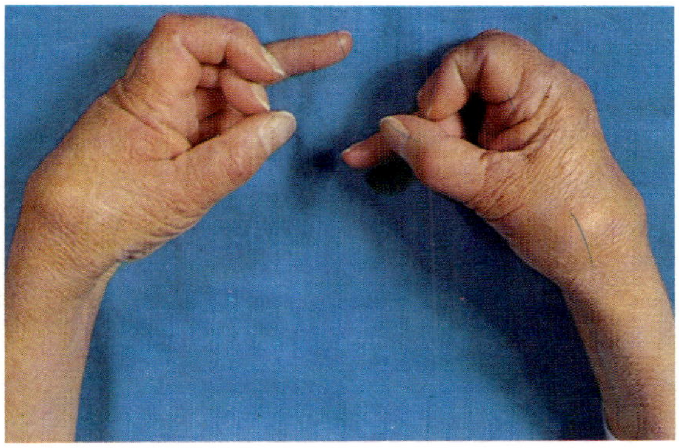

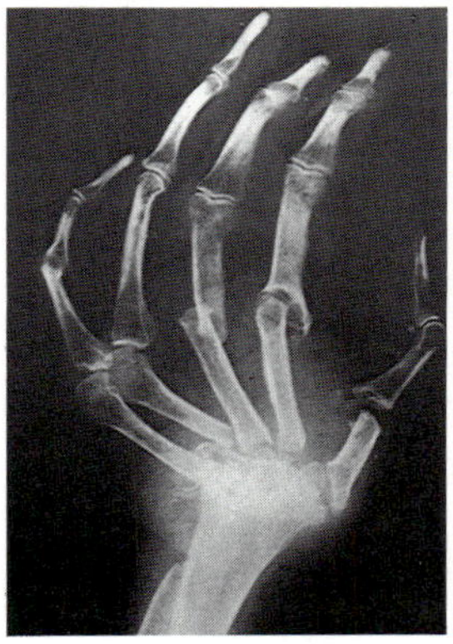

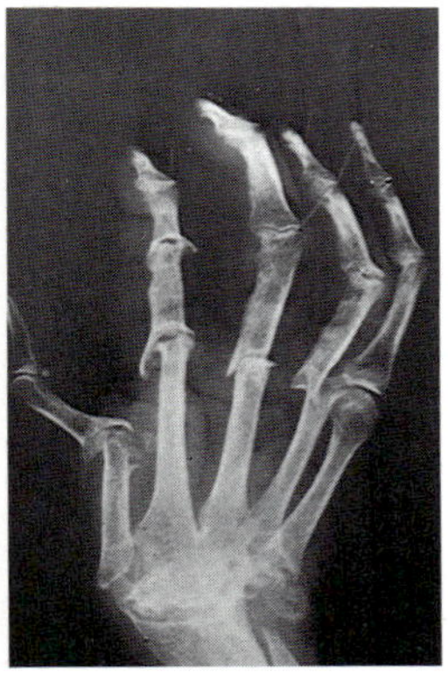

751–754 Rheumatoid arthritis of the wrist and fingers. These joints are often the first clinically affected in rheumatoid disease. The metacarpophalangeal joints are commonly affected. Destructive arthropathy is seen in the radiographs. A profile view of the hands shows that the flexor tendons of the little fingers of the hands have suffered spontaneous rupture.

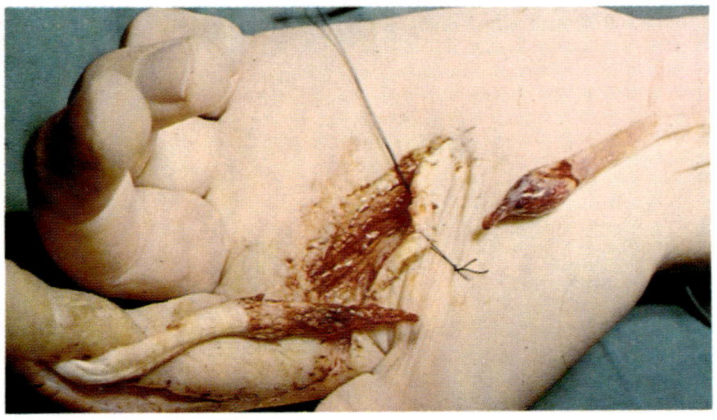

755 Ruptured flexor digitorum profundus to the index finger. Rupture of flexor tendons occur at the wrist in rheumatoid arthritis, although it is less common than rupture of extensor tendons. Vascularisation of the diseased tendon preceding rupture can clearly be seen.

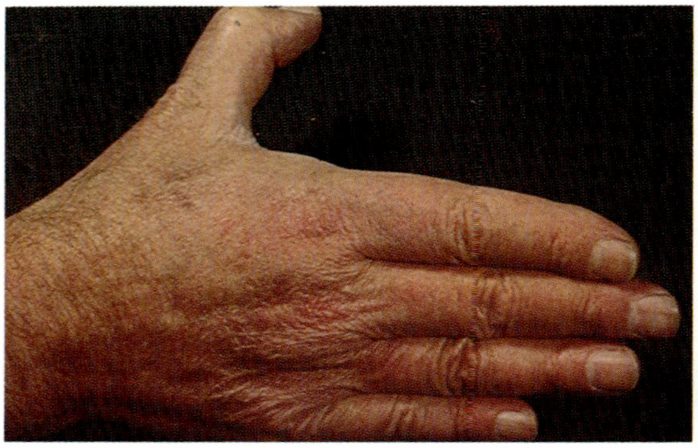

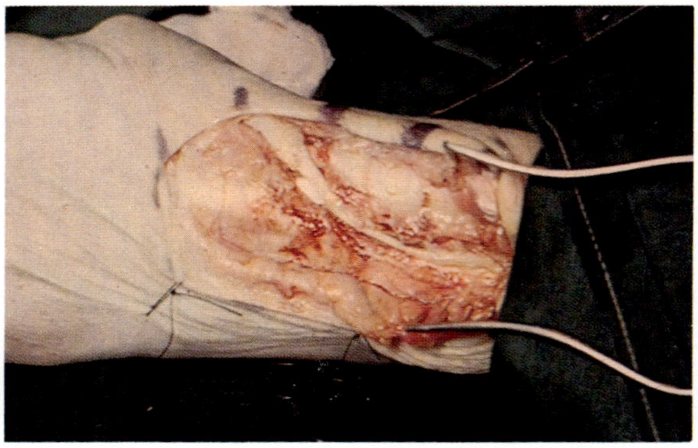

756 & **757** Ruptured Extensor pollicis longus tendon. The rupture most commonly occurs at the level of Lister's tubercle, as shown in the operative picture. It occurs in rheumatoid arthritis or as a complication of a Colles' fracture. In the latter situation the problem typically presents at 6 weeks after a minimally displaced or undisplaced fracture. Contrary to popular belief, rupture does not occur because of attrition over bony fragments at the fracture site but because of avascular attrition, the tendon being supplied by terminal branches of the anterior interosseous artery. Treatment is by the very successful extensor indicis transfer.

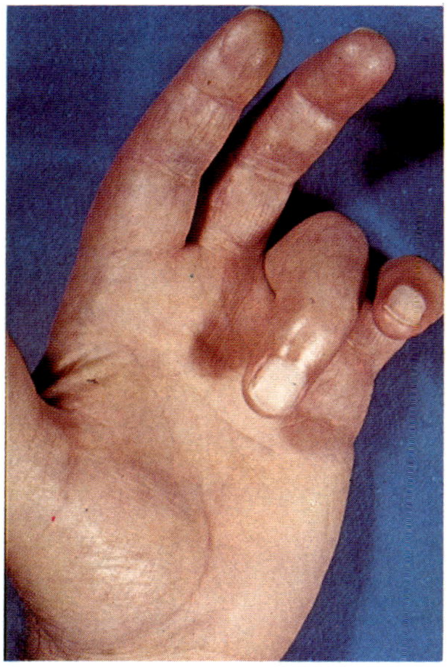

758 Trigger finger. Stenosing tenovaginitis at the entrance to the fibrous flexor sheath causes a fibrous nodule to develop in the long flexor tendons. The swelling snaps to and fro through the mouth of the sheath causing the finger to trigger. It may be an early manifestation of rheumatoid disease, but is seen most commonly as an isolated constitutional condition caused by degenerative changes and narrowing of the fibrous sheath.

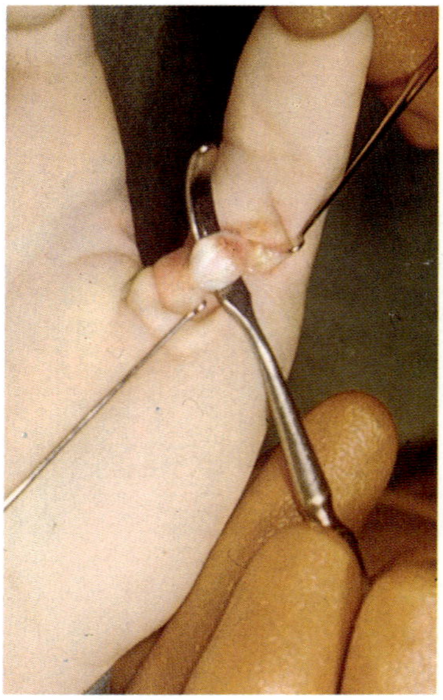

759 Trigger thumb. The flexor pollicis longus is displayed at the entrance to the fibrous flexor sheath. It occurs in the newborn owing to the foetal position of the thumb clasped into the hand, other causes are the same as those for trigger finger.

Deformities of the fingers

The structure of a finger, made up of a row of phalanges is inherently unstable, particularly in compression. Stability is dependent upon the integrity of the joint surfaces, capsule and ligaments and the fine balance between flexor and extensor activity. Disruption of any of these elements by disease, e.g. rheumatoid arthritis, or trauma will lead to a collapse of the finger, producing a zig-zag deformity.

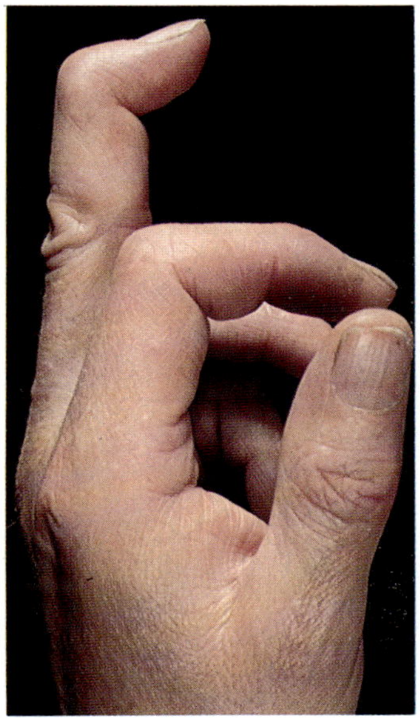

760 Mallet finger. Caused by a stubbing injury to the fingertip in which the terminal extensor slip is ruptured sometimes with a fragment of bone. In more severe cases hyperextension at the PIP joint occurs producing a 'swan-neck' deformity.

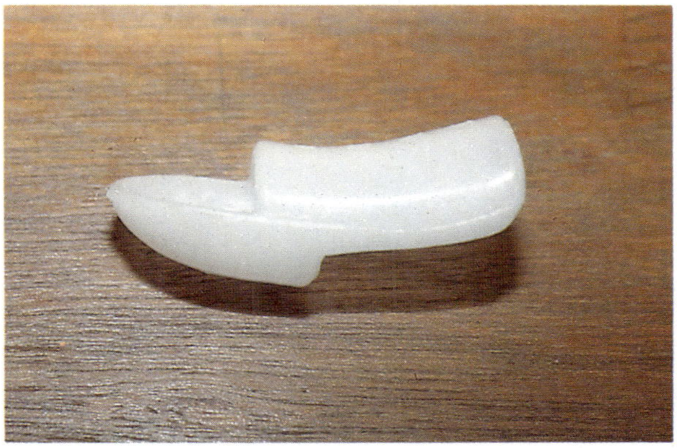

761 The Stack splint. Splinting the distal joint in extension allows healing over a period of weeks thus restoring tendon balance.

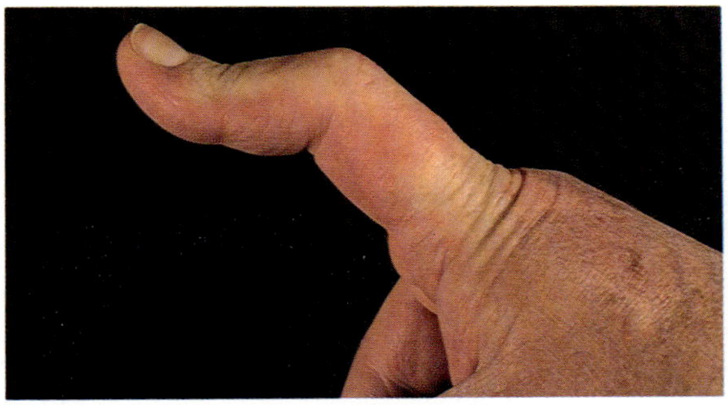

762 Boutonnière deformity. Rupture of the central slip of the extensor tendon over the PIP joint, allowing the head of the proximal phalanx to buttonhole through the dorsum. The lateral slips of the extensor mechanism slowly displace palmarly, worsening and maintaining the deformity.

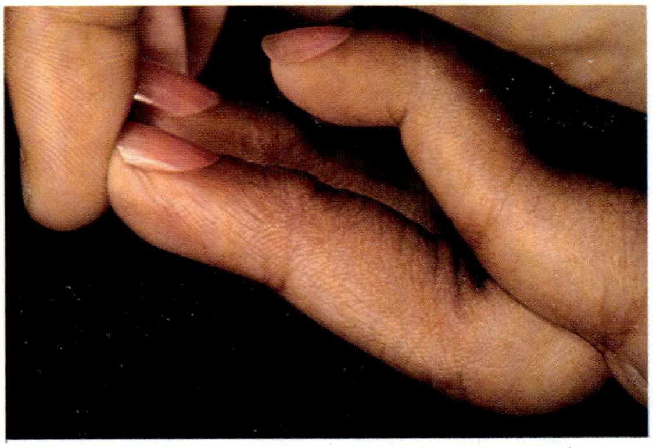

763 'Swan-neck' deformity. This may develop following a mallet injury, a PIP joint volar plate injury or rupture of flexor sublimis insertion.

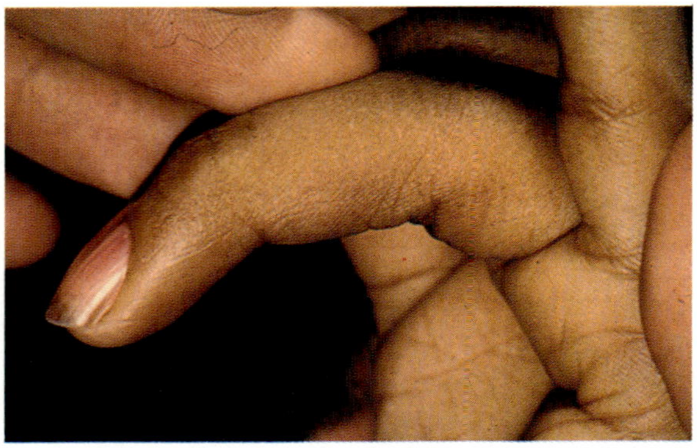

764 The deformity is correctable by passive flexion of the PIP joint, although with time the PIP joint and the deformity may become fixed.

Dupuytren's disease

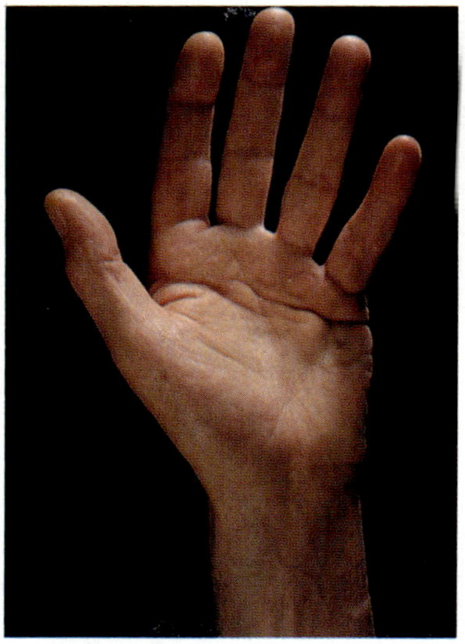

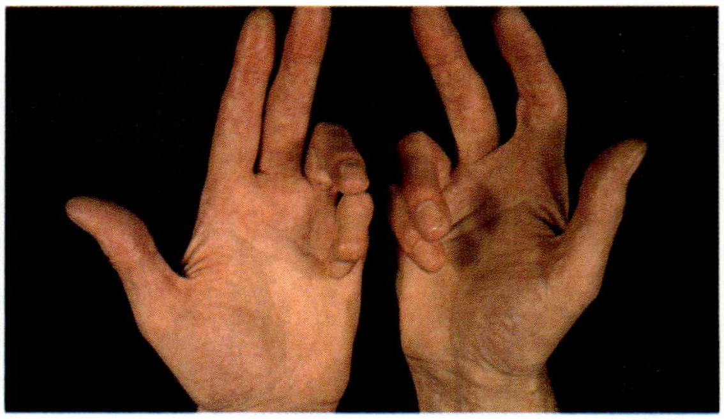

765 & **766** Dupuytren's contracture. Thickening and contracture of the palmar fascia, frequently involving the skin and running across the proximal joints of the fingers causes fixed contracture. Ring and little finger involvement is the commonest pattern. It is ten times commoner in men and is probably of sex-linked dominant inheritance. The association of the condition with alcoholism and liver disease is likely due to the fact that these conditions act as a metabolic trigger to earlier manifestation of the disease in susceptible individuals.

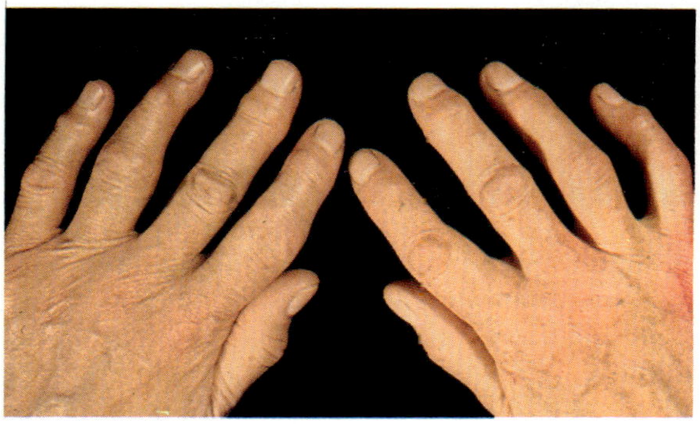

767 Garrod's pads. Knuckle pads or thickening of the subcutaneous tissue on the dorsum of the PIP joints is often seen in association with Dupuytren's contracture. Frequently the knuckle pads precede the development of palmar disease but are a sure indicator that the condition will ultimately develop.

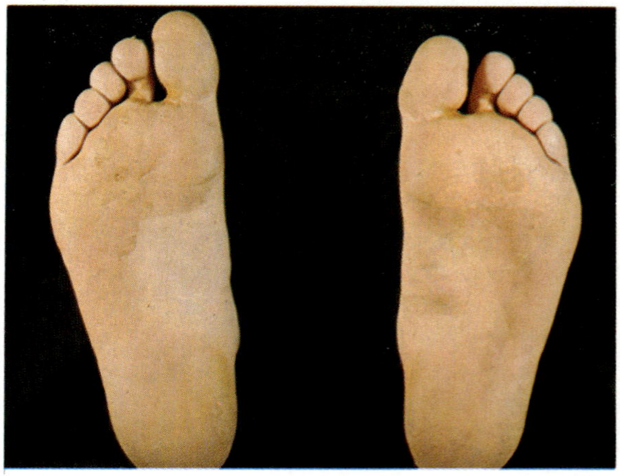

768 Fibrous nodular thickening is sometimes seen in the plantar fascia. Involvement of this site is more frequently seen in patients with a 'Dupuytren's diathesis' exhibiting a strong family history and onset of the disease at an early age.

Volkmann's ischaemic contracture

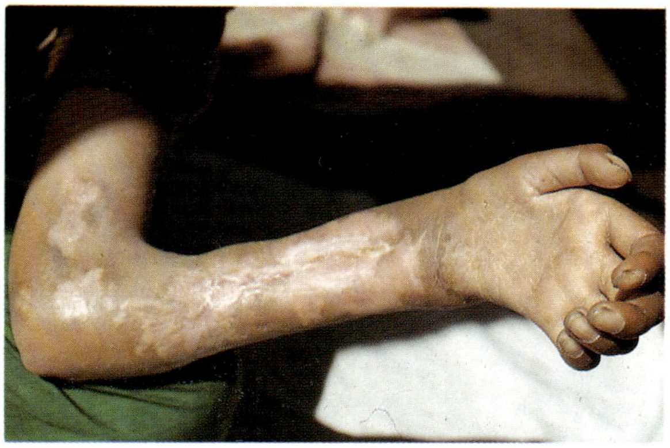

769 Ischaemic necrosis of the forearm muscles can arise after crushing injuries to the forearm or fractures around the elbow or forearm in which direct damage to vessels supplying the muscles occur or bleeding and oedema into closed fascial compartments leads to an increased pressure and ultimate vascular embarassment.

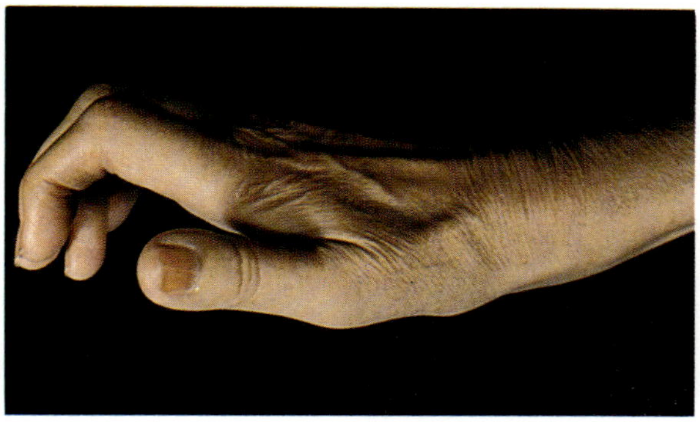

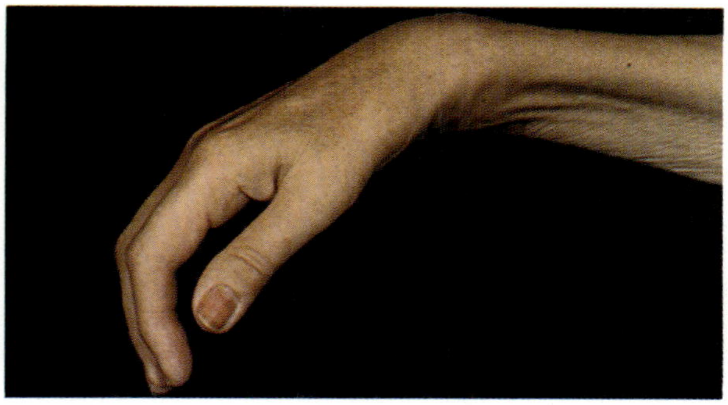

770 & **771** When the wrist is extended the fingers are strongly forced into flexion by the shortened flexor muscles; when the wrist is flexed the fingers can be straightened.

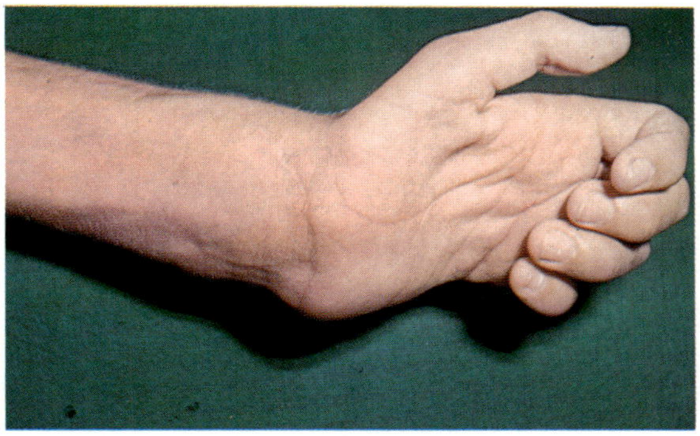

772 Ischaemia of the forearm muscles and nerves. The fingers are flexed and there is marked wasting of the intrinsic muscles of the hand.

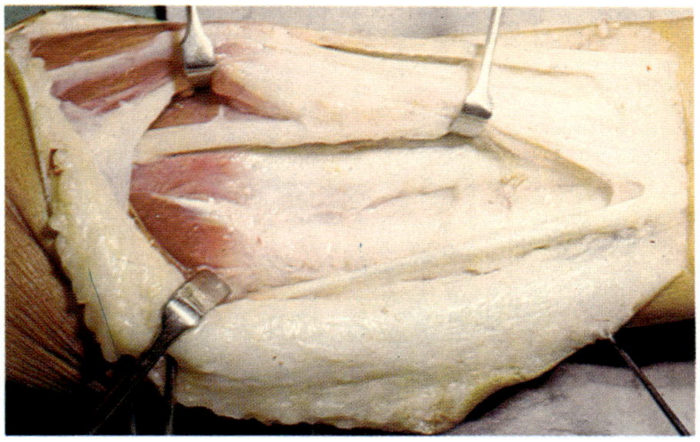

773 The forearm muscles seen at operation. A segment of the muscle bulk has been replaced by scar tissue.

Lumps and tumours

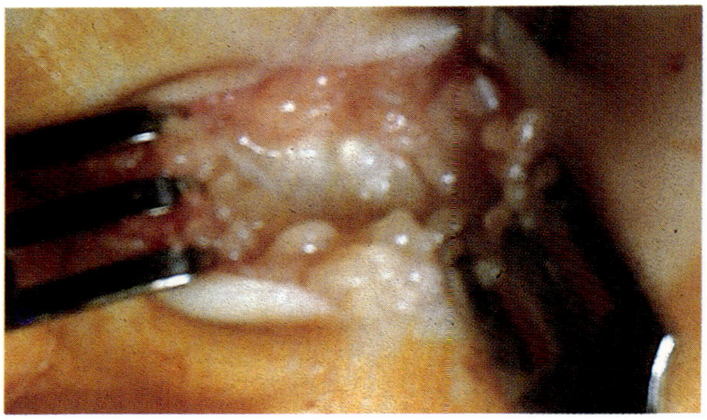

774 Flexor tendon sheath ganglion. These lesions are frequently small (frequently called seed ganglion) and arise from the synovium of the flexor tendon sheath characteristically at the level of the proximal finger crease. Pressure during grasping or holding bags draws attention to them owing to discomfort.

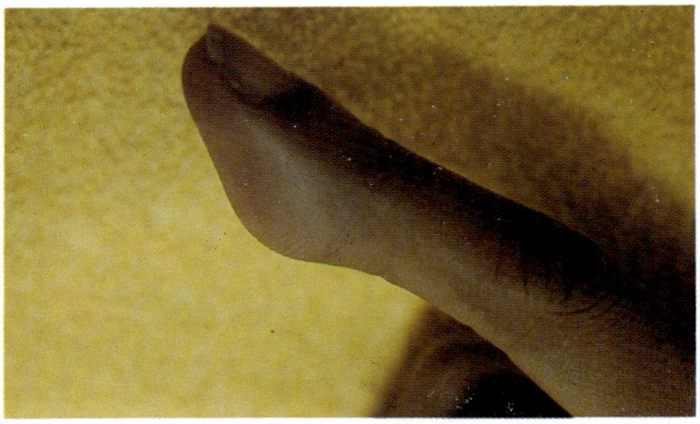

775 Epidermoid inclusion cyst. Although much less common than ganglia these are the most common tumour masses found in the hand. An episode of trauma drives a fragment of keratinising epithelium into the subcutaneous tissues where it survives and forms an epithelium-lined cyst.

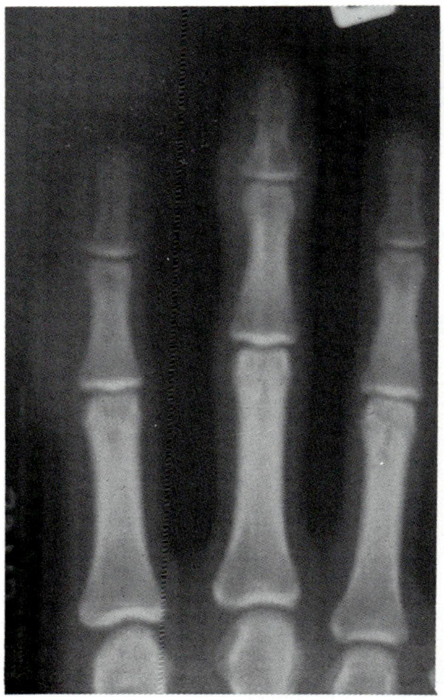

776 Epidermoid inclusion cyst. In the finger tip bone may be involved in the process.

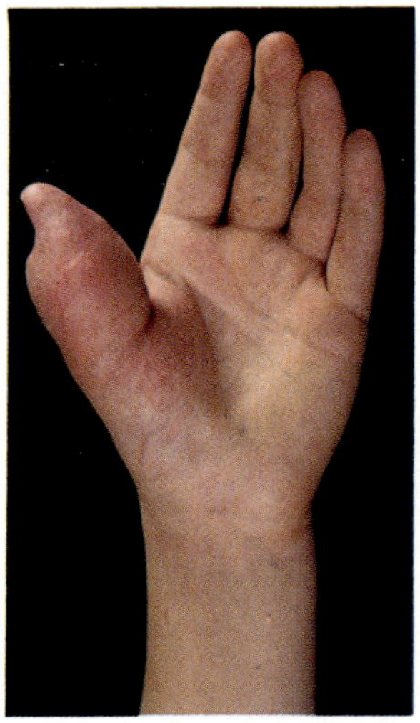

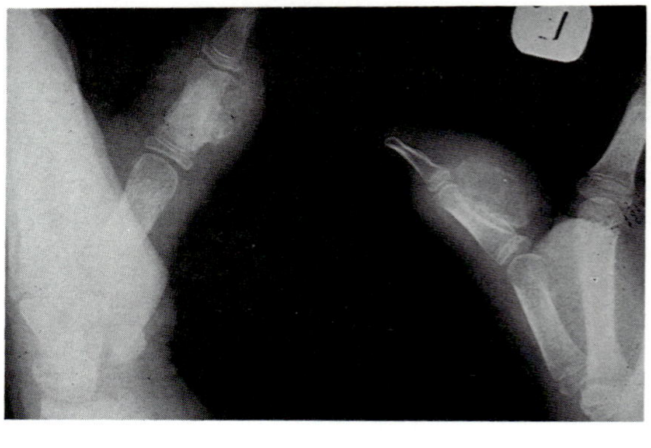

777 & **778** Implantation dermoid cyst. These cysts are also post-traumatic, although the episode may not be remembered. A cyst forms around implanted debris. In this case a calcified mass, which appears to have eroded the proximal phalanx, can be seen in the radiograph.

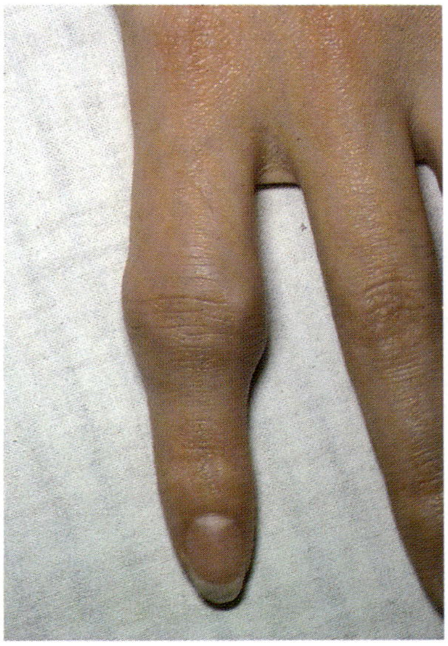

779 **779** Pigmented villonodular synovitis. Also called giant-cell tumour of tendon sheath, this is not a true tumour, but is second only to ganglia for producing a tumourous mass in the hand.

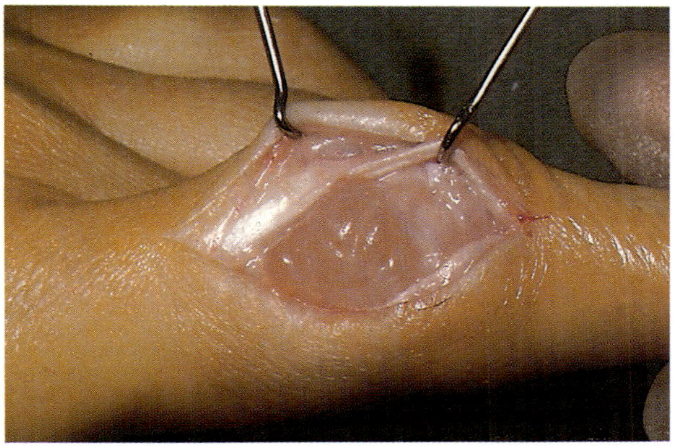

780 At operation the lesion frequently exhibits a yellowish or orange colouration.

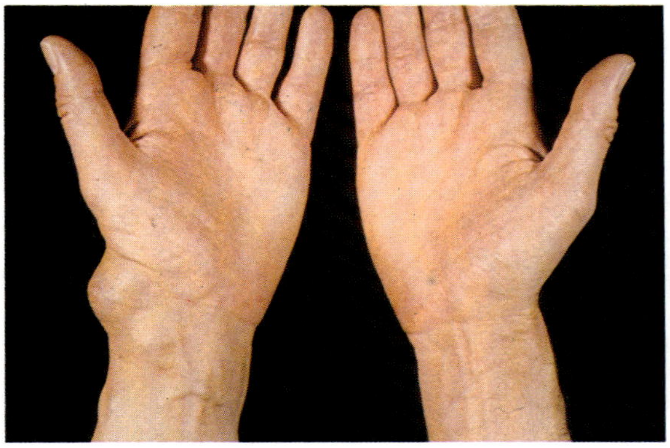

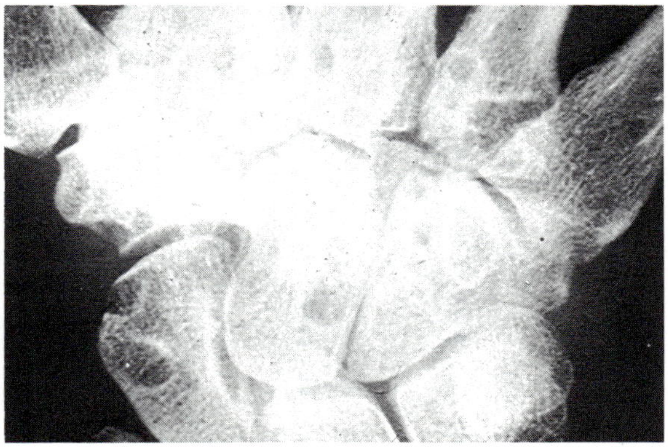

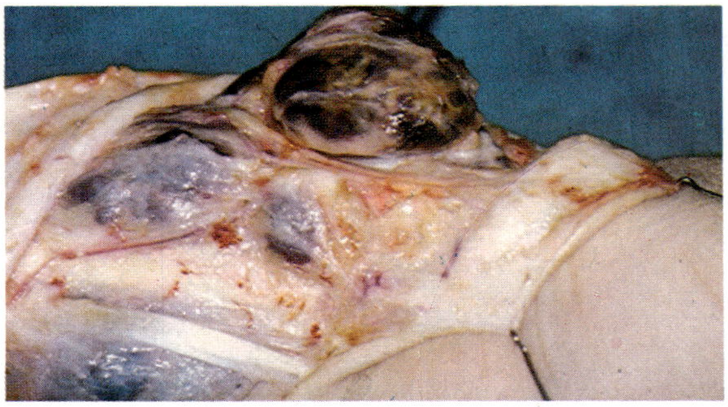

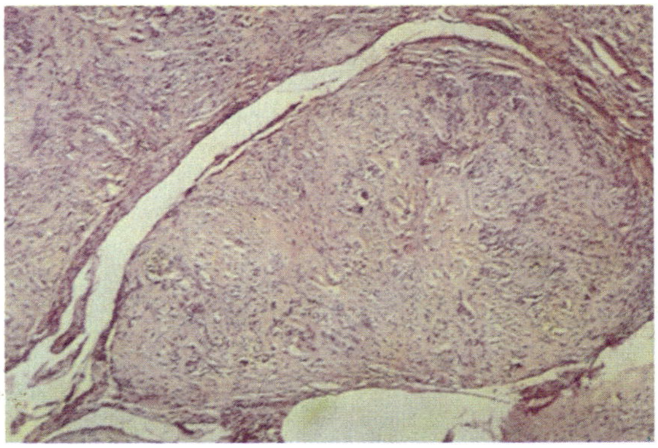

781–784 Pigmented villonodular synovitis of the wrist.

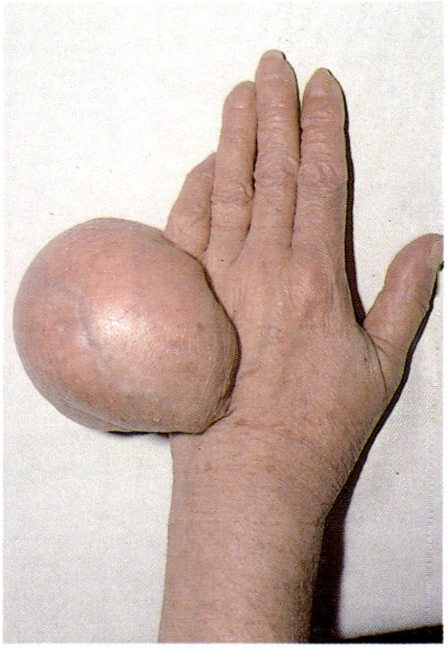

785 Lipoma. Lipomas are among the commonest truly new growths to be found in the hand.

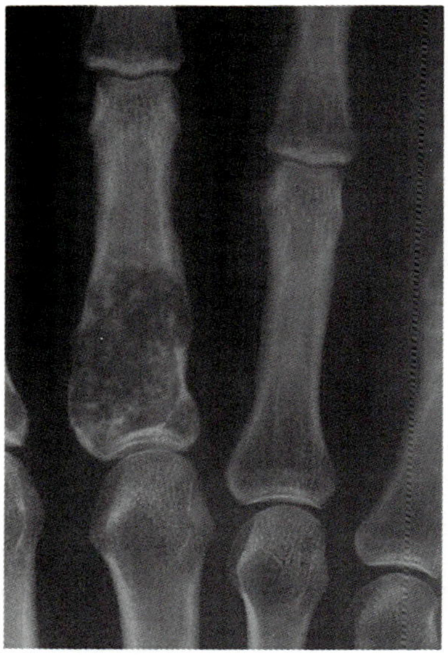

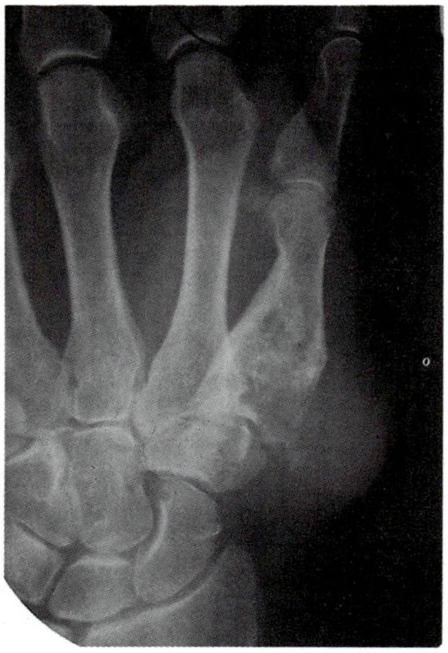

786 & **787** Enchondroma. Enchondromas are the commonest bony tumours. Very rarely malignant change can result in chondrosarcoma.

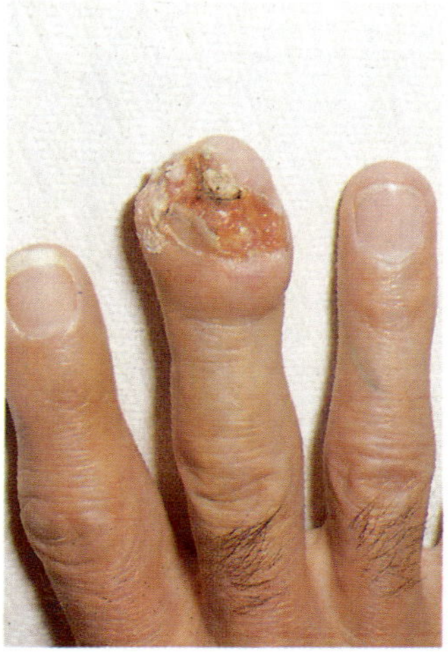

788 Squamous cell carcinoma is one of the commonest malignancies to be found in the hand.

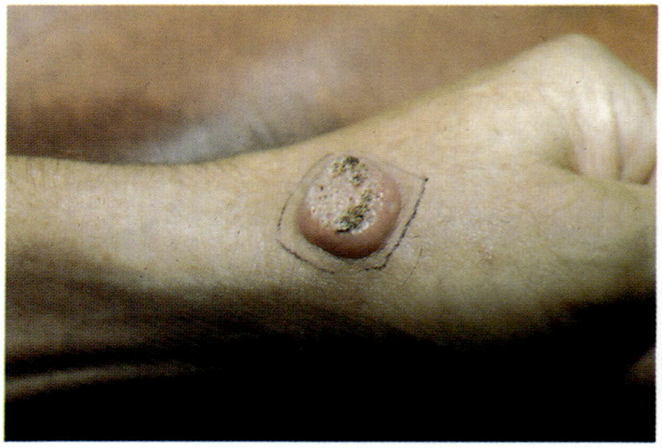

789 Keratoacanthoma. The true behaviour of this lesion is still not certain. Differentiation from squamous or basal cell carcinomas is only possible histologically.

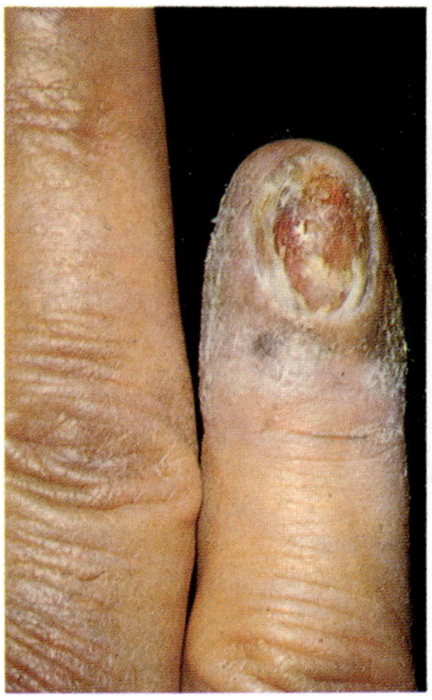

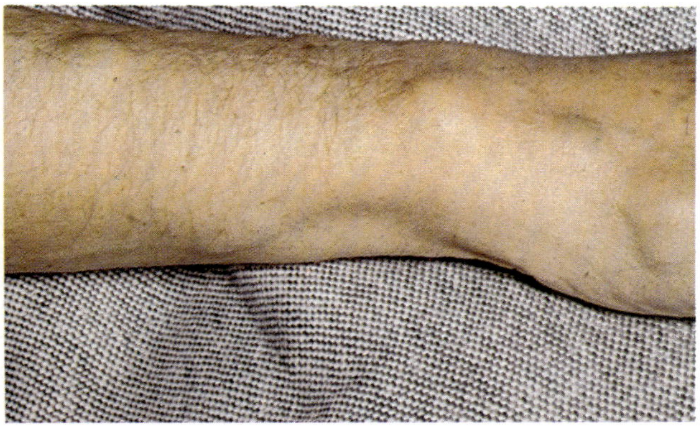

790 & **791** Malignant melanoma arising from the nail-bed of the little finger. The malignant melanoma has spread along the lymphatics and a secondary tumour has developed on the dorsum of the lower forearm.

Raynaud's phenomenon

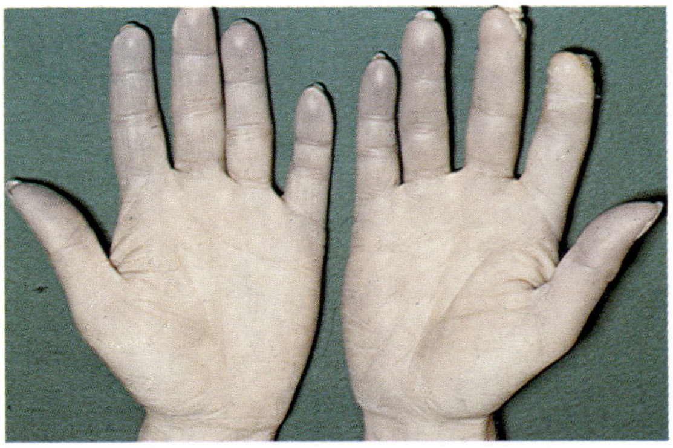

792 Raynaud's phenomenon. Intermittent spasm of the small peripheral arterioles initiated by cold, causing blanching of fingers and toes. It may be due to a variety of causes. In severe cases, trophic changes and even gangrene may supervene. One cause is the prolonged use of vibrating tools.

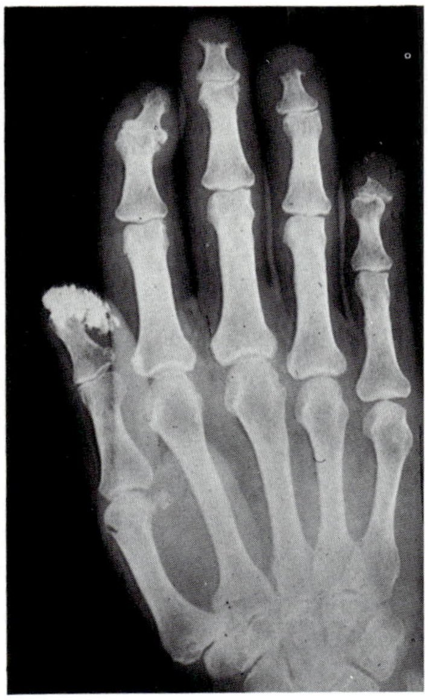

793 Soft tissue calcification and atrophy of terminal digits are seen both in cryopathy and chronic Raynaud's phenomenon.

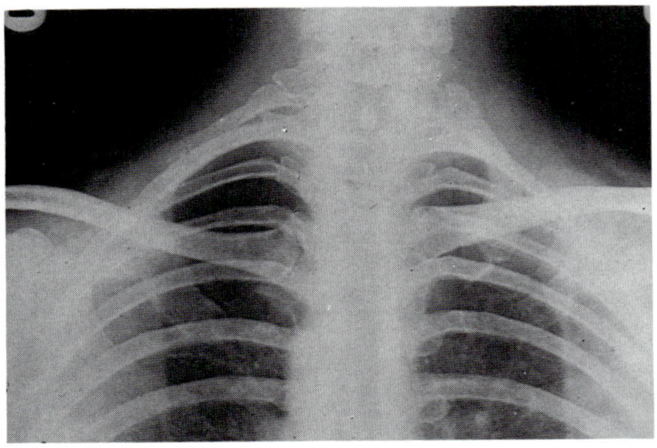

794 Bilateral cervical ribs causing irritation of the cervical sympathetic fibres was established as the cause in the radiograph.

Peripheral nerve lesions affecting the hand

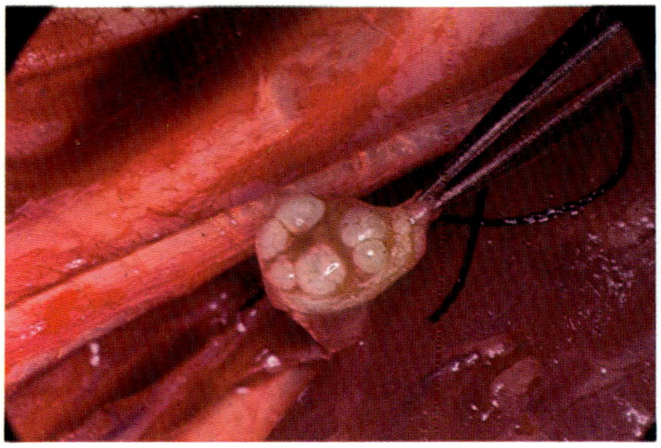

795 Normal nerve bundles in cross-section.

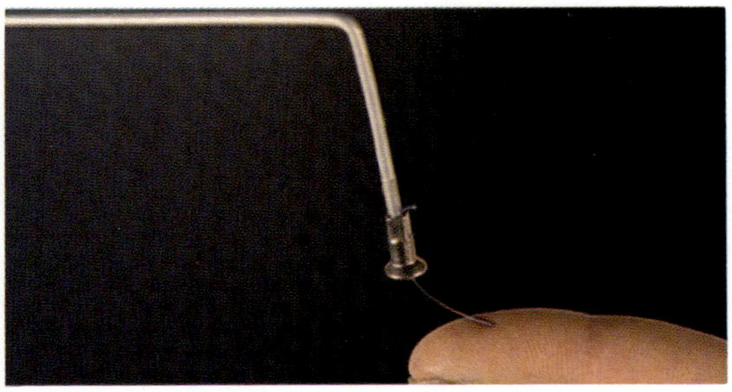

796 Sensory testing of the skin is of critical importance in nerve injuries of the hand. A simple device consists of a piece of O-calibre nylon fixed into a bicycle spoke which has been curved to a right-angle. A pressure equivalent to 1g von Frey hair deforms the nylon.

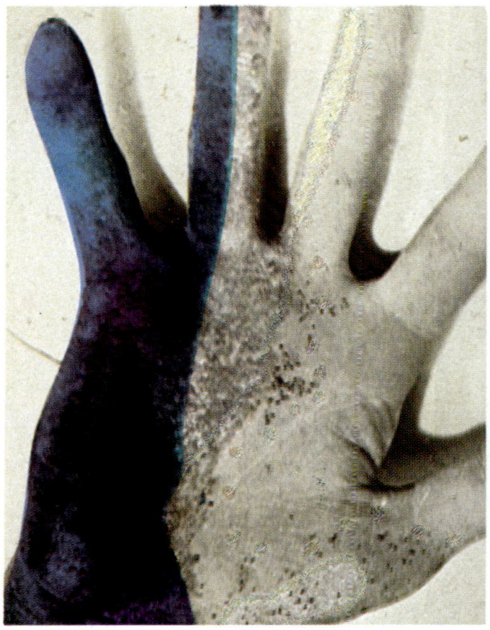

797 Quinizarine powder turns deep blue when it is moistened by sweat. The area which remains unchanged has therefore been deprived of its normal pseudomotor nerve fibres which are carried in the sensory nerve to their destination. The test outlines the insensitive area of skin in a complete median nerve lesion.

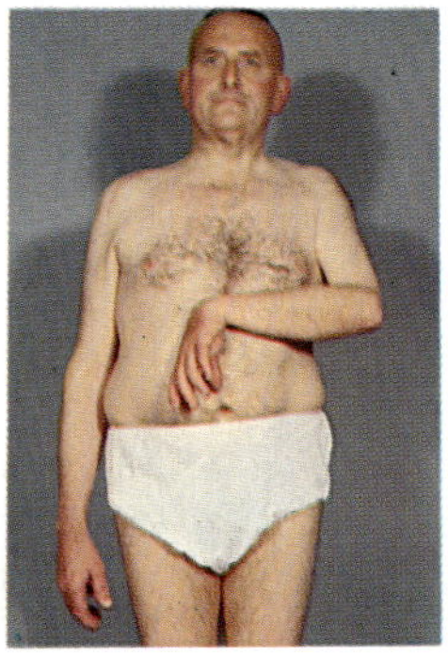

798 Birth injury: upper arm type (Erb's palsy). The arm is held to the side with the forearm in full pronation due to paralysis of the shoulder abductors and forearm supinator muscles supplied by the upper trunk of the brachial plexus C5/6/(7). The unaffected stronger muscles produce the deformity. The typical 'waiter's tip' position.

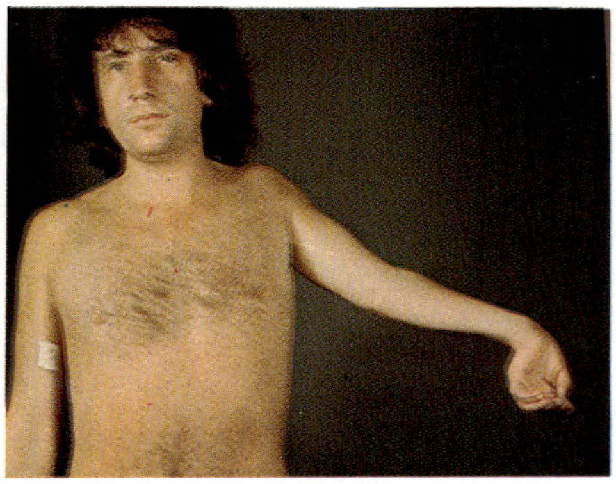

799 Birth injury: lower arm type (Klumpke). This less common birth injury of the brachial plexus (C8/T1) usually results from a breach delivery with the arm forced above the head. Abduction of the shoulder is possible and the forearm is held in full supination with clawing of the fingers.

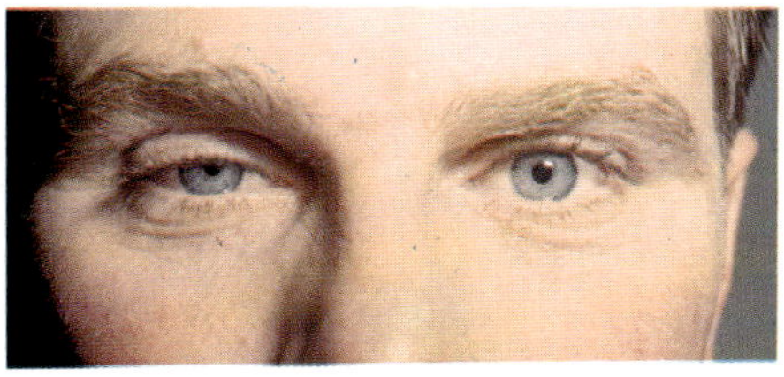

800 Horner's syndrome. The cervical sympathetic fibres traverse the T1 nerve root and may be damaged in lower arm palsy, causing ptosis of the eyelid, a constricted pupil, and enophthalmos.

Median nerve lesions

A high median nerve lesion causes loss of flexion of the proximal and distal interphalangeal joints of the index and middle fingers. In high median nerve paralysis both long flexors of index and middle fingers fail to flex at the interphalangeal joints on grasping.

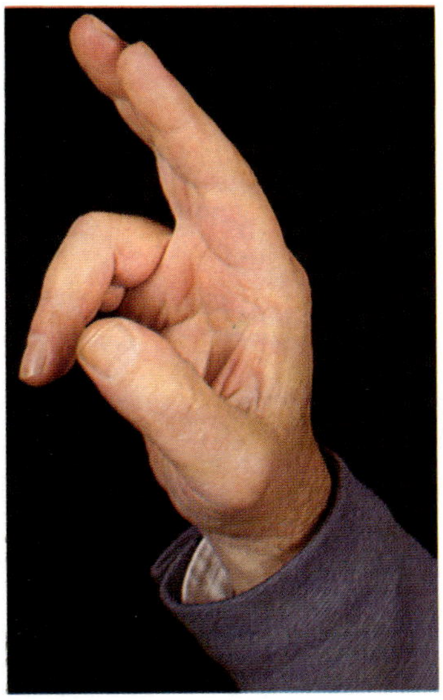

801 The hand of benediction.

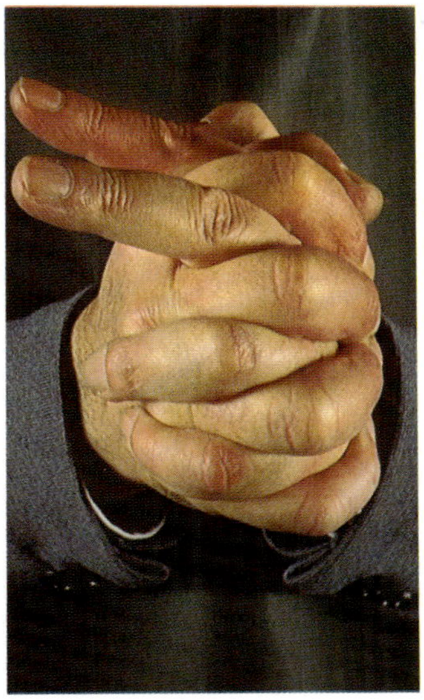

802 Ochsner's clasping test.

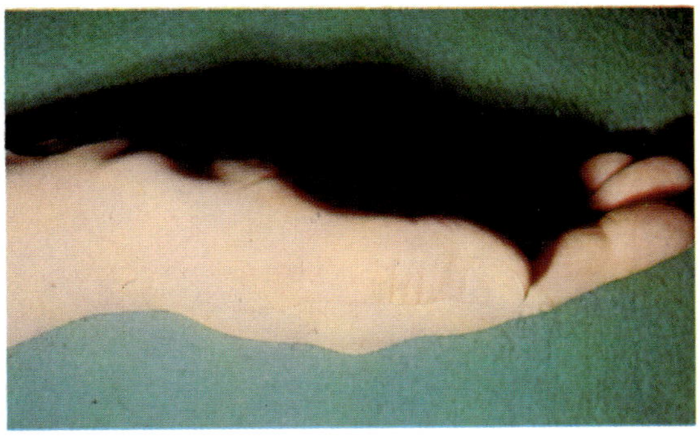

803 Thenar wasting. In the hand the median nerve supplies the radial two lumbrical muscles, opponens pollicis, abductor pollicis brevis and flexor pollicis brevis. Variations do occur but the abductor pollicis brevis is always median-nerve innervated. Special lighting shows the wasting of APB, a valuable sign in median nerve lesions.

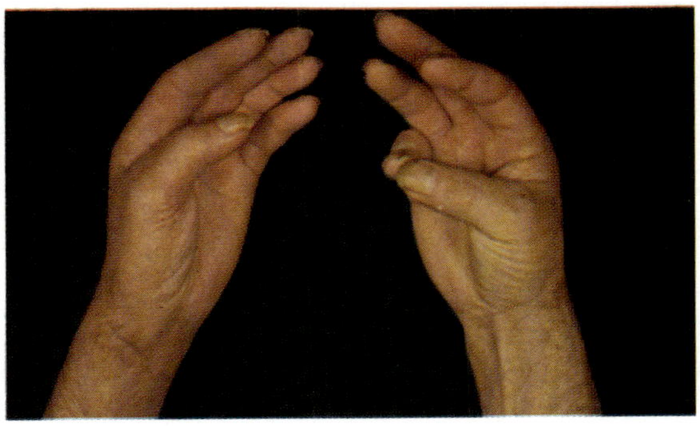

804 Opposition of the thumb. An early and reliable sign of median nerve damage. Note that the right thumb opposes fully to the little finger, whereas on the left side it fails to do so and less of the thumb nail is visible owing to impaired rotation.

Median nerve compression neuropathy

Three distinct entrapment syndromes of the median nerve are described.

The pronator syndrome

Presents with pain in the proximal forearm, worsened by activity. Loss of sensation or paraesthesiae in the median distribution but with a negative Phalen's test. There are four potential sites of entrapment.

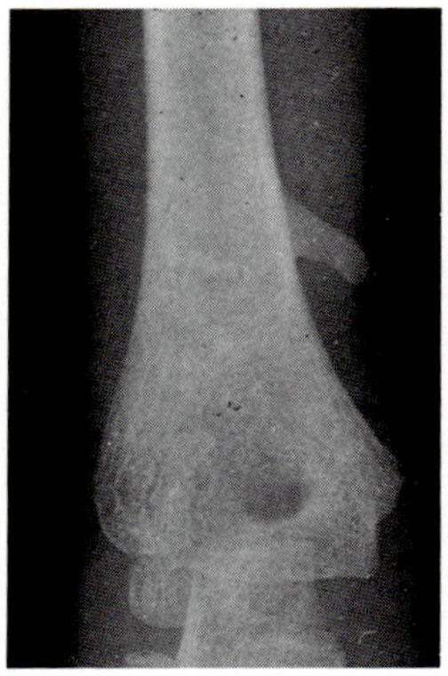

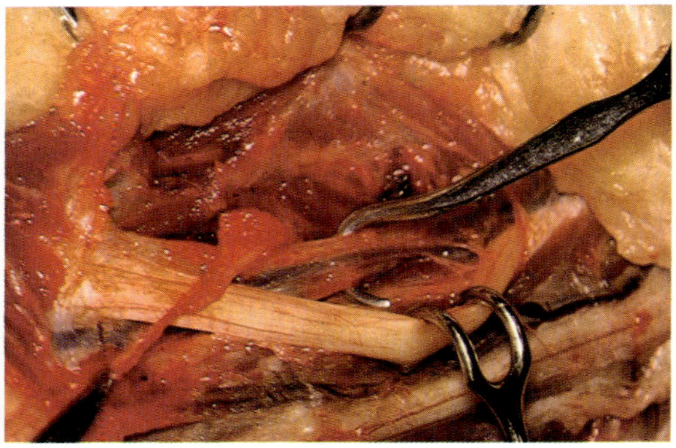

805 & **806** Supracondylar spur and Ligament of Struthers. The area displayed at operation shows the ligament running downwards crossing the median nerve.

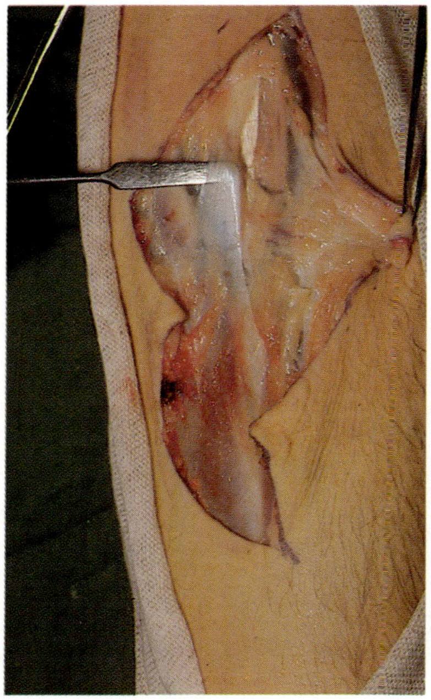

807 The lacertus fibrosus. Aggravation of symptoms on flexion of the elbow with the forearm pronated may suggest this as a site of compression.

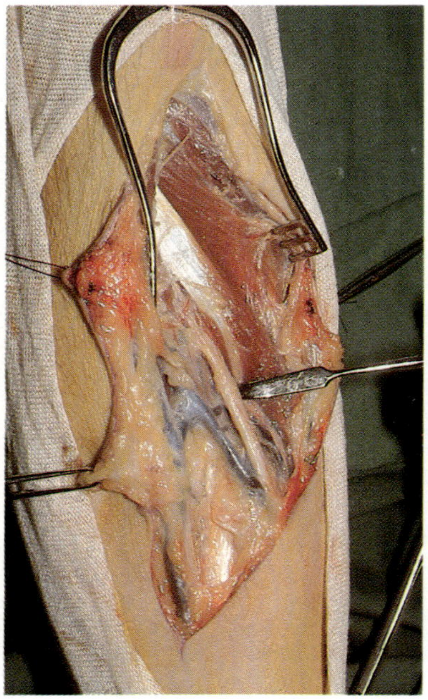

808 The pronator teres muscle. The median nerve enters the forearm between the two heads of pronator teres. Compression by muscle hypertrophy or by fascial bands between the two heads is thought to occur.

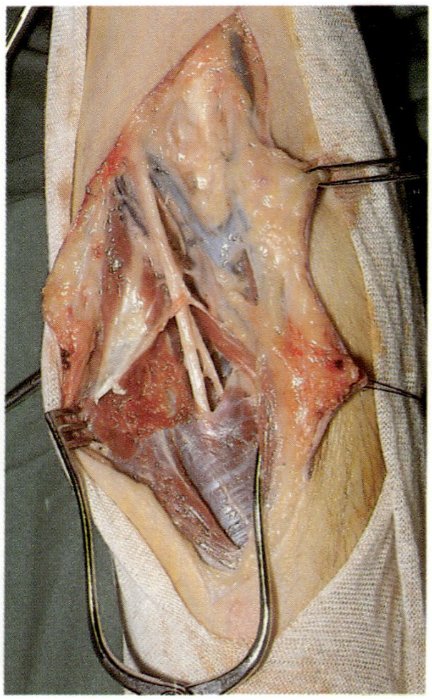

809 Fibrous arch of flexor digitorum superficialis.

Anterior interosseous syndrome

Characterised by aching pain in the proximal forearm, weakness or paralysis of the index profundus, flexor pollicis longus and pronator quadratus.

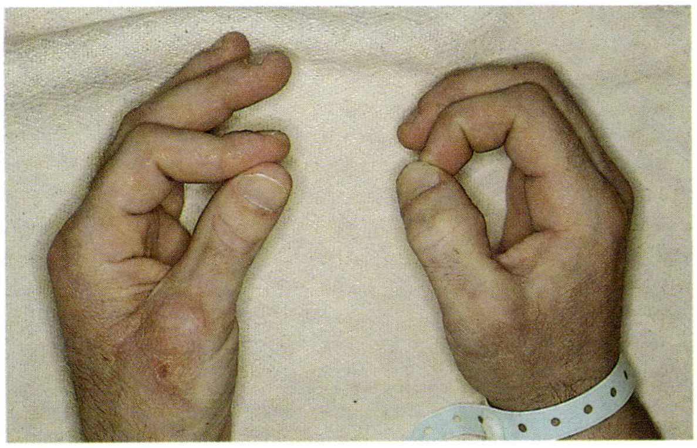

810 The patient is unable to make a circle between index finger and thumb. There are no sensory symptoms.

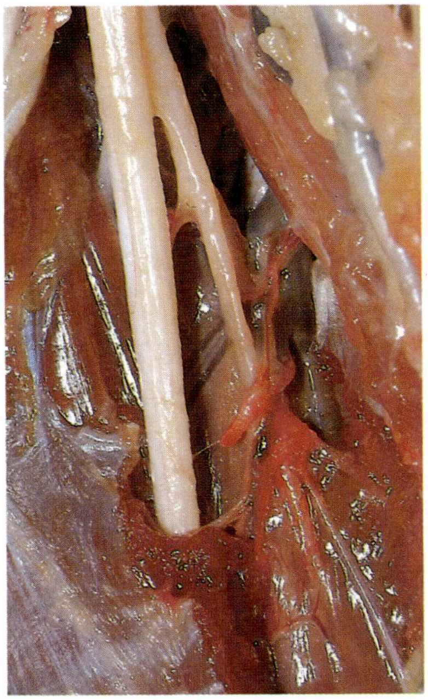

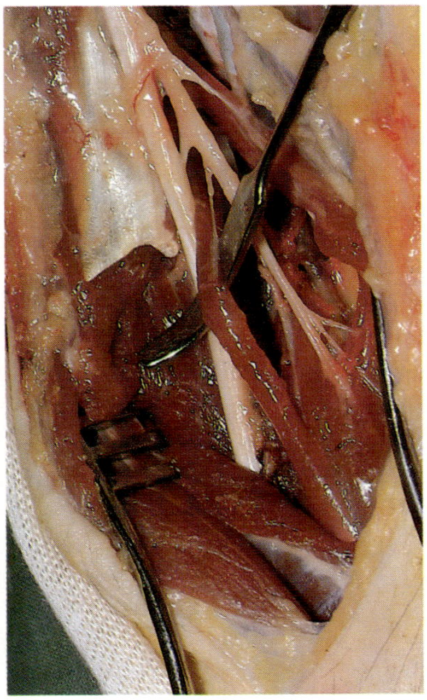

811 & **812** Compression has been attributed to fascial bands, thrombosed or aberrent vessels, bursae and accessory muscle units. In this case a leash of vessels crosses the nerve (**811**) and an accessory head of flexor pollicis longus, Gantzer's muscle, is present (**812**). Neither has obviously compressed the nerve. Some authorities are of the view that this syndrome is a local neuralgic amyotrophy rather than a compression syndrome.

Carpal tunnel syndrome

This is by far the commonest site of median nerve entrapment and is usually idiopathic. Typically, patients complain of burning parasthesiae in the hands which wakes them at night. Motor symptoms and signs occur late. Examination may show little abnormality though paraesthesiae may be produced by tapping over the median nerve at the wrist crease (Tinel's sign).

The commoner conditions that may cause carpal tunnel syndrome are:

- Flexor synovitis – e.g. Rheumatoid arthritis.
- Fluid retention – e.g. pregnancy, hypothyroidism, menopause.
- Trauma – e.g. Colles' fracture.
- Ganglion.
- Aberrant muscles.
- Chronic renal failure – ? AV shunt, amyloidosis.

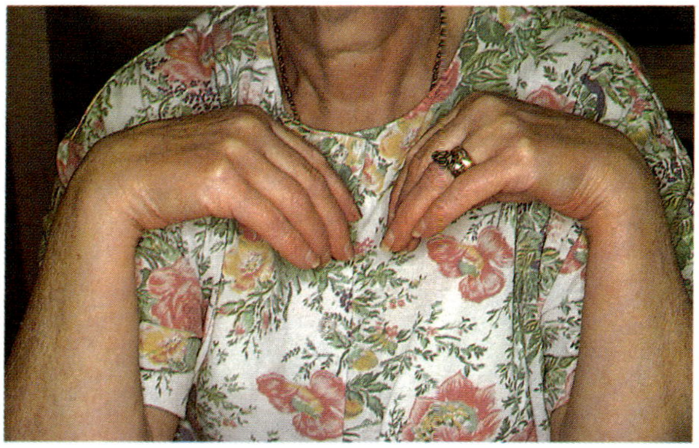

813 The most useful and reliable confirmatory test has proved to be Phalen's test where unforced flexion of the wrists rapidly induces symptoms.

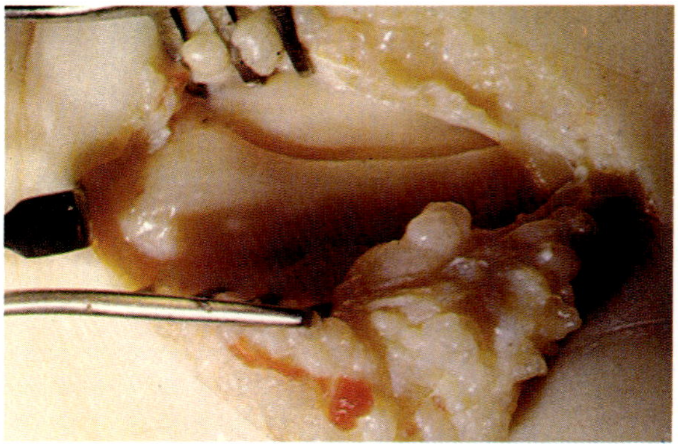

814 Carpal tunnel syndrome. Compression of the median nerve is clearly seen once the fibrous carpal tunnel has been divided. Immediately proximal to the compression the nerve is considerably enlarged by a neuroma – in fact a glioma – of the nerve owing to endoneural fibrosis. The blades of the retractor indicate the level of the carpal ligament.

Ulnar nerve lesions

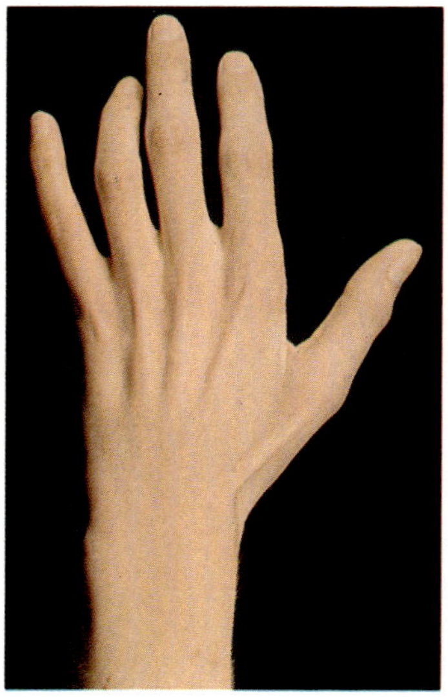

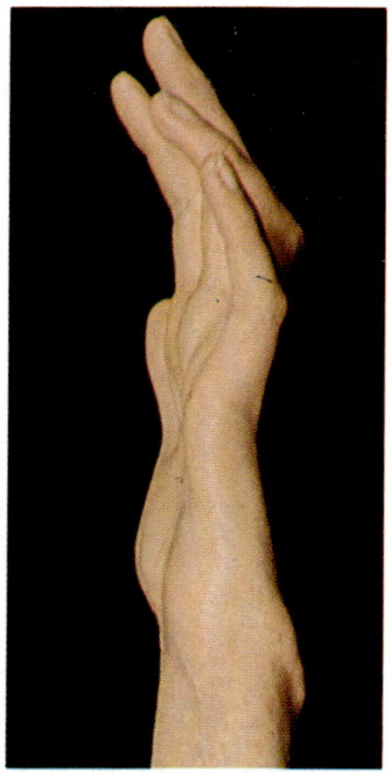

815 & **816** Wasting of the interosseous muscles. The ulnar nerve is motor to all the small muscles of the hand except those supplied by the median nerve. Marked guttering between the extensor tendons is evident with a particular loss of bulk in the thumb web caused by wasting of the first dorsal interosseous and the adductor pollicis. In profile hypothenar wasting is clear.

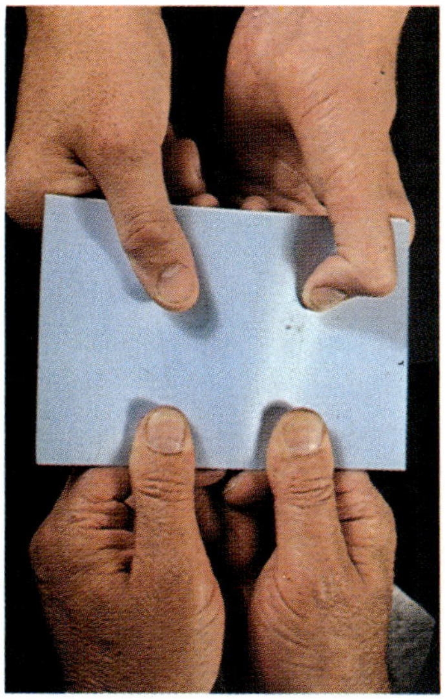

817 Froment's test. When the patient attempts to grasp the paper between thumb and index finger the interphalangeal joint of the thumb flexes to grasp the paper. The test confirms weakness or paralysis of the adductor pollicis, the median innervated flexor pollicis being subconsciously recruited to prevent loss of grip.

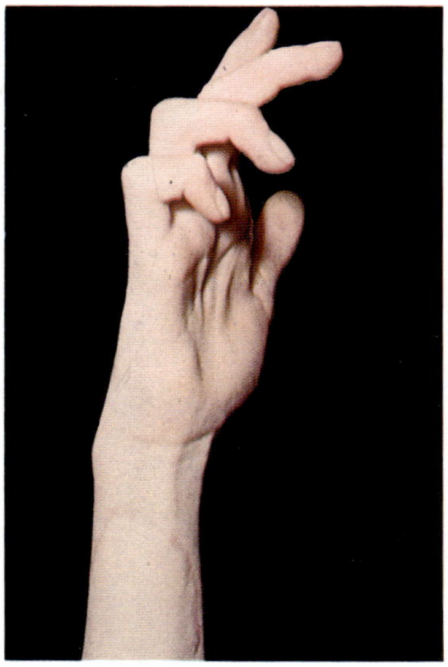

818 Ulnar claw hand. There is hyperextension of the MP joints and flexion of the IP joints owing to paralysis of intrinsic muscles and consequent unopposed action of the long flexors and extensors. Middle and index fingers are less affected because their lumbricals are median innervated. Contrary to the effects of most nerve lesions, in ulnar nerve lesions, a low injury, shown here, produces a more severe deformity than a high injury. This is due to the fact that in high ulnar nerve injuries the flexor digitorum profundus to little ring fingers are paralysed and therefore the clawing is less. This explains the so called 'ulnar paradox'.

Ulnar nerve compression neuropathy

There are two main sites of ulnar nerve compression. The commonest is in the cubital tunnel already described in the section on the elbow. The second is at the wrist where the nerve passes through Guyon's canal.

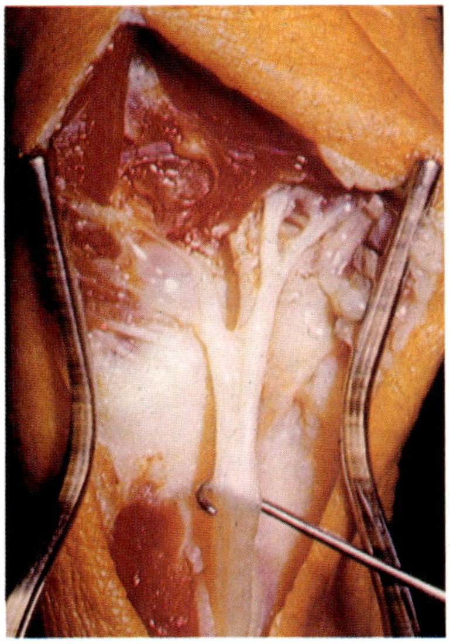

819 Guyon's canal. The canal has been deroofed. Distally the ulnar nerve divides into superficial (mainly sensory) and deep (motor) branches. A ganglion can be seen pressing on the deep branch just distal to the hook of hamate.

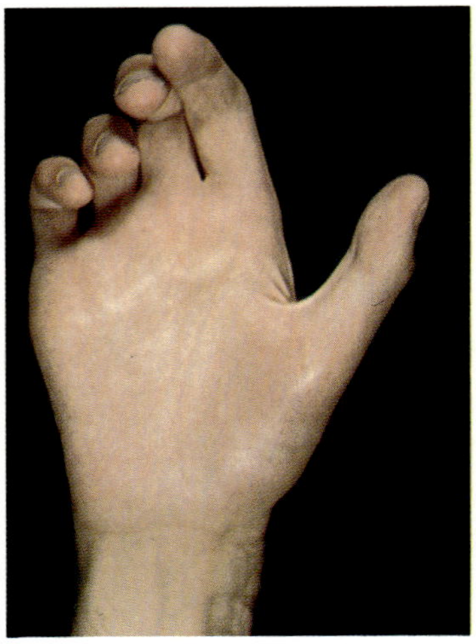

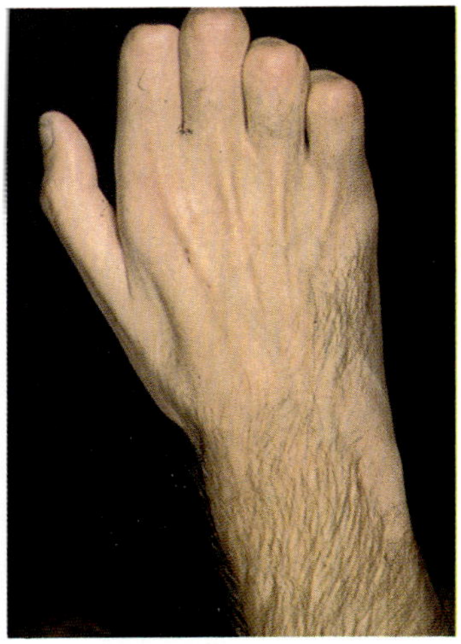

820 & **821** Combined low median and ulnar nerve injury produces the worst form of clawhand. The fixed clawed position of the fingers with thin and atrophic skin is evident. There is severe wasting of all the intrinsic musculature.

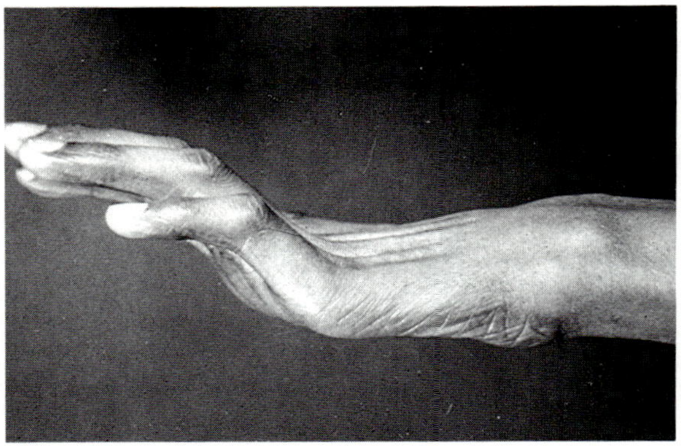

822 Intrinsic muscle paralysis following poliomyelitis in infancy. Hyperextension at the MP and flexion at the proximal IP joints results from the unopposed action of the long extensor and flexor muscles.

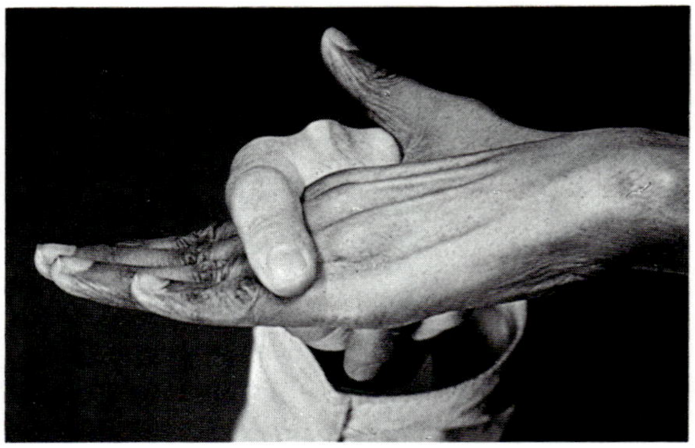

823 The fingers can extend fully when the paralysed intrinsic muscles are passively simulated by the examiner's hand.

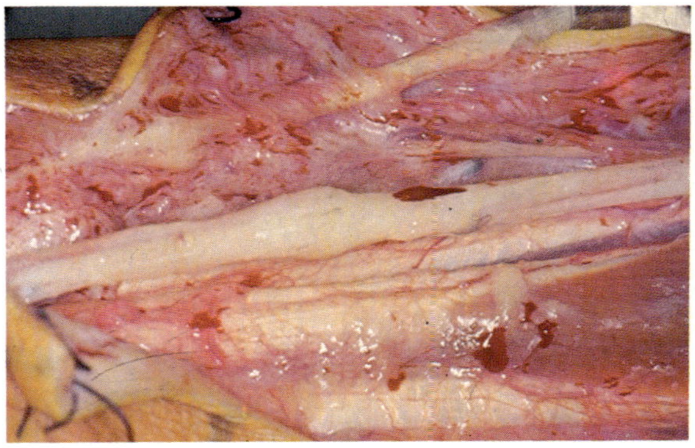

824 'Neuroma'. A lesion in continuity of the ulnar nerve immediately above the wrist. The nerve has been crushed but the perineurium remains intact. At the site of injury the nerve is narrowed, but immediately proximal to the injury it is enlarged by a traumatic 'neuroma'.

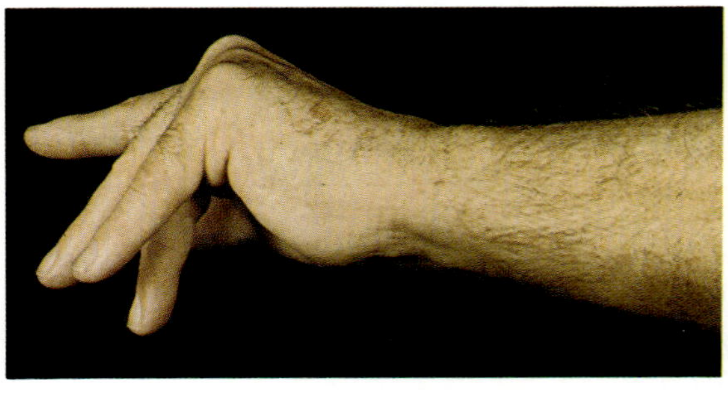

825 Hysterical contraction of the hand. An analysis of the balancing forces of muscle required to produce this attitude shows that it is anatomically impossible to explain by any form of nerve damage. It bears some resemblance to Trousseau's sign (main d'accoucher). The condition was, however, unilateral and there was no suggestion of tetany. It is an example of motor hysteria.

Hip joint

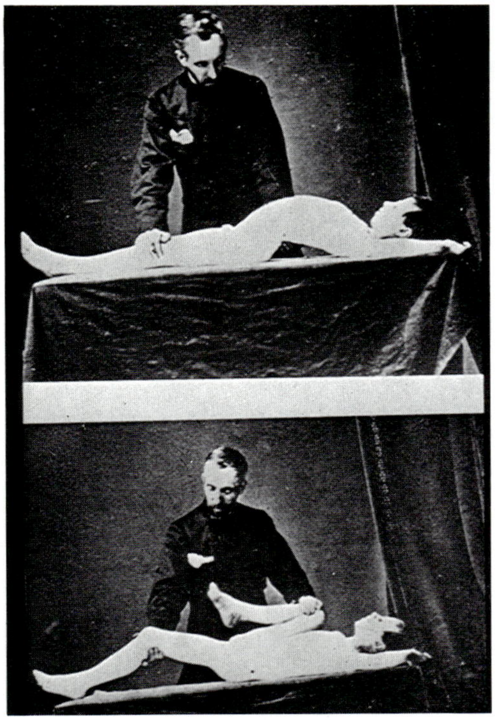

826 Hugh Owen-Thomas demonstrating his test to display hidden fixed flexion deformity.

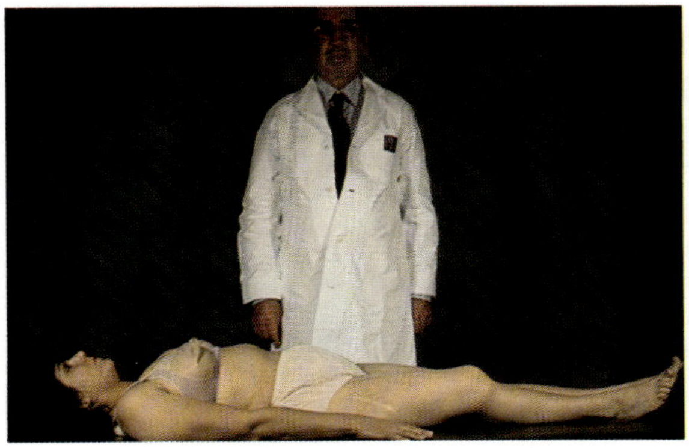

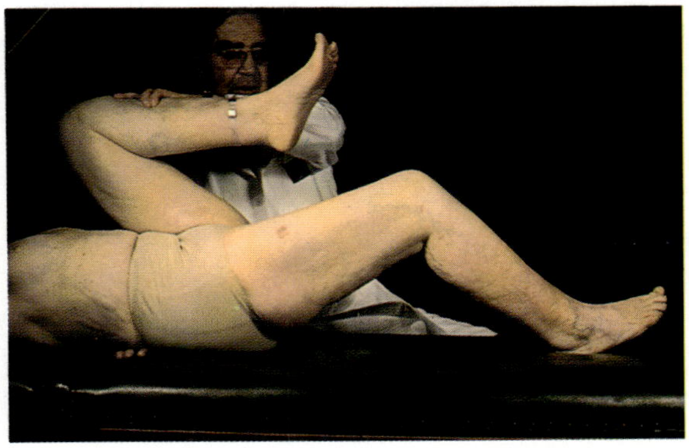

827 & **828** Thomas' test. The patient lies flat on the couch, any fixed flexion deformity is hidden by pelvic tilt increasing the normal lumbar lordosis. When the opposite hip is flexed to obliterate the lumbar lordosis (note the examiner's hand under the lumbar spine to check this) any hidden flexion deformity of the hip becomes apparent.

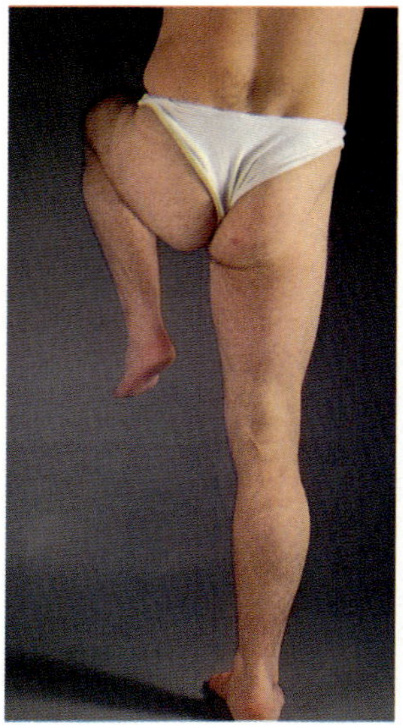

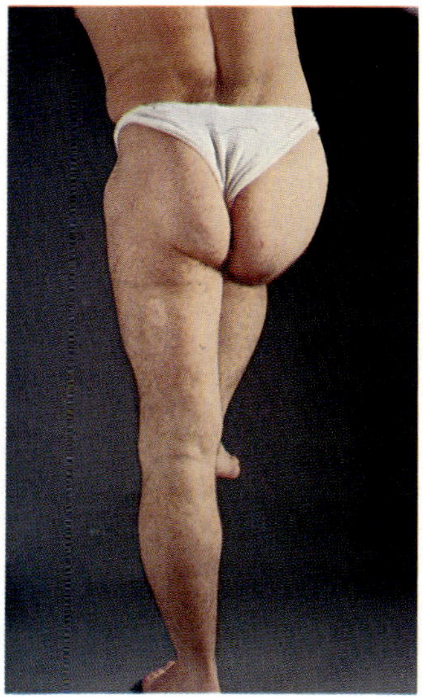

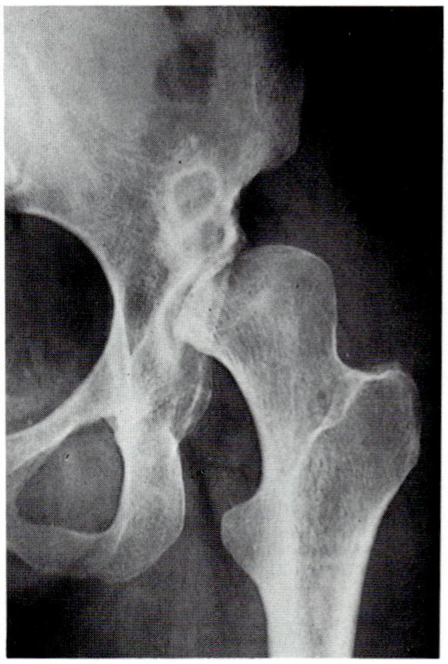

829–831 Trendelenburg's test. When the patient stands on one leg, the stability of the hip depends upon two principal factors: effective muscles between pelvis and greater trochanter, and a stable, centrally placed femoral head. When this mechanism fails for any reason, the test is positive.

The patient stands on the normal leg: his trunk inclines towards the same side, and the pelvis tilts and is stabilised towards the same side, causing the other buttock to rise.

Note the position of the gluteal folds. The right hip is stable: the test is negative.

The patient then stands upon the affected side. The stabilising mechanism has failed and the buttock on the opposite side droops downwards; the left hip is unstable: the test is positive.

The cause of failure in this case is subluxation of the hip joint so that the fulcrum for the action of the pelvifemoral muscle is lost.

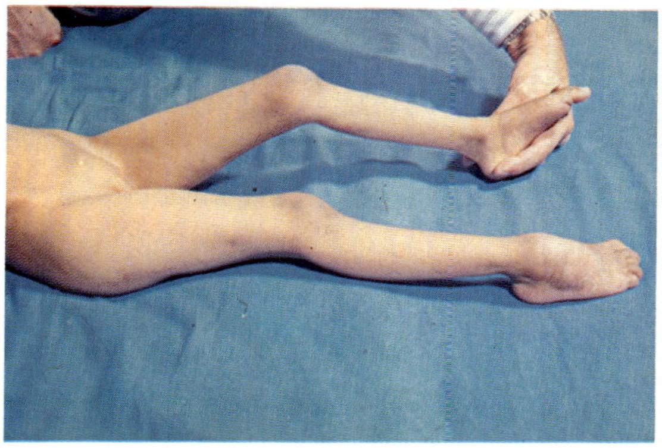

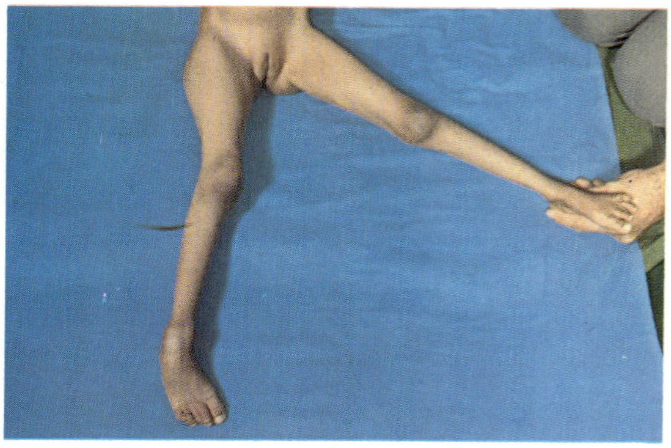

832 & **833** Yount's test. This child has a flexion deformity of both the left hip and knee due to a contracted tensor fascia latae muscle straddling across the hip and knee joints. By abducting the hip to relax tensor fascia latae, the apparent flexion deformity of both the hip and knee diminishes.

Leg length inequality

Inequality of the length of the legs may be due to a wide variety of causes. In its simplest form, it is caused by shortening in any part of one leg, or lengthening in any part of the other.

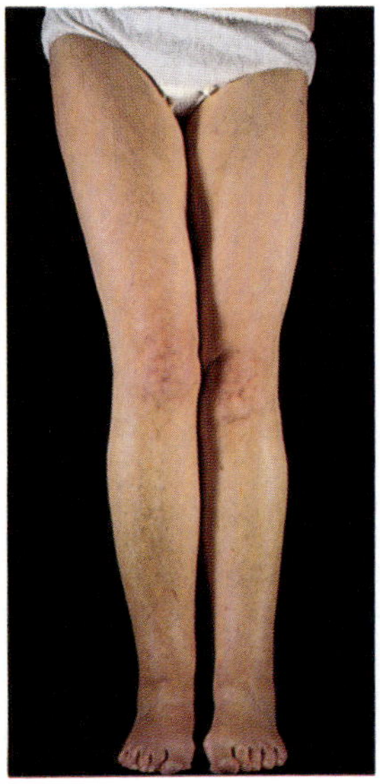

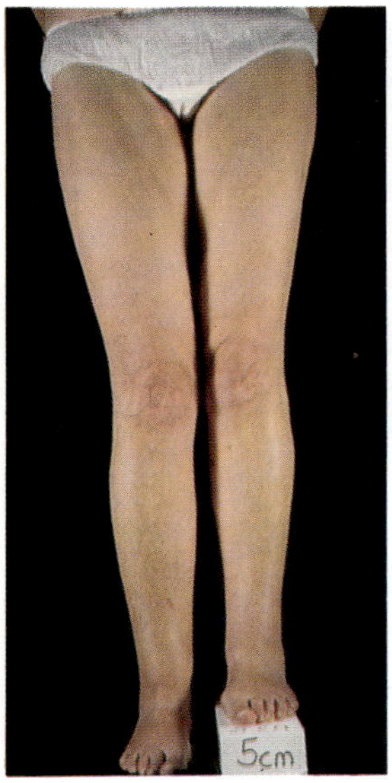

834 & **835** True shortening. When the patient stands erect, the pelvis is tilted owing to shortening of the left leg. A 5 cm block underneath the left leg squares the pelvis, indicating true difference in the length of the legs.

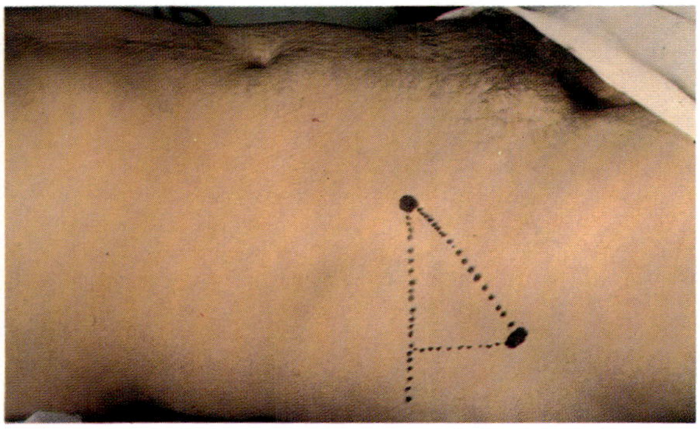

836 Bryant's triangle. Shortening may occur either above or below the greater trochanter, i.e. in the femoral neck and hip joint, or below it. The relationship between the anterior superior iliac spine and the tip of the greater trochanter is assessed by drawing lines from the anterior superior iliac spine vertically downwards and to the tip of the greater trochanter. The base of the triangle is a guide to the neck-shaft angle of the femur. Normally it is more or less an isosceles triangle. In practice, Bryant's triangle does not require to be marked out, but is readily assessed by palpation with the thumb on the anterior superior iliac spine and fingertips on the top of the greater trochanter, the two sides being simultaneously compared.

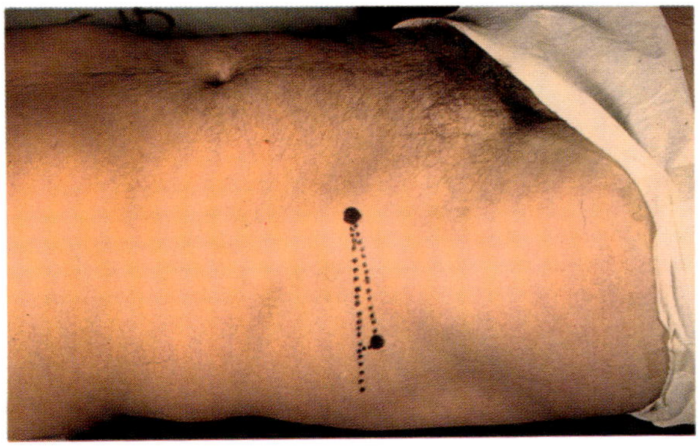

837 True shortening. The fact that the shortening is sited above the trochanter level is evidenced by the fact that the base of the triangle has been diminished and the trochanter now lies almost vertically below the iliac spine.

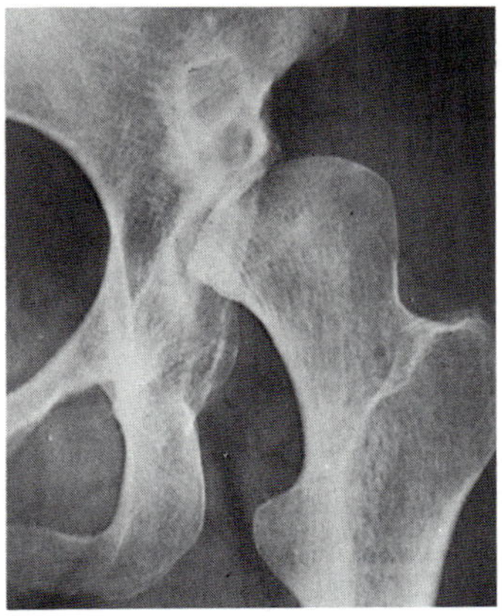

838 Radiograph shows the shortening caused by upward displacement of the femoral head.

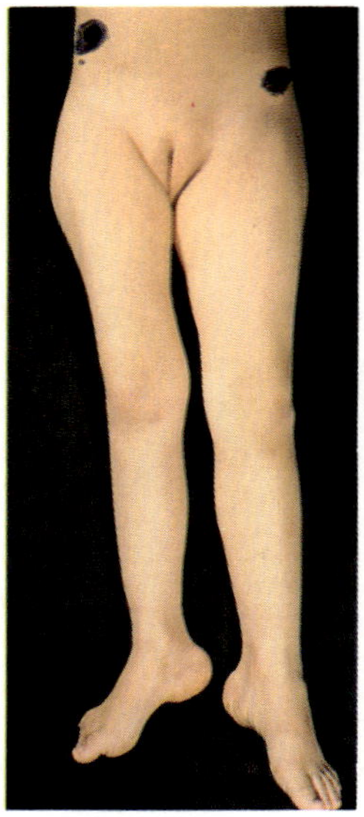

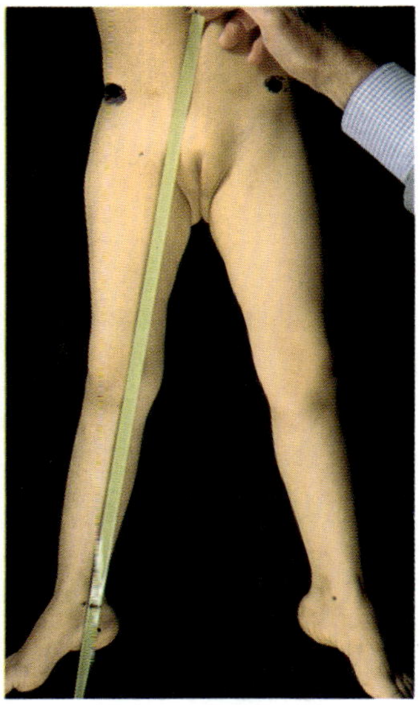

839 & **840** Apparent lengthening. Leg length inequality may be apparent only; fixed adduction deformity at the hip causes apparent shortening, whereas fixed abduction causes apparent lengthening. This child has a fixed abduction deformity of the left hip caused by muscle contracture following poliomyelitis. There is apparent lengthening of the left leg. When the right leg is measured in the same degree of abduction as the left, the leg lengths are seen to be equal.

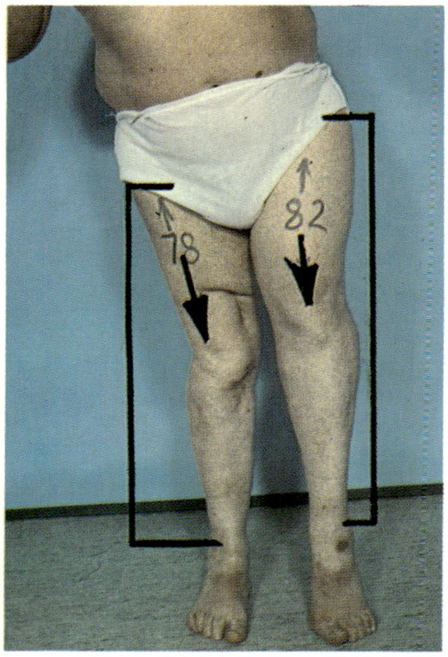

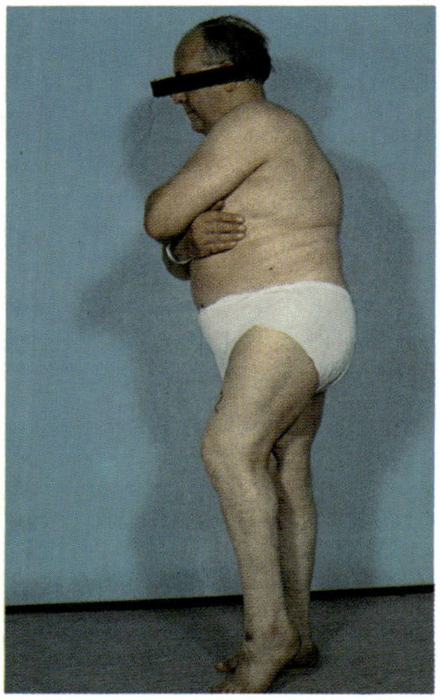

841 & **842** Complex leg inequality. The cause of leg length inequality may be complex; true shortening of one leg may be masked or exceeded by apparent shortening owing to fixed deformity of the other hip. This patient stands on the tip of the left toe, suggesting shortening of the left lower limb. The right leg is, in fact, the shorter. A severe adduction deformity of the left hip more than compensates for the difference.

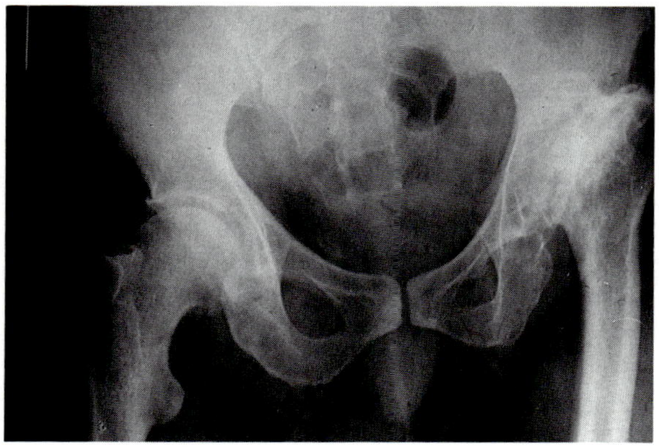

843 Radiographs showing severe adduction deformity of the left hip. This caused an apparent shortening of the left leg whereas it was, in fact, the longer of the two.

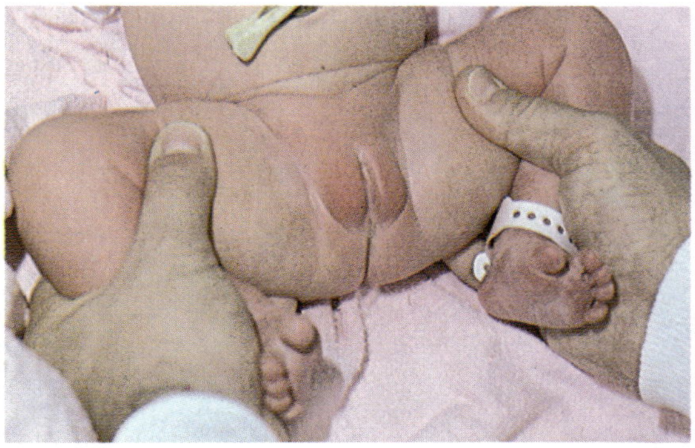

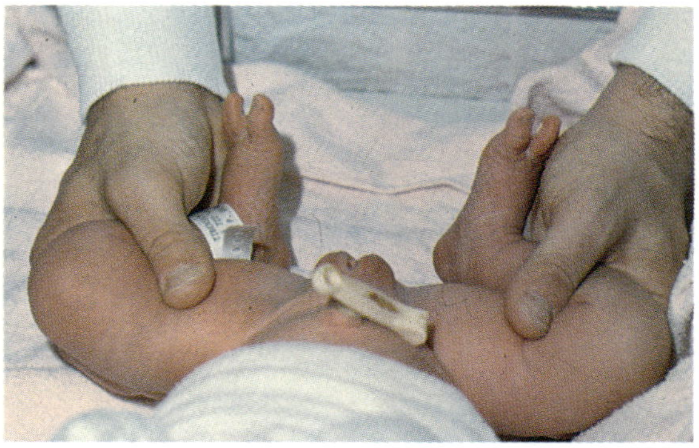

844 Congenital dislocation of the hip. Barlow's test. Newborn infants should be examined for congenital dislocation or instability of the hip by one of a number of tests. In Barlow's test the upper femur is grasped between index and middle fingers over the greater trochanter and the thumb in the groin. The femoral head can be levered in and out of the joint confirming instability.

845 Ortolani's test is a test of reduction of a dislocated hip. The examiner applies forward pressure with the fingers from behind with the hips maintained in abduction by the thumbs. A positive test is dependant upon a clunk of re-entry as the femoral head is relocated in the acetabulum.

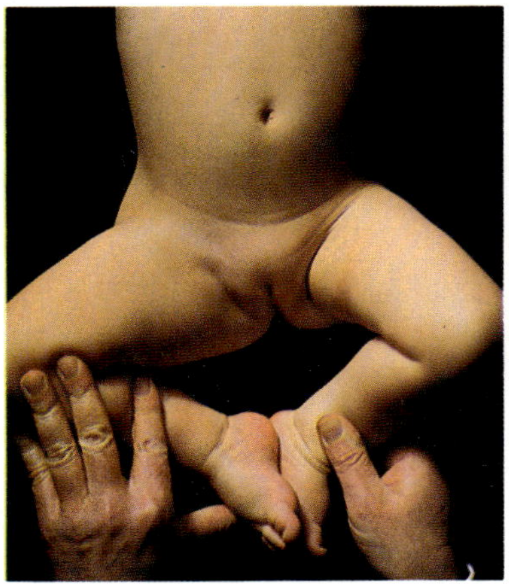

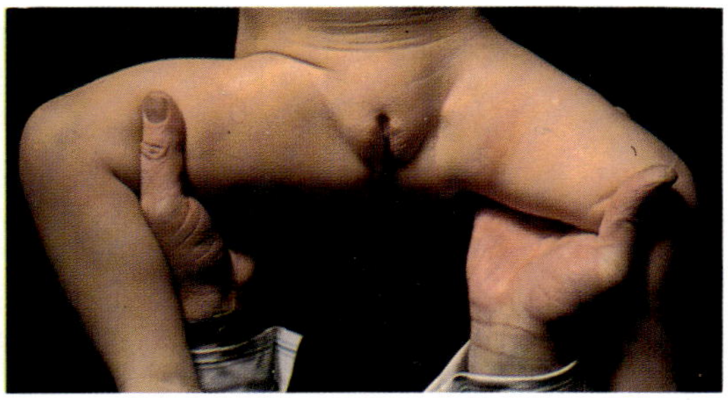

846 & **847** Congenital dislocation of the left hip in a somewhat older infant. There is obvious loss of full abduction in flexion. An unsuccessful attempt to relocate the hip by the Ortolani manoeuvre.

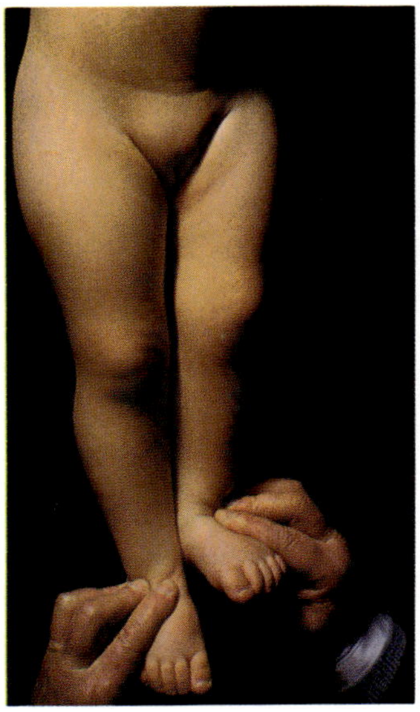

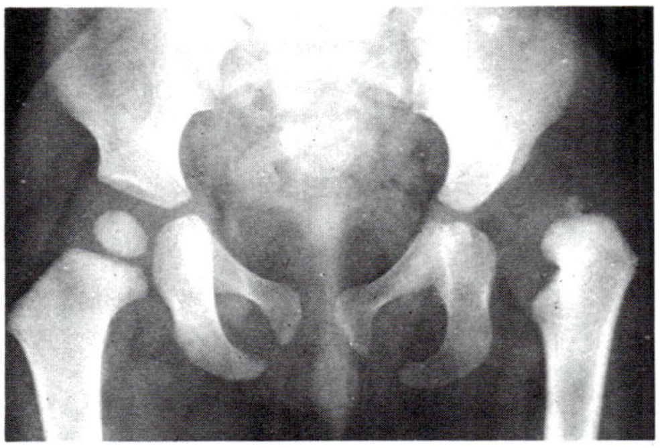

848 & **849** Congenital dislocation of the hip in an older child, illustrating telescoping: the left leg is shortened when the hip is pushed upwards and backwards. This test is probably better done with the hips in the flexed position.

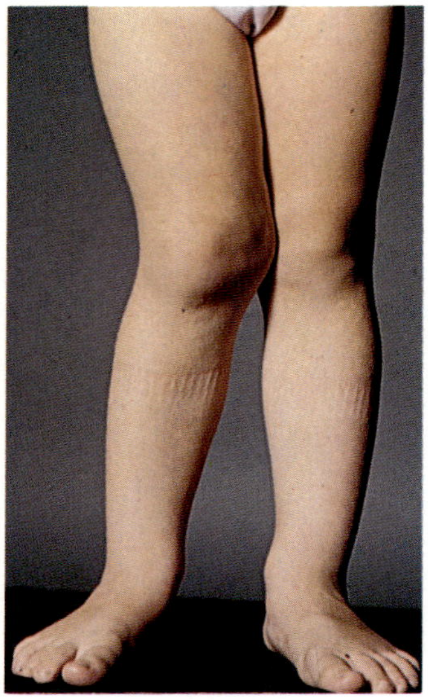

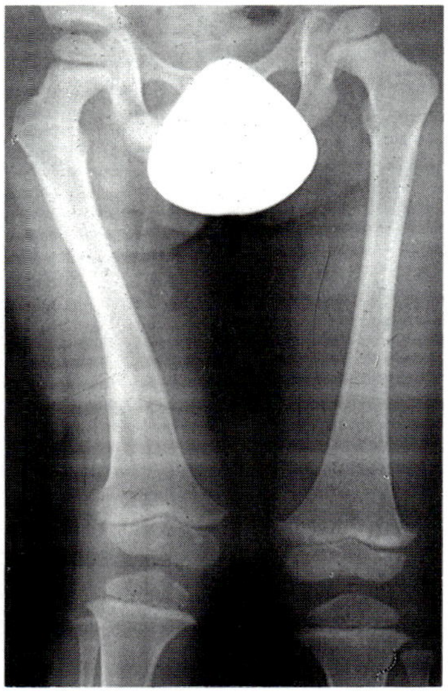

850 & **851** Congenital short femur. The affected leg is on the left. The child prefers to flex his right knee for comfort when standing, because it is relatively too long. The condition varies considerably from almost complete absence of the femur, to relatively slight shortening and alteration of bone texture, as shown on this radiograph.

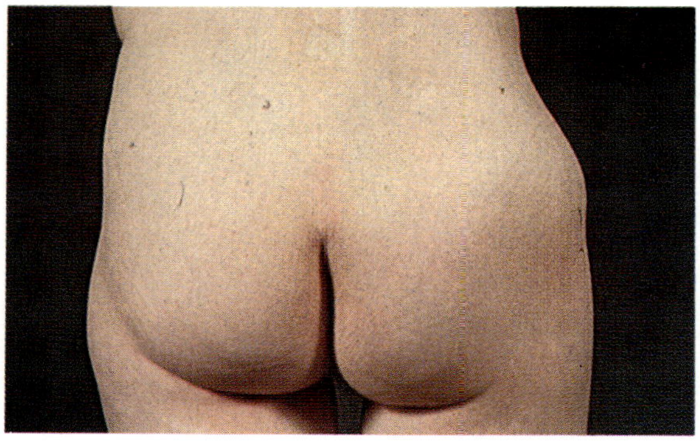

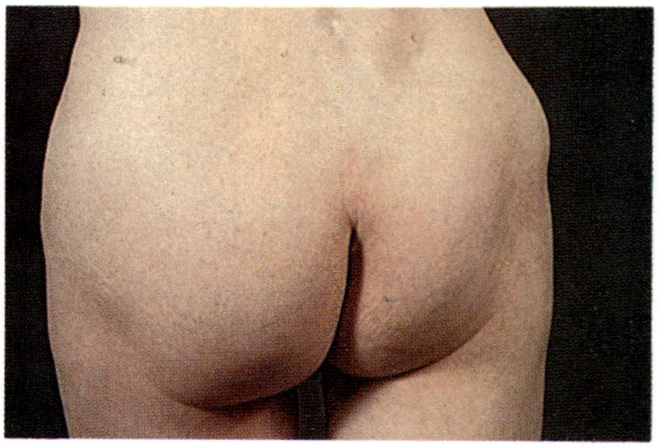

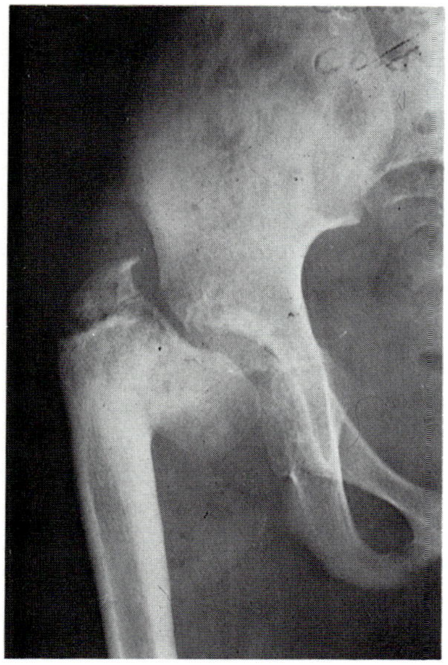

852–854 Congenital coxa vara. This is possibly part of the same spectrum of disorders classified as congenital proximal femoral deficiency.

The Trendelenburg test (**852–853**) demonstrates positive instability of the right hip. The patient now takes weight on the abnormal right leg, causing the buttock on the opposite side to droop.

Owing to the raised position of the greater trochanter (**854**), the pelvifemoral muscles are relatively ineffective and fail to stabilise the hip. This accounts for the positive Trendelenburg test.

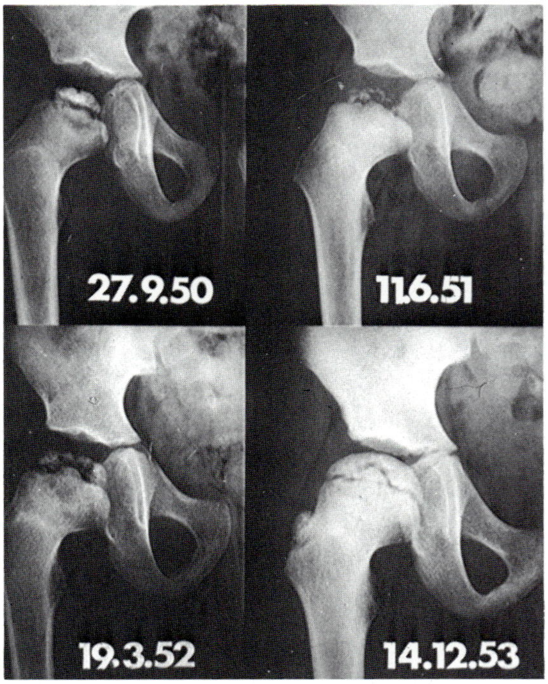

855 Perthes' disease (Coxa plana) results from avascular necrosis of the capital epiphysis of the femur in childhood. It is commonest at a mean age of 5 years and is commoner in boys. It is transient and self-limiting, but alteration of the final shape of the femoral head may lead to degenerative changes in later life. The series of radiographs shows creeping substitution of avascular bone over a 3-year period.

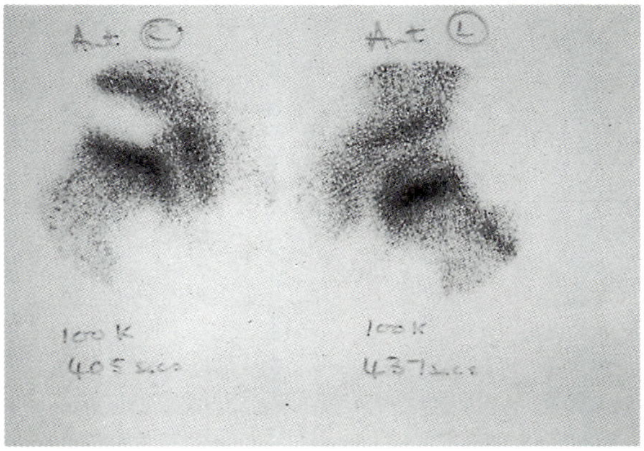

856 A bone scan carried out in the early stages of Perthes' disease when the child presented with an 'irritable hip'. Failure of isotope uptake in one half of the capital epiphysis indicates avascularity.

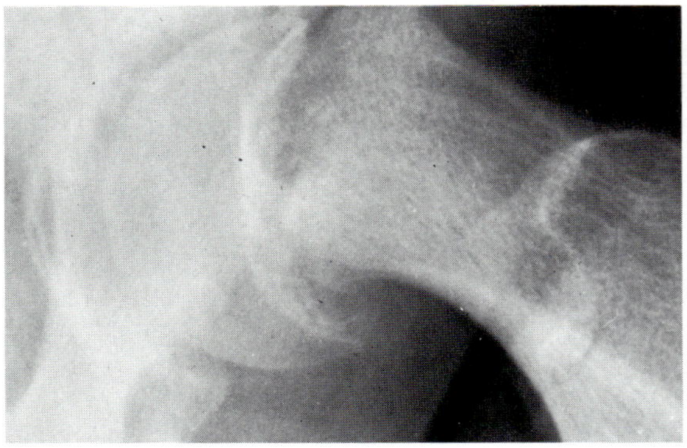

857 Slipped upper femoral epiphysis (Adolescent coxa vara). Impairment of maturation of the upper femoral epiphysis allows the capital epiphysis to slip postero– inferiorly on the femoral neck. The slip can occur acutely or gradually. With major slips the affected leg is short, adducted and externally rotated.

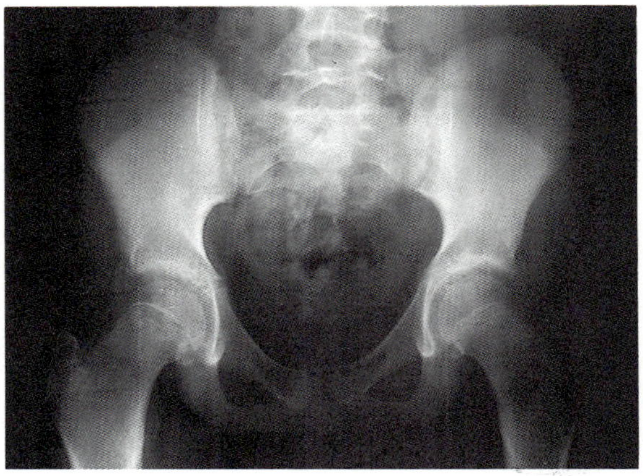

858 Affected adolescents frequently complain of referred pain in the knee and clinicians should be aware of this and remember to examine the hip. Radiographic signs of an early slip may be subtle and easily missed. In the radiograph shown the slip is in the right hip. If a line is traced along the superior aspect of the femoral neck, on the affected right side its runs straight on to the head of the femur. On the normal left side there is a step up on to the femoral head (Trethowan's sign).

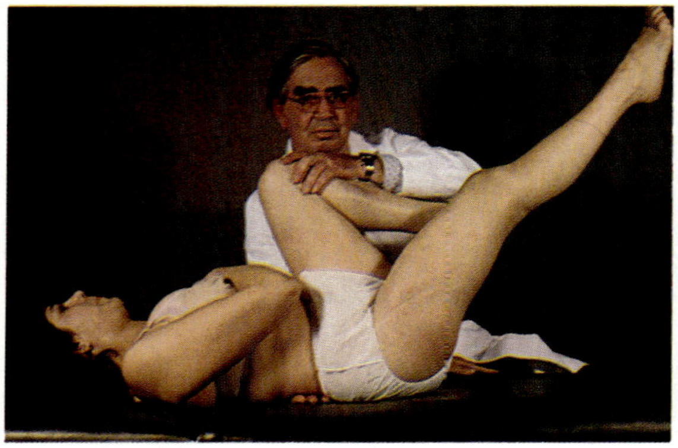

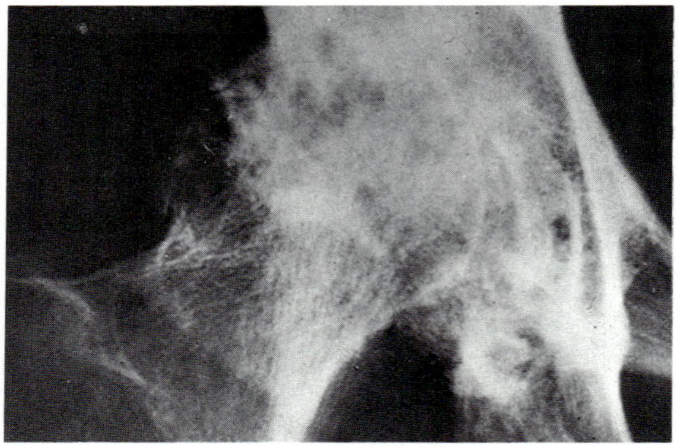

859 & **860** Osteoarthritis of the hip joint. This middle-aged lady had pain in the groin and buttock, with referral to the right knee. She also had a limp. Thomas' test was positive, showing a fixed flexion deformity of the right hip. The radiograph shows that she had severe degenerative osteoarthritis associated with segmental avascular necrosis of the femoral head. Its cause was undetermined.

Table 4. Causes of avascular necrosis

- Idiopathic.
- Post traumatic.
- Alcoholism.
- Steroid therapy.
- Caisson's disease.
- Sickle cell disease.
- Gaucher's disease.

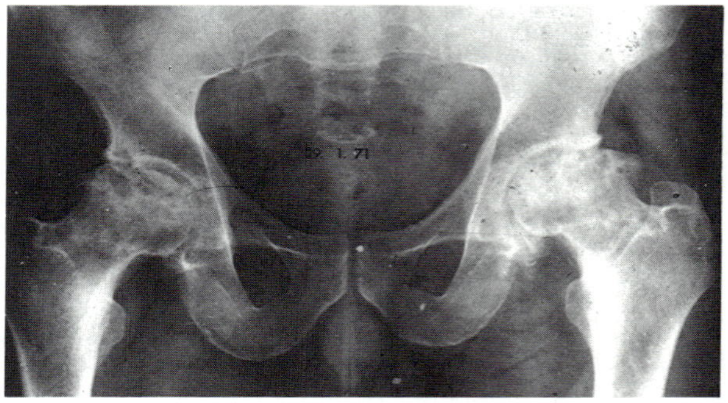

861 Avascular necrosis. Although the aetiology of osteoarthritis of the hip joint is uncertain in the majority of patients, a number of aetiological factors have been established. The radiograph showed typical bilateral osteoarthritis with patchy avascular necrosis in a severe alcoholic.

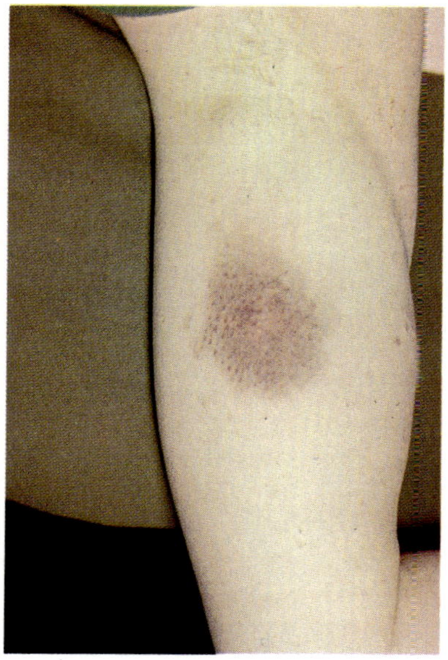

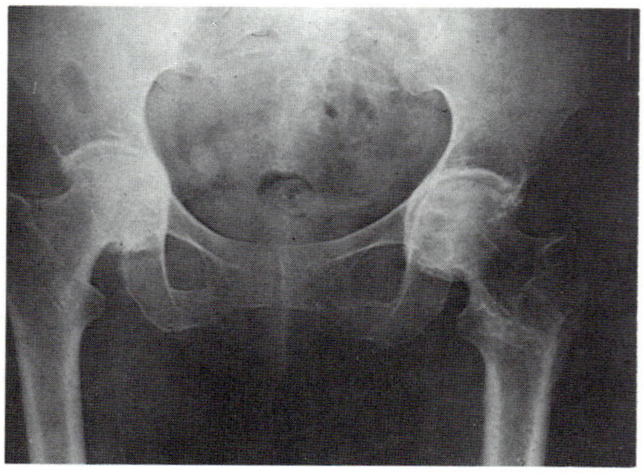

862 & **863** Thrombocytopenic purpura: a rare cause of osteoarthritis of the hip. There is marked loss of joint space and patchy avascular necrosis throughout the femoral heads associated with impaired blood supply due to purpura.

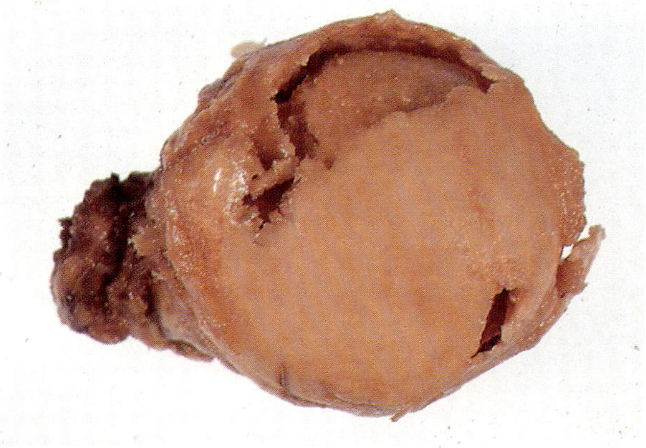

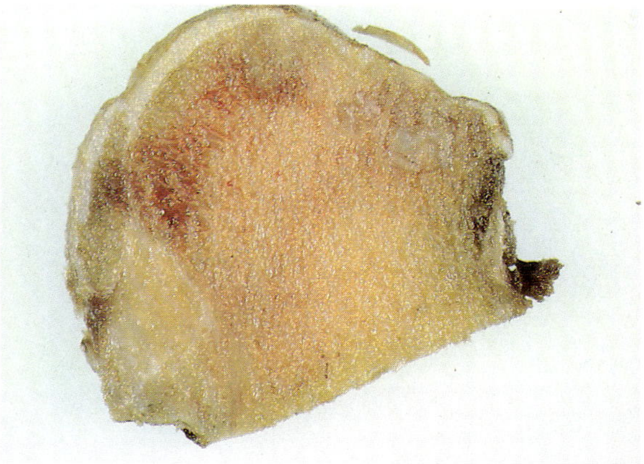

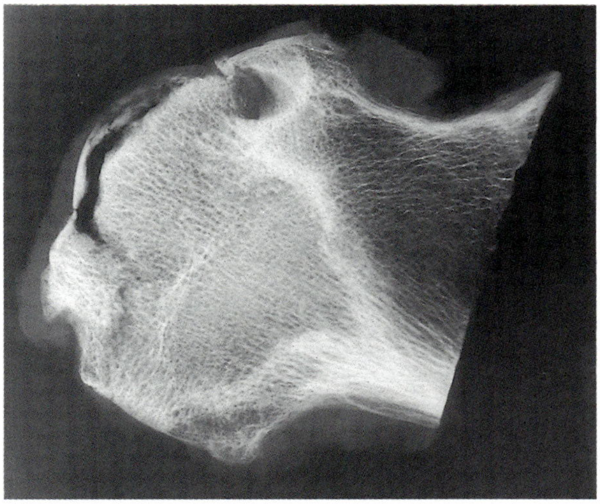

864–866 Excised femoral head with avascular necrosis and separation of the articular cartilage with segmental collapse of the weight-bearing area of the femoral head.

Some complications of hip arthroplasty

Arthroplasty of the hip has now been performed for over 25 years and has revolutionised the management of osteoarthritis of the hip. Some of the problems of the procedure are now being seen in orthopaedic clinics.

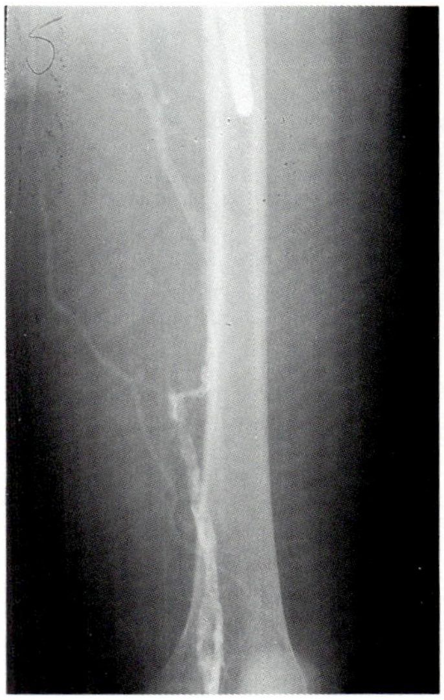

867 Venous thrombosis probably occurs in up to 80% of patients undergoing hip replacement. In many it may only be calf veins that are involved, but some 30% may develop clots in the femoral segment, which are a greater threat to propagation and embolisation.

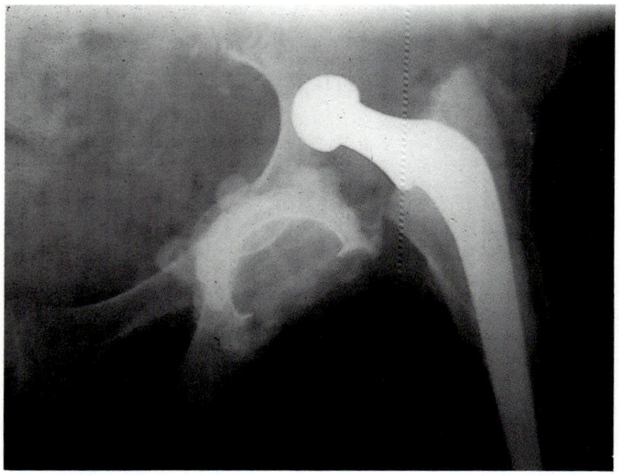

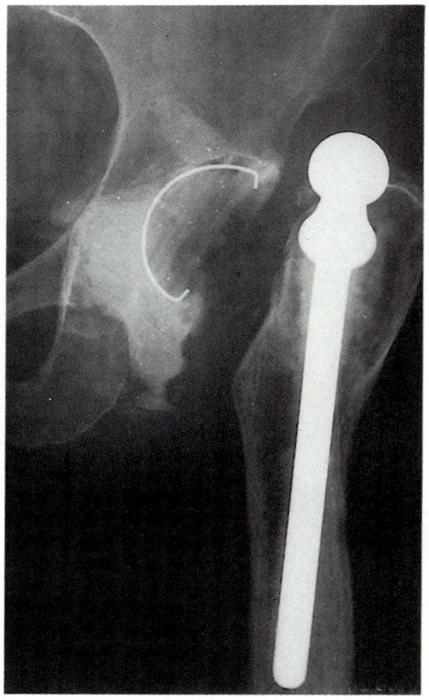

868 & **869** Dislocation of the prosthesis may occur early or late. Early dislocation is usually due to malposition of the leg in the early post operative-period. After reduction progress may subsequently be uneventful. Late and recurrent dislocations are a problem and usually there are other factors involved such as malposition of components (in **869** the cup is too vertical) or trochanteric detachment.

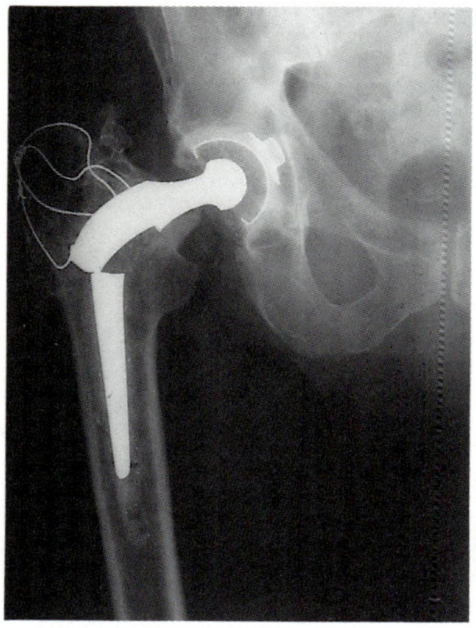

870 Fatigue fracture of components is now less common with improvements in implant composition.

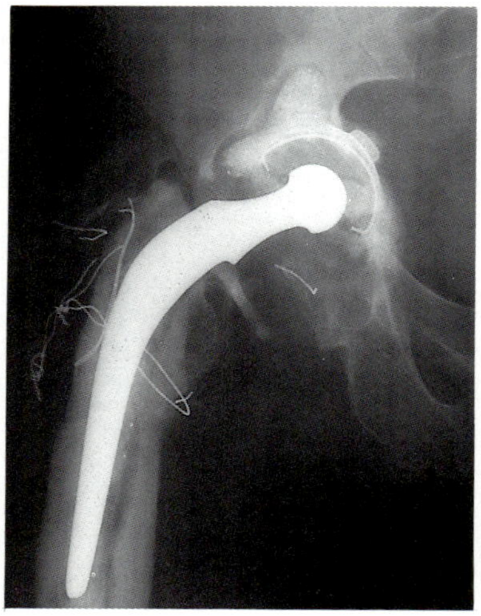

871 Loosening and migration of components may occur mechanically or as a result of infection.

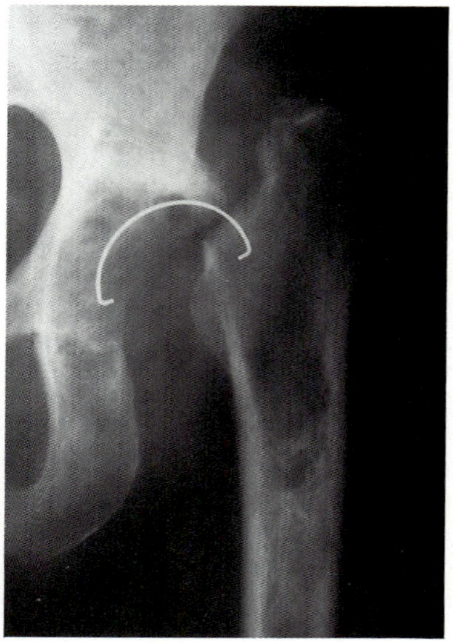

872 An excision arthroplasty may be the ultimate salvage procedure.

Knee joint

Rotational abnormalities of the lower limbs are chiefly due to the angle of anteversion of the femoral necks. In the foetus the femoral necks point almost directly forwards at 90°; by the time of birth the anteversion is 25–30° and in adult life 16–18°. Persistence of excessive anteversion of the femoral necks (PFA) is the usual cause of rotational deformity of the lower limbs.

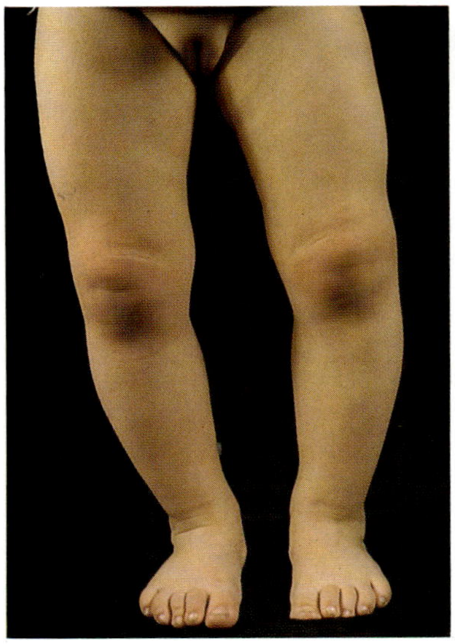

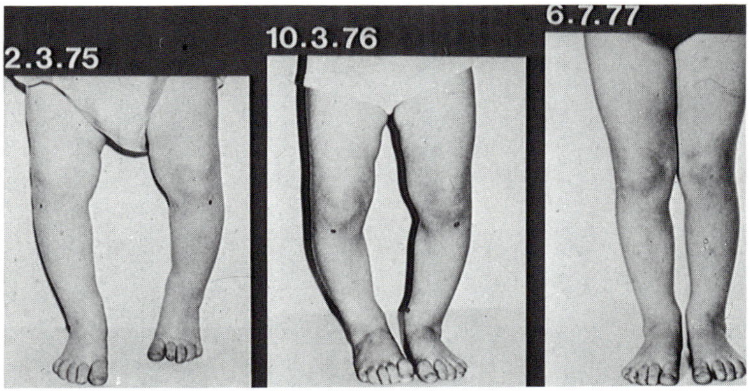

873 & **874** Genu varum. Physiological bow legs in a 2-year-old infant. Note the symmetry of the bowing. It is almost always due to transient abnormalities of rotation of the lower limbs. Bow legs under the age of 3 years are usually physiological and self-correcting.

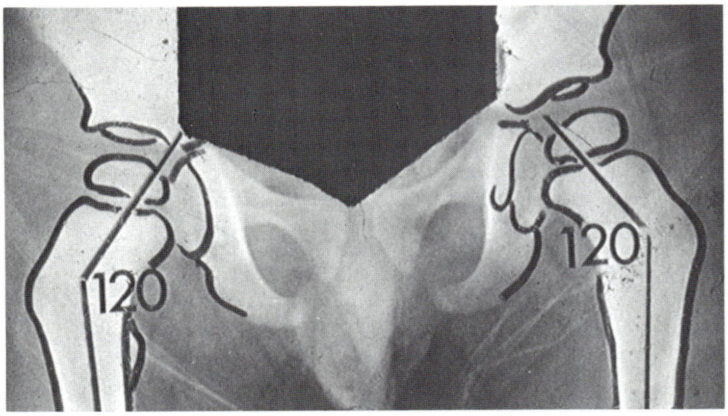

875 Normal neck-shaft angle of the upper end of the femora.

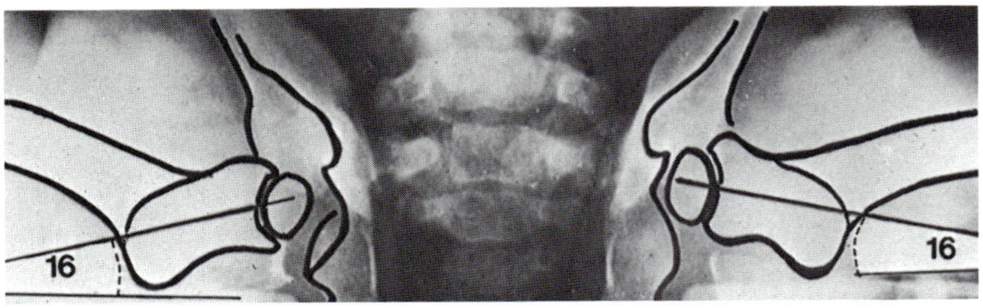

876 Normal anteversion angle of the femoral necks.

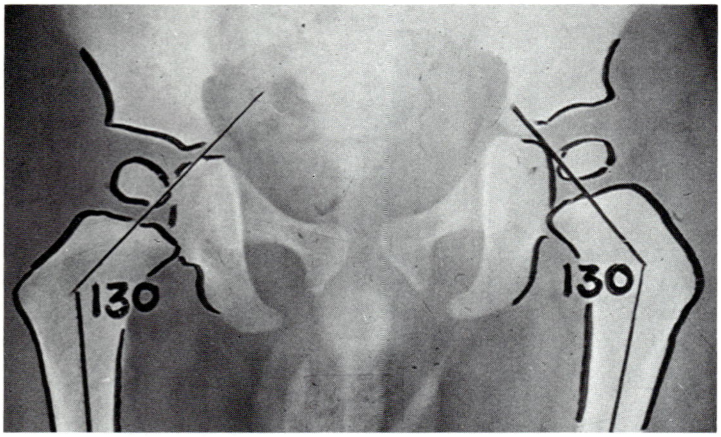

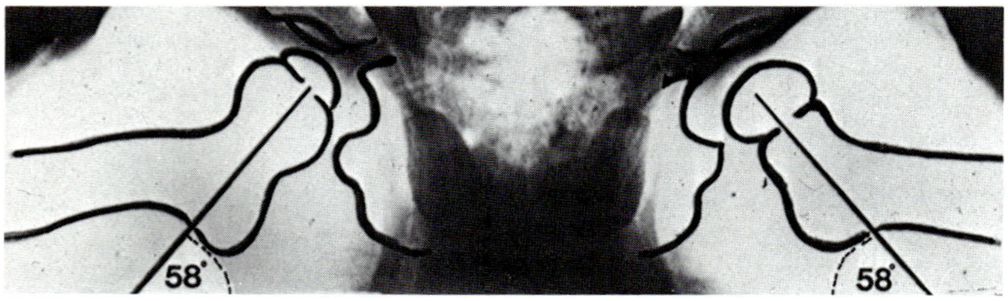

877 & **878** Although the anteroposterior view shows a neck-shaft angle within the normal range, the special projection lateral view shows that the degree of anteversion of the femoral neck is in considerable excess of the normal.

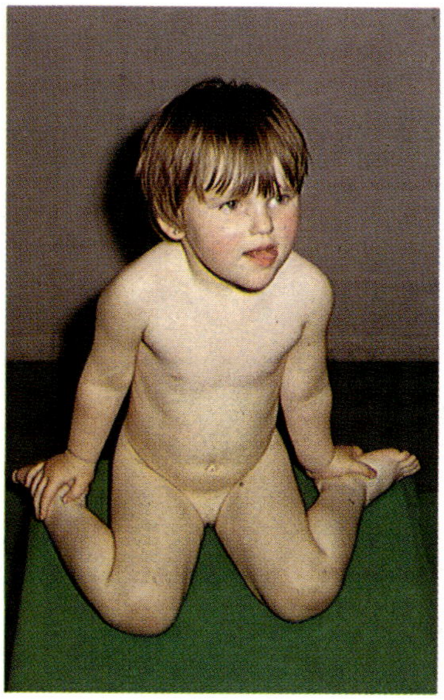

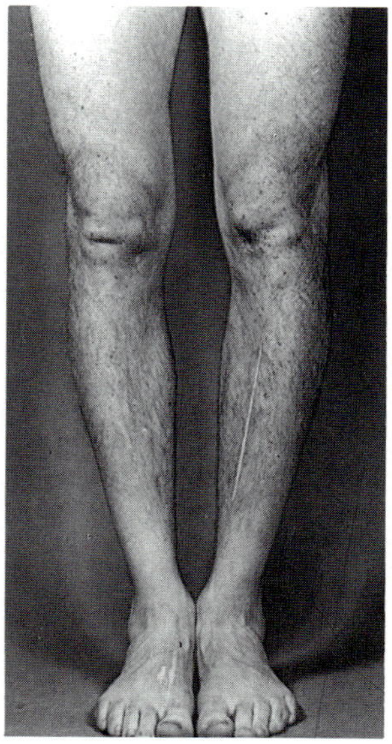

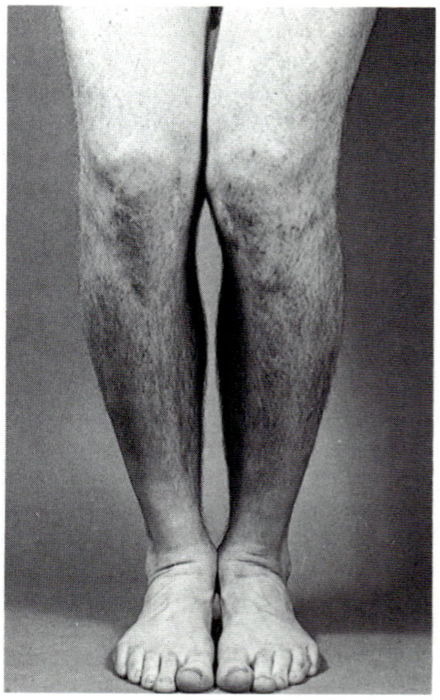

879 Persistent femoral anteversion. Children often elect to sit in this 'television position', comfortably relocating their hips.

880 & **881** Apparent bow legs: this young man has apparent symmetrical bowing of his legs. When he slightly rotates his hips inwards, the apparent bowing disappears. It is caused by persistent femoral anteversion.

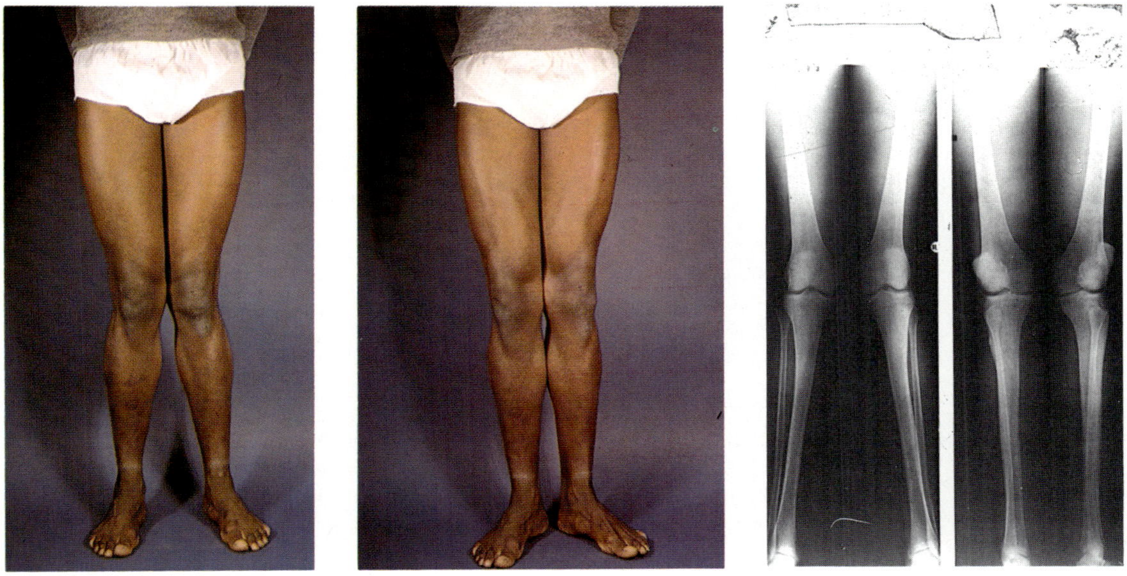

882–884 Apparent knock-knees: This young man's deformity disappears when he simply rotates his hips outwards. Note the position of the patellae. His knock-knees are due to an abnormality of anteversion of the femoral necks. In his case it is diminished.

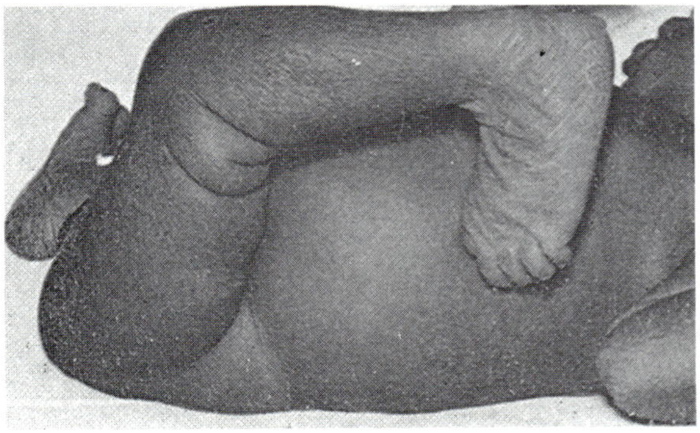

885 Congenital genu recurvatum. This deformity is due to the abnormal intrauterine posture of a basically normal limb. The prognosis after treatment is therefore very good.

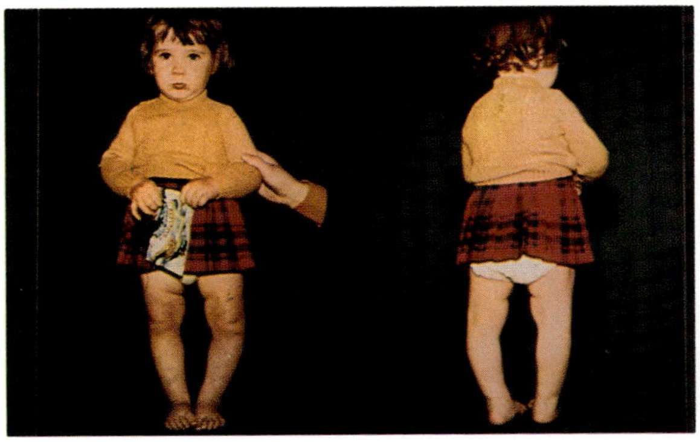

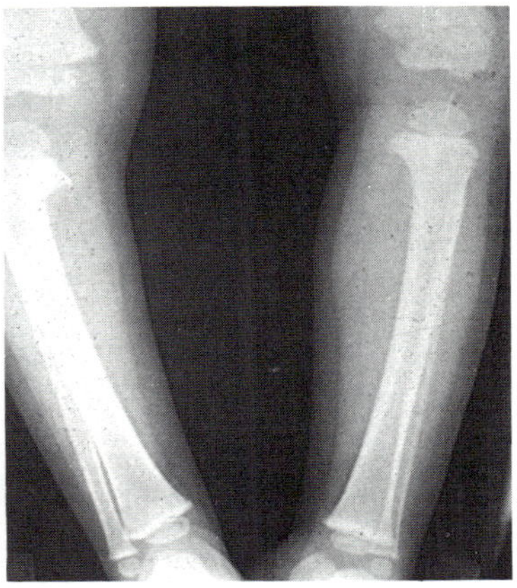

886 & **887** Tibia vara. A very small number of children have bow legs which persist. They are usually children who have walked very early and the bowing is usually not symmetrical. One leg is obviously more affected than the other. Distinctive 'beaking' on the medial side of the proximal tibial growth plates is apparent.

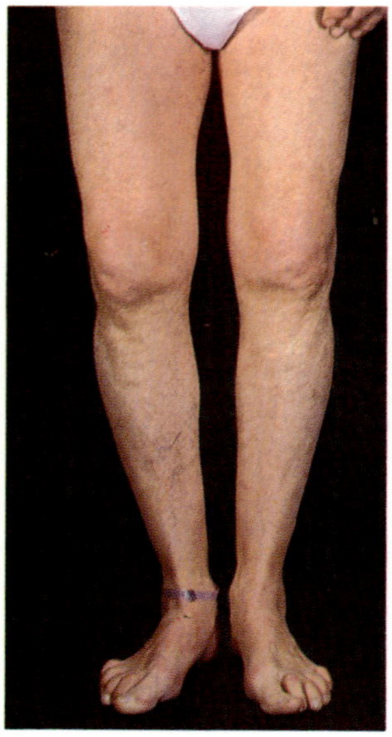

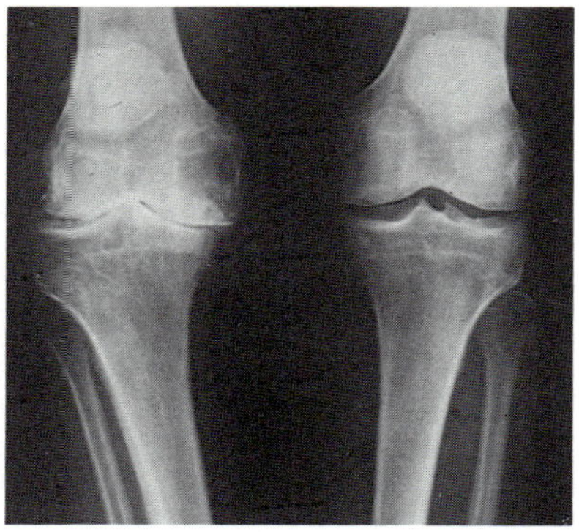

888 & **889** Genu varum in the adult. This man had straight legs and developed genu varum in middle age. The condition is unilateral. There is a history of a football injury 20 years previously causing degenerative arthritis, affecting principally the medial compartment of the right knee – almost certainly secondary to an old meniscus injury.

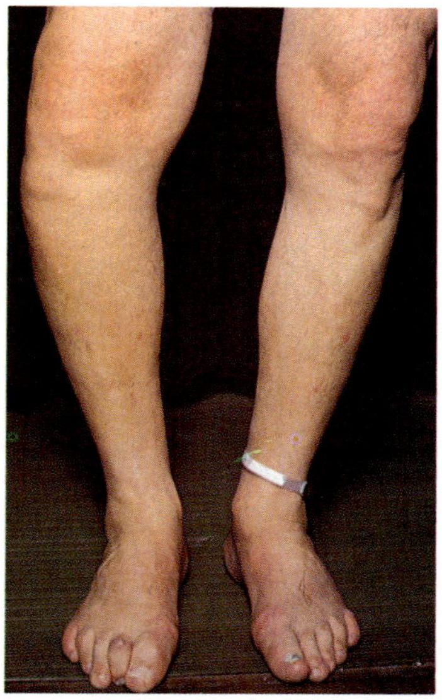

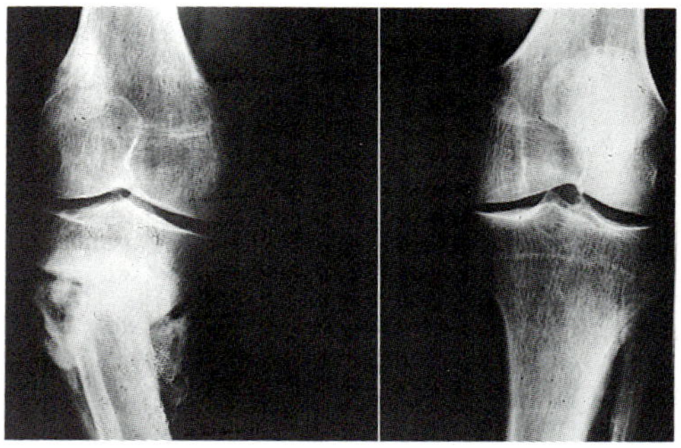

890 & **891** Post-traumatic genu varum following a major injury 1 year previously. The deformity is due to a malunited fracture of the upper end of the tibia and fibula.

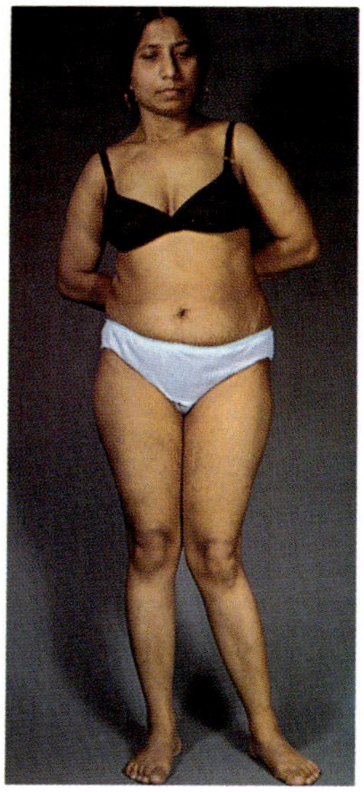

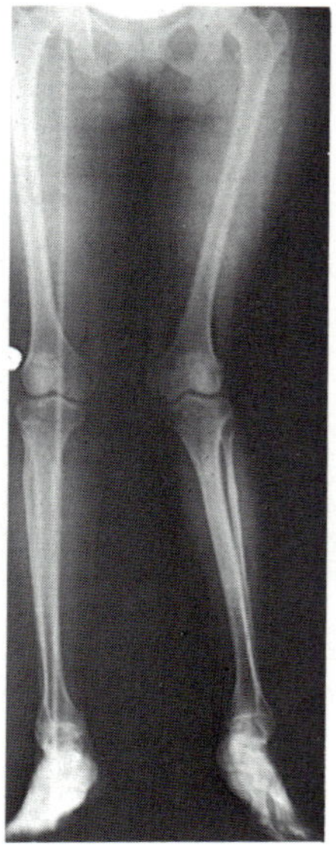

892 & **893** Unilateral genu valgum. No history of injury could be recalled, but the premature arrest on the lateral side of the upper tibial growth plate was almost certainly caused by trivial injury.

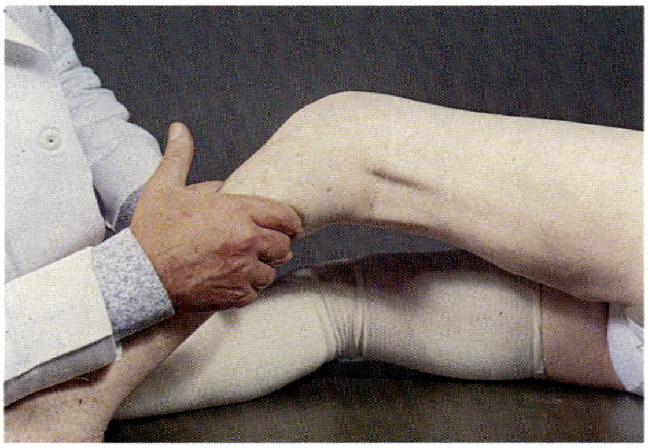

894–897 'Frame' knee. This is now rarely seen as a complication of the treatment of tuberculosis of the hip on an abduction frame. There is general ligamentous laxity, and there may be premature epiphyseal arrest.

894 Anterior cruciate laxity indicated by the 'anterior draw sign'.

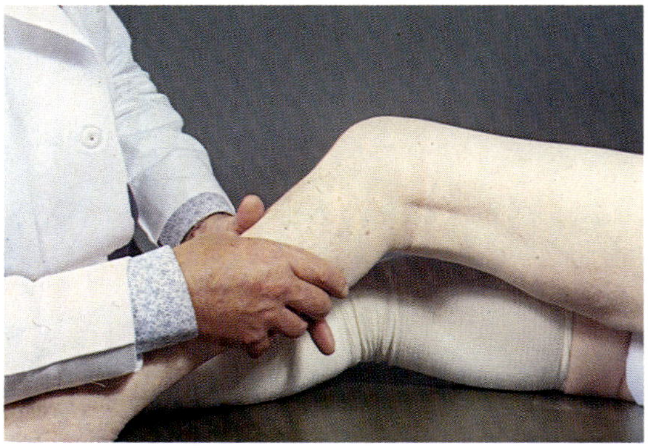

895 Posterior cruciate ligament laxity indicated by the 'posterior draw sign'.

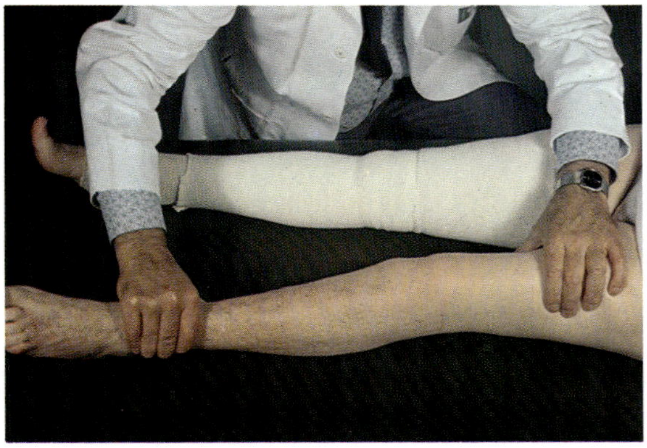

896 There is laxity of the lateral ligament and joint capsule so that the extended knee can be forced passively into varus.

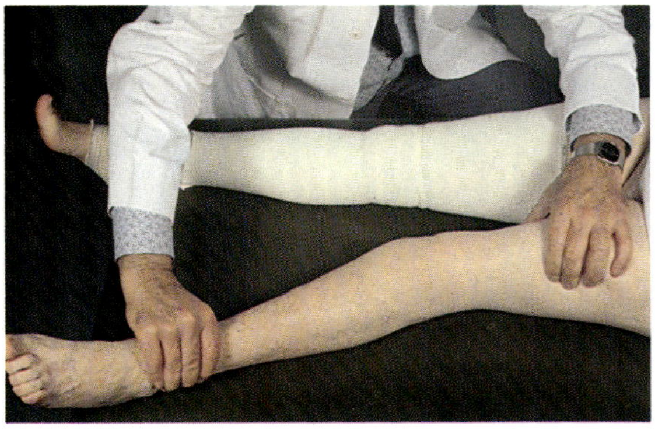

897 There is laxity of the medial ligament and joint capsule so that the knee can be passively forced into valgus.

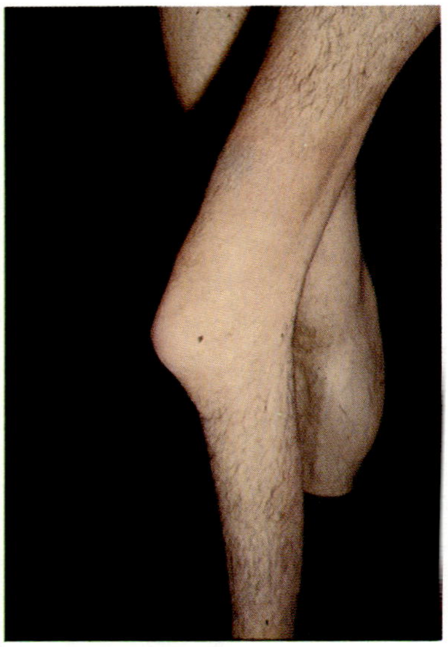

898 'Triple deformity' of the knee is seen as a consequence of muscle imbalance. It may follow poliomyelitis in childhood. The three deformities are posterior subluxation, external rotation and valgus.

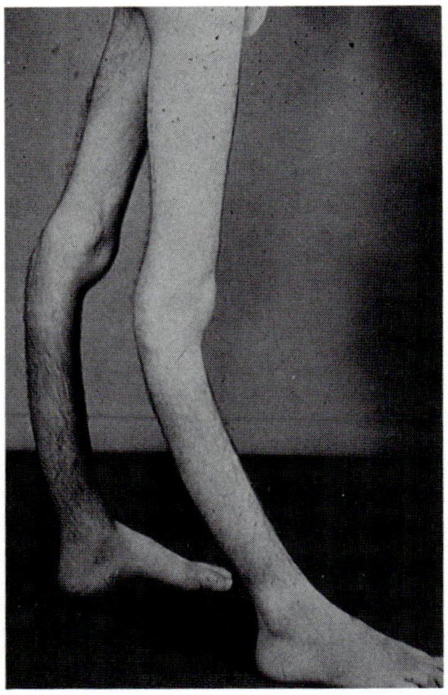

899 Genu recurvatum. This young man had an attack of poliomyelitis in infancy. Despite the excessive extension of the knees, both quadriceps muscles are paralysed. He was able to stand with the knees locked back passively for stability. The deformity is of considerable advantage to the patient. It is either functionally acquired, or deliberately produced by surgery.

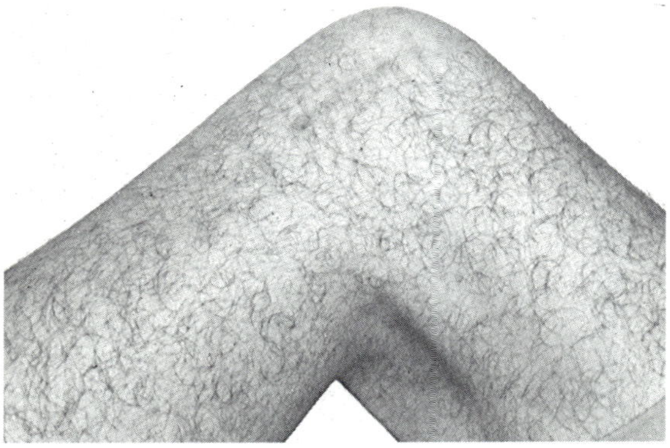

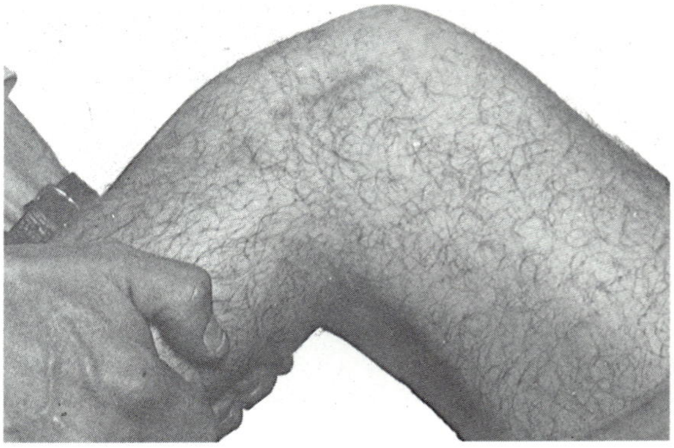

900 & **901** Chronic rupture of the anterior cruciate ligament of the knee. There is no abnormality seen with the knee in flexion at rest. The 'anterior draw sign' is markedly positive.

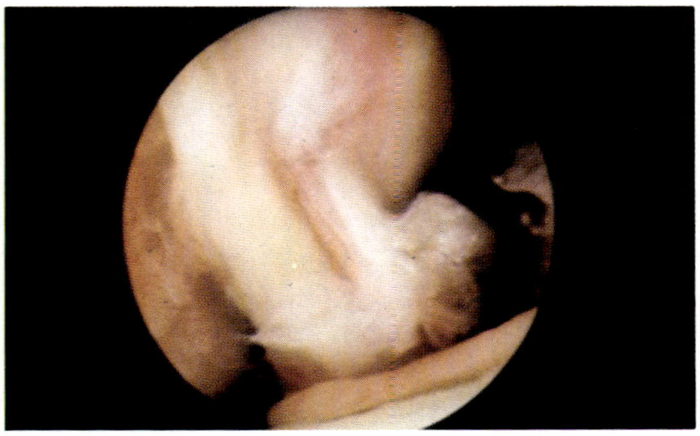

902 Disruption of the anterior cruciate ligament is seen on arthroscopy.

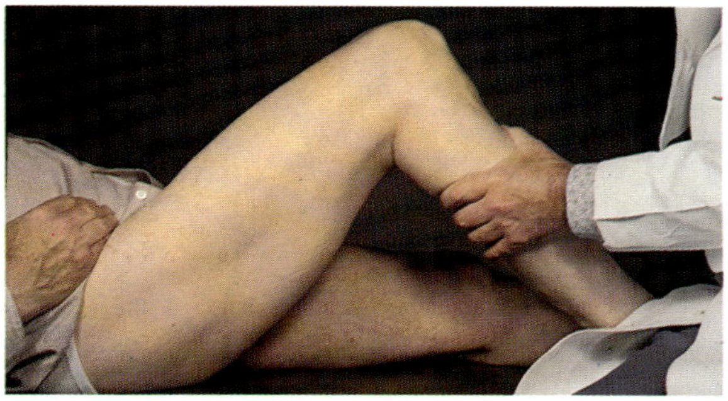

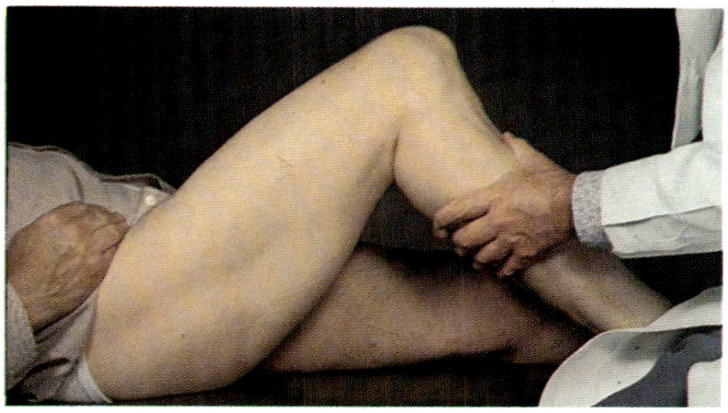

903 & **904** Chronic rupture of the posterior cruciate ligament. At rest in flexion the upper end of the tibia is subluxated backwards on the femur. The subluxation is passively increased by backward pressure.

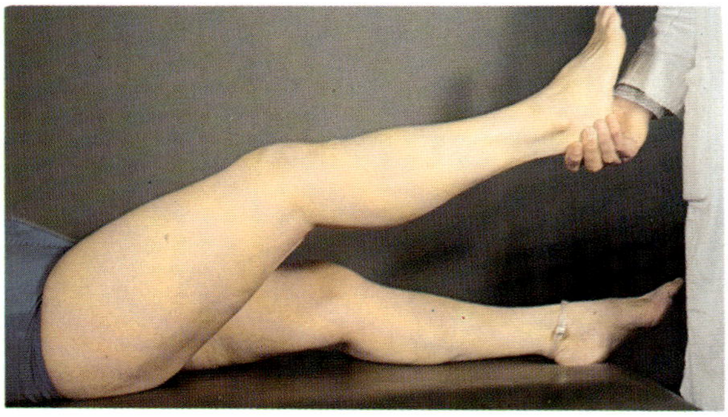

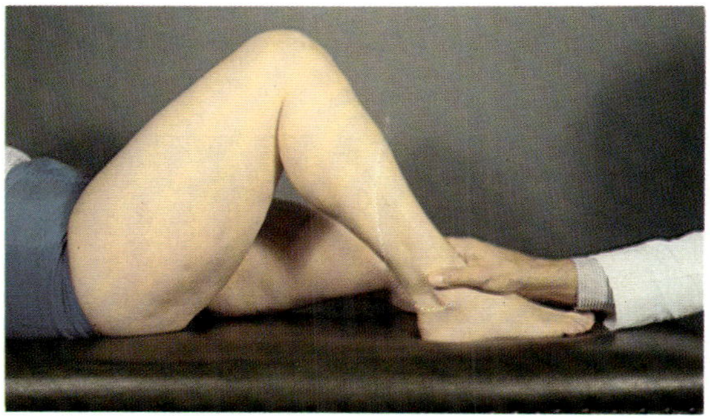

905 & **906** 'Locked knee'. This term is used to imply lack of normal extension of the knee following injury. With the leg hanging fully dependent on the examiner's hand, the knee stops some 20° short of full extension. It should be compared with the opposite side. The knee is not truly locked because a good range of flexion remains. The locked knee may be due to a loose body, but it is usually caused by injury to one or other meniscus.

907

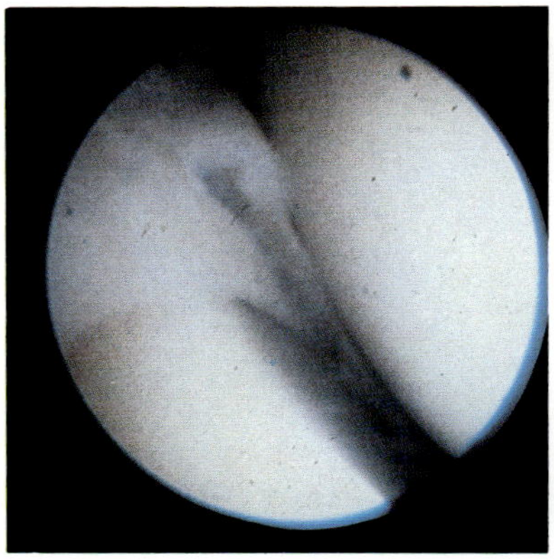

908

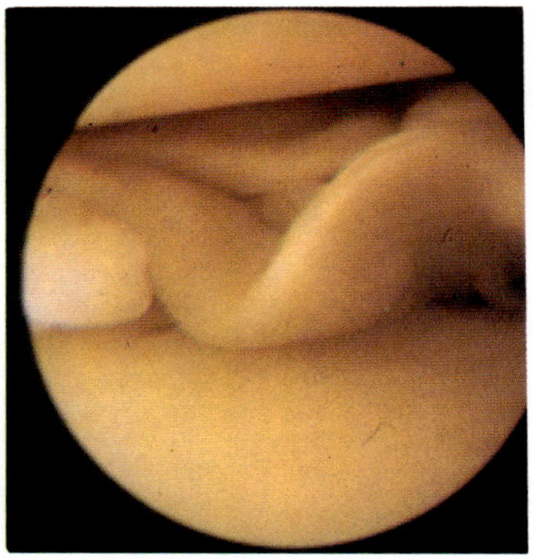

909

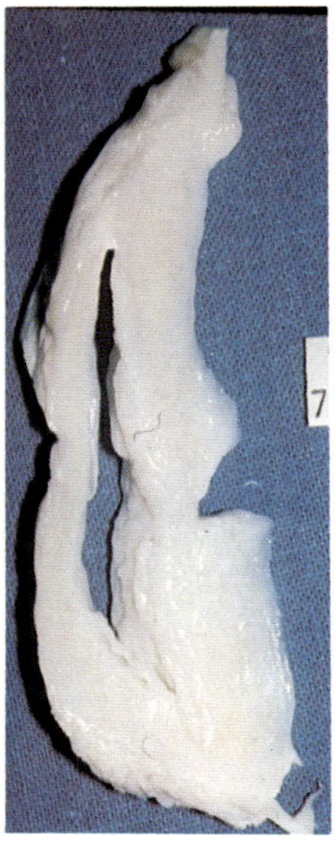

907–909 Ruptured medial meniscus. The arthroscopic examination is seen in **907** and **908**, and the operative specimen, a bucket-handle rupture, in **909**.

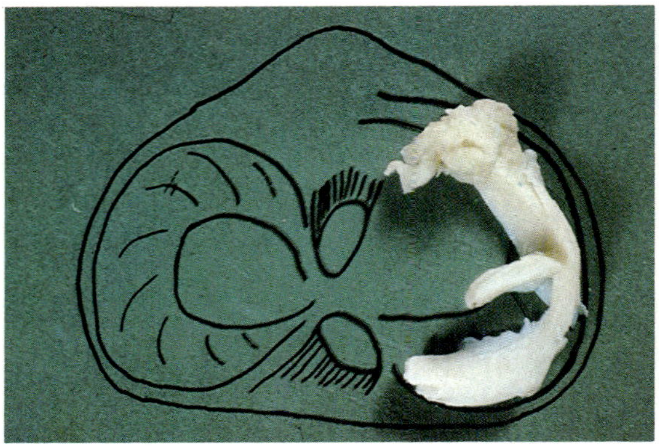

910 Ruptured medial meniscus, showing a posterior tag, one of the common varieties of medial meniscus rupture.

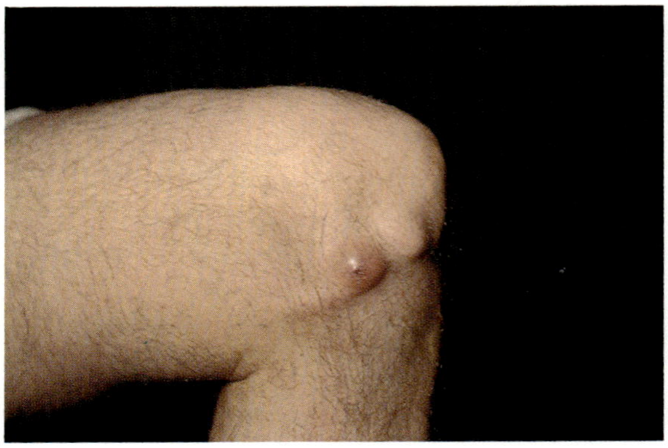

911 Multilocular cyst. Two soft swellings on the medial aspect of this man's left knee. They cause minimal pain and little impairment of function.

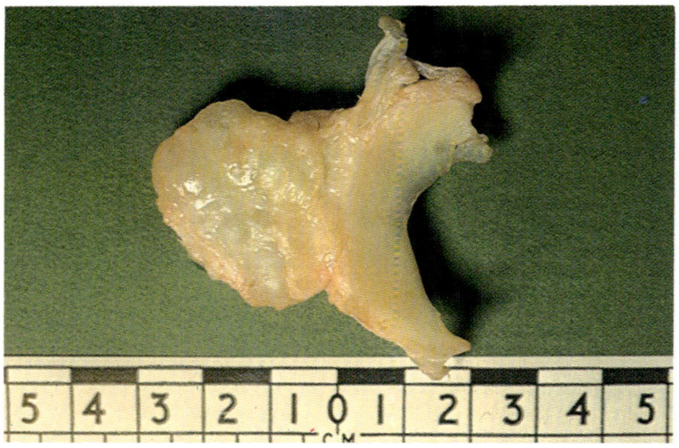

912 Multilocular cyst. Operative specimen arising from the perimeter of the medial meniscus.

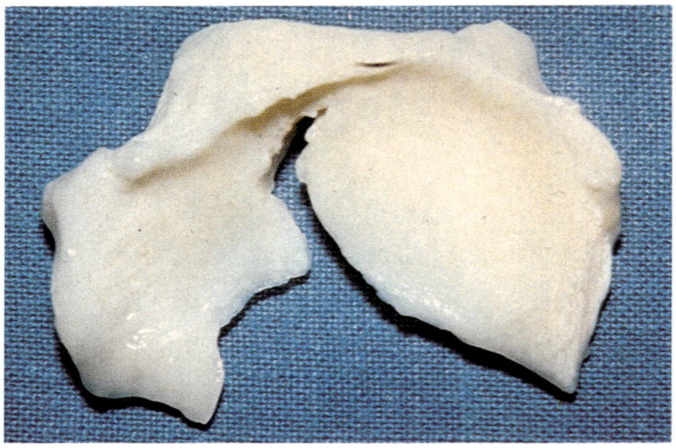

913 Rupture of lateral meniscus. This more often ruptures transversely. The pattern of such a transverse rupture can be structured like a parrot's beak.

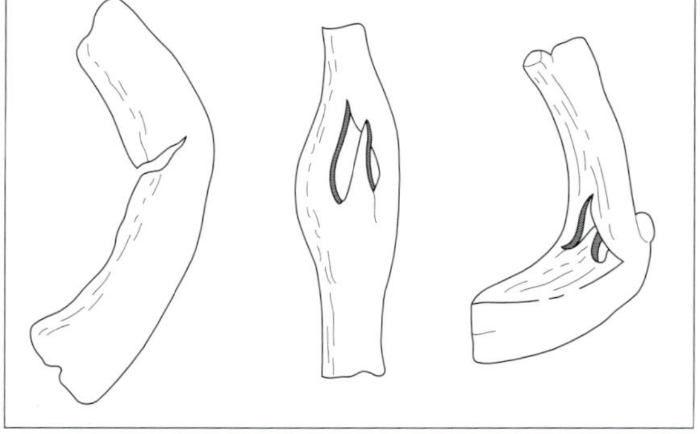

914 'Parrot-beak' rupture of the ateral meniscus.

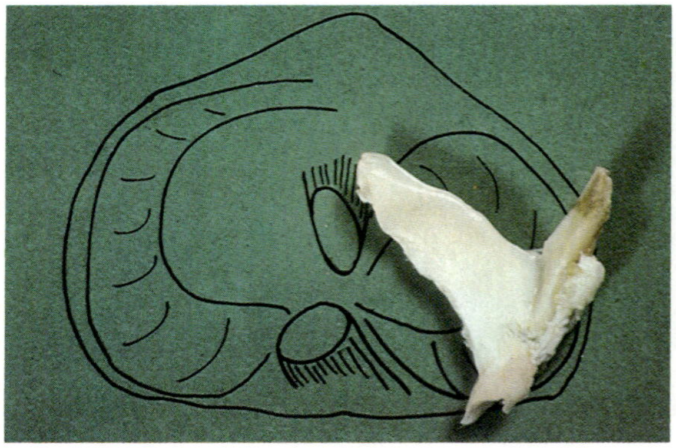

915 Another pattern of rupture of lateral meniscus causing locking of the knee.

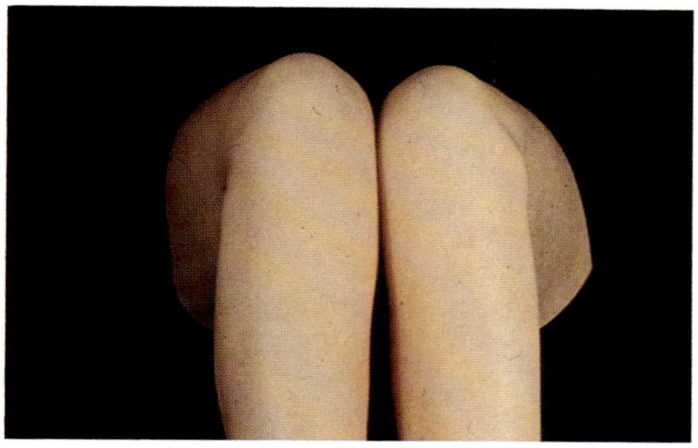

916–919 Cyst of the lateral meniscus. This is at least six times more common than a cyst of the medial meniscus. There is often a history of previous injury.

916 A small lateral meniscus cyst can best be seen with the knee in the semiflexed position.

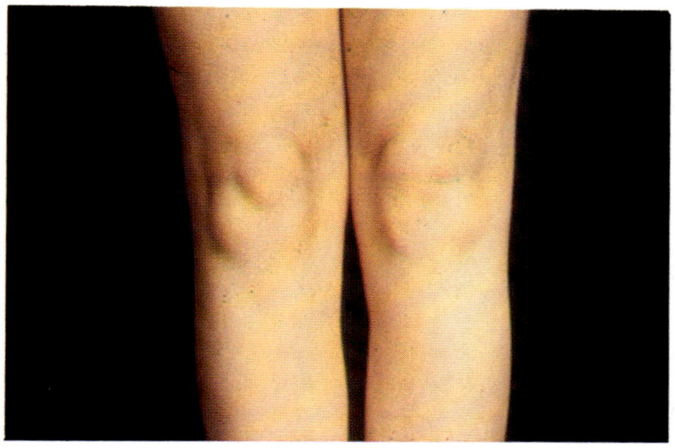

917 When the knee is straight the swelling cannot be seen.

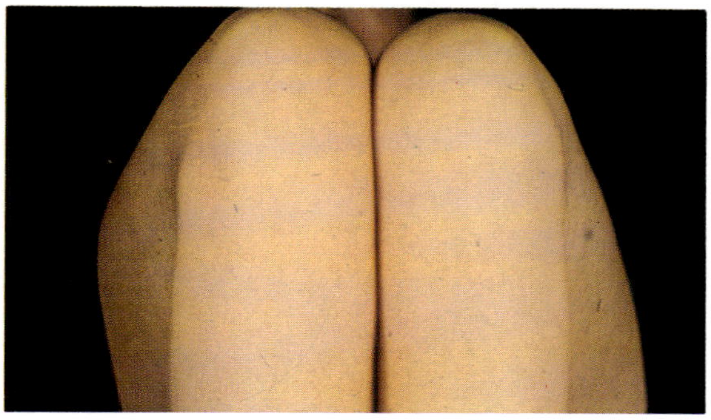

918 When the knee is fully flexed the swelling cannot be seen.

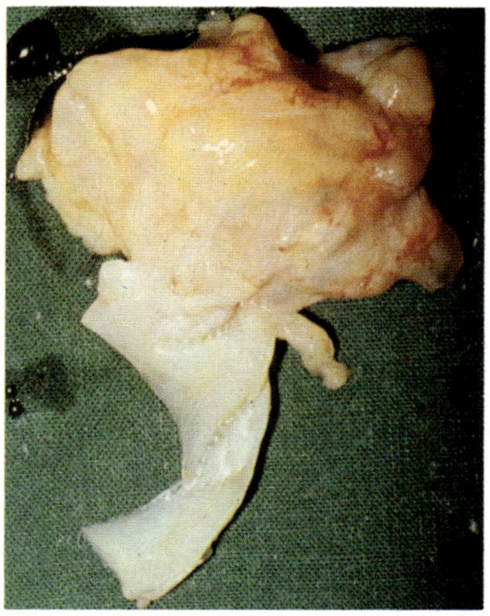

919 The lateral meniscus removed with its attached cyst.

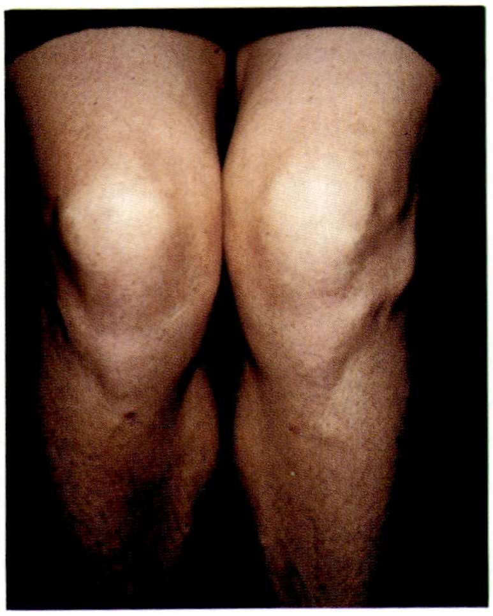

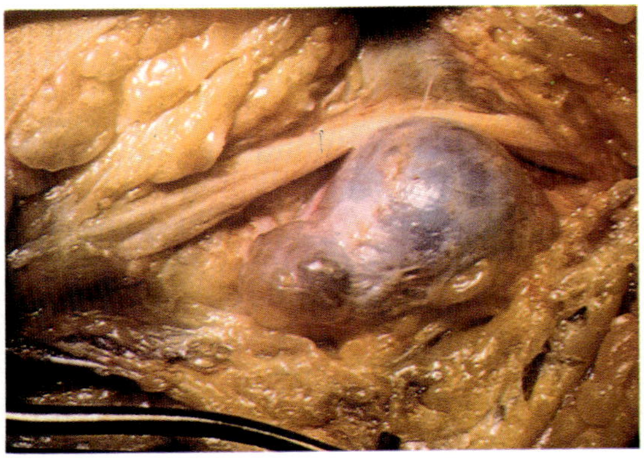

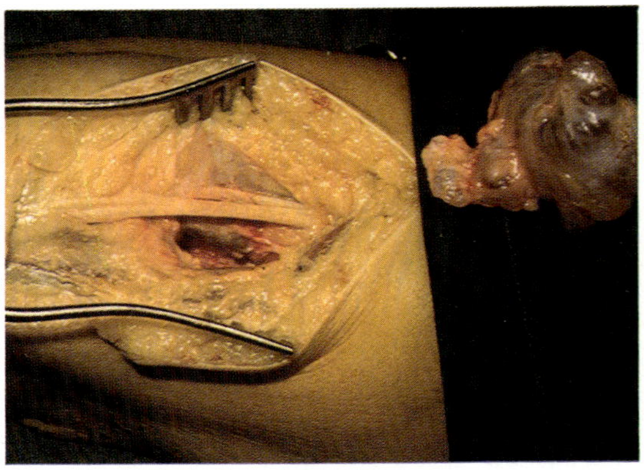

920–922 Multilocular ganglion. Swelling on the outer aspect of the left knee which does not disappear on full extension and flexion may be due to a ganglion arising from the superior tibiofibular joint. A multilocular ganglion is seen in close association with the common peroneal nerve.

922 The ganglion is dissected free from the nerve.

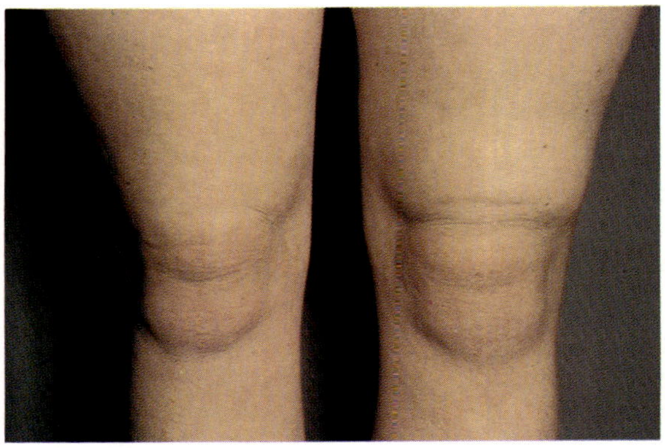

923 Rupture of the quadriceps muscle. This may occur after a trivial injury as the final insult in a degenerate tendon. It has been described as the presenting symptom in a patient suffering from diabetes or, classically, tabes dorsalis.

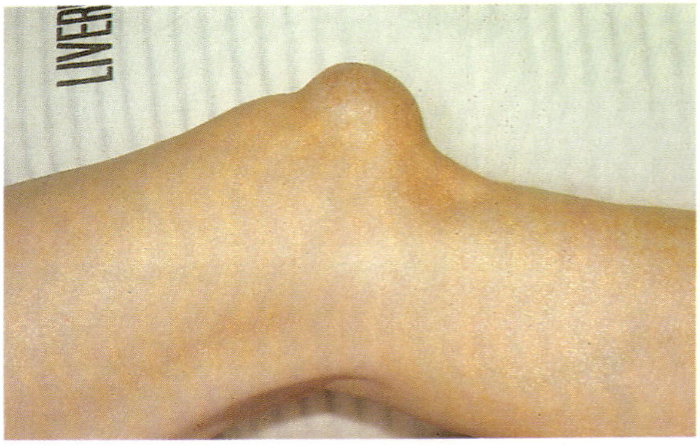

924 Prepatellar bursitis. Swelling of the prepatellar bursa may be caused by occupational pressure from constant kneeling; inflammation can arise from minor trauma to the front of the knee or from inflammatory diseases such as rheumatoid arthritis.

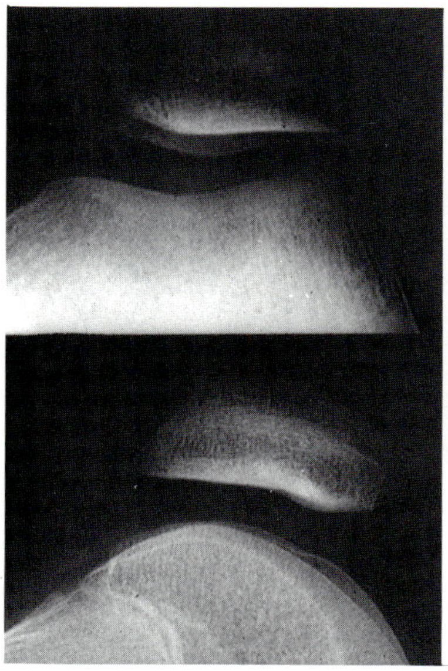

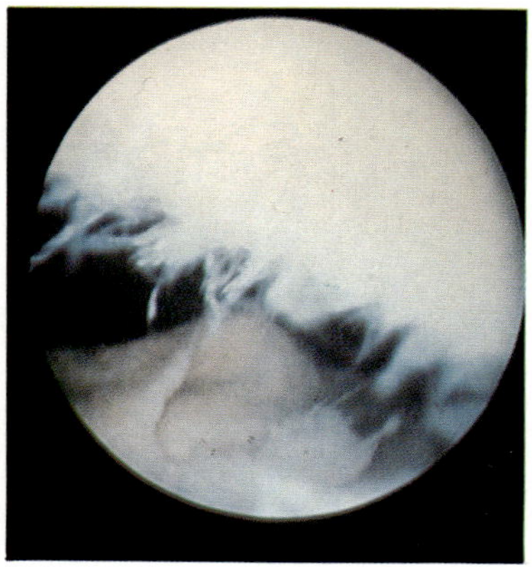

926 Fibrillation of articular cartilage seen through an arthroscope. Occasionally, the condition becomes progressive and unequal pressures upon the articular cartilage of the patella produces pathological changes.

925 Chondromalacia patellae. Patellofemoral pain is a very common symptom, particularly in adolescent girls. It is probably caused by transient malalignment of the extensor mechanism at the knee resulting in unequal pressure on the patellar facets.

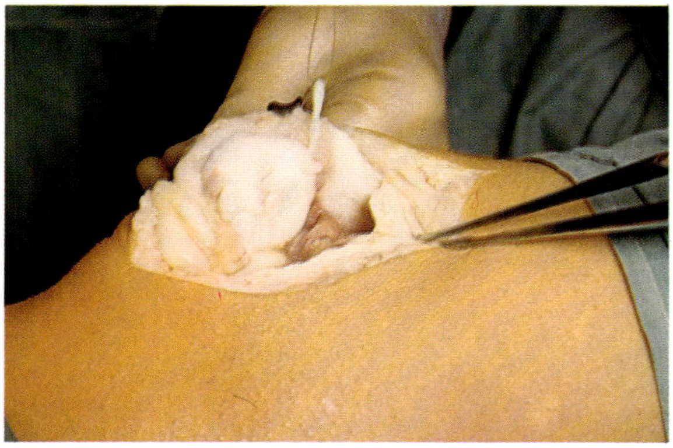

927 Condition of the patella seen at operation.

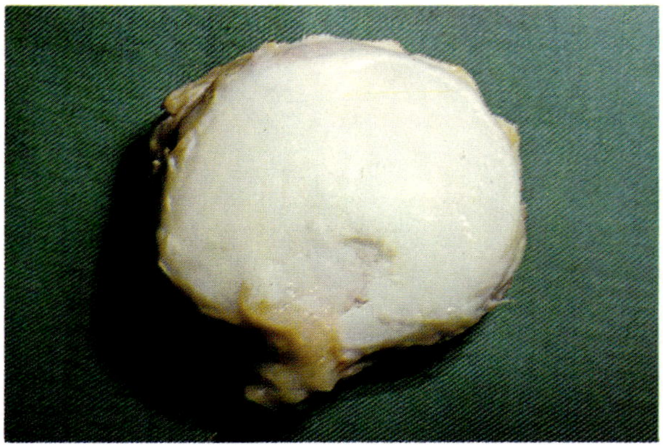

928 The lesion is initially almost entirely confined to one facet – usually the lateral.

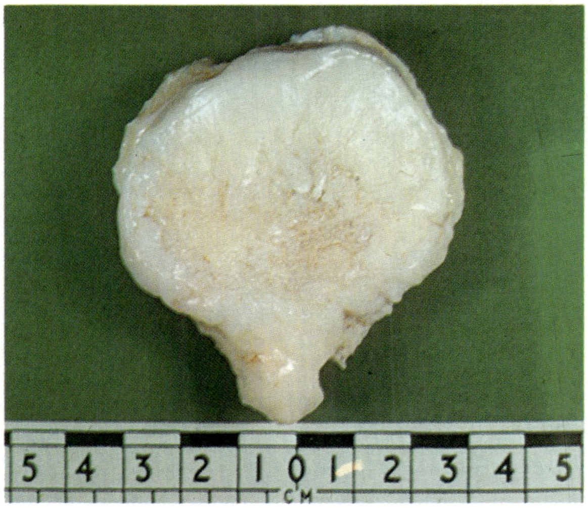

929 The entire articular surface of the patella has become involved in this more advanced case.

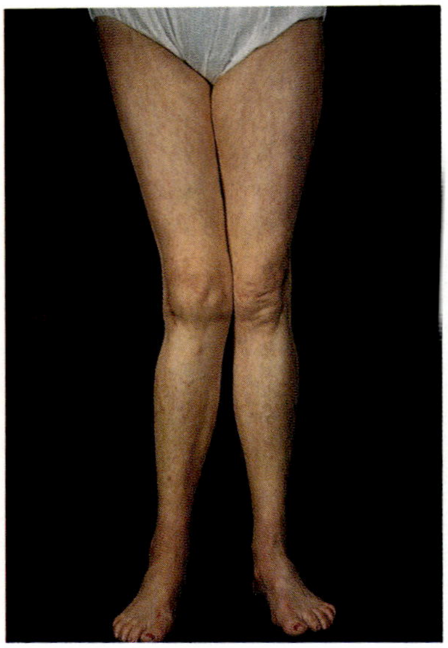

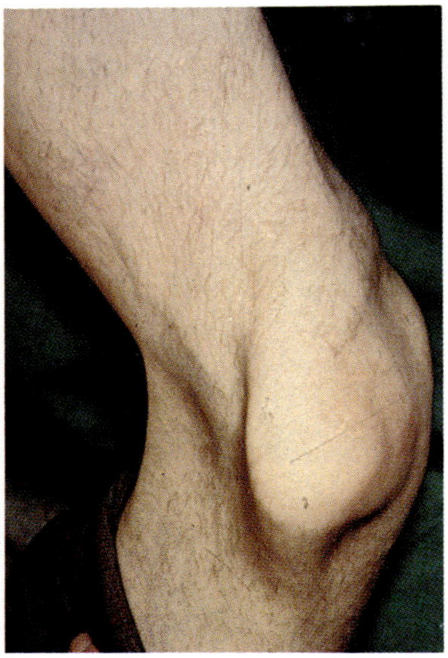

930 & **931** Patellar instability. Post-traumatic unilateral genu valgum in a young girl leads to malalignment of the extensor mechanism and lateral instability of the patella. Recurrent dislocation of patella occurred.

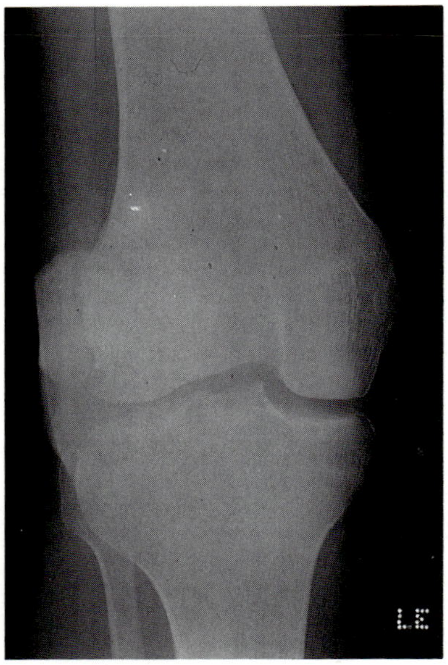

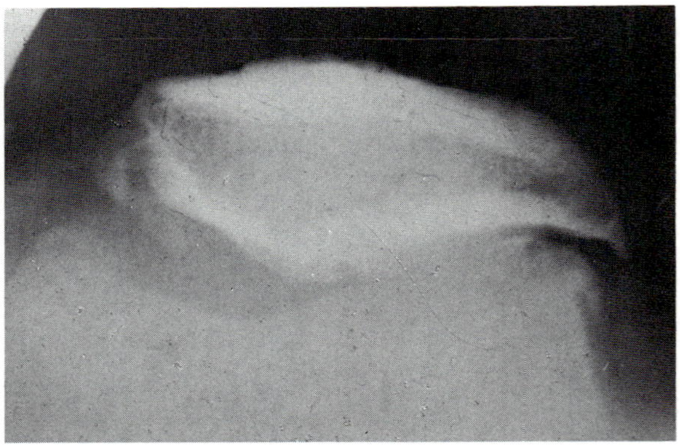

932 & **933** Radiograph taken at the time of dislocation. An anteroposterior radiograph shows the lateral dislocation. The skyline view shows degenerative changes in the patellofemoral joint, affecting principally the lateral facet. Such changes are seen either as the end result of chondromalacia patellae, or after recurrent dislocation of the patella.

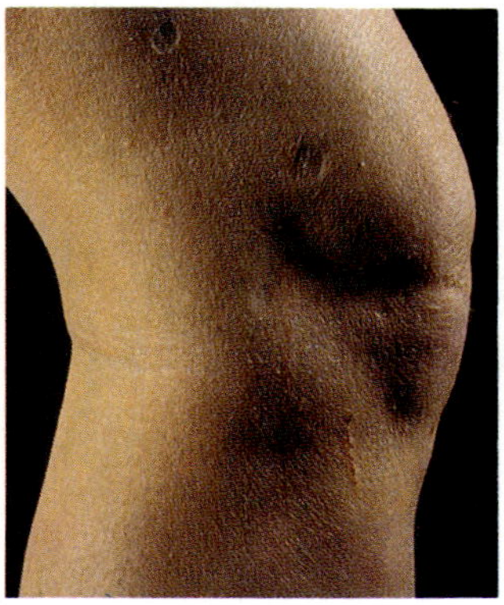

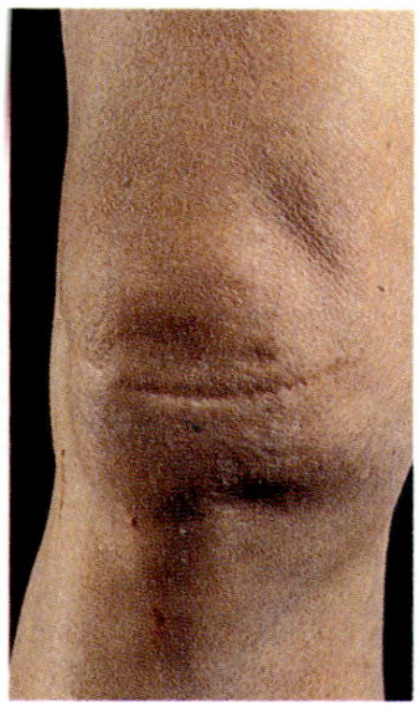

934 & **935** Excision of the patella. Note the virtually normal appearance of the knee except for the scar. Patients are often unnecessarily concerned by the prospect of disfigurement from this operation.

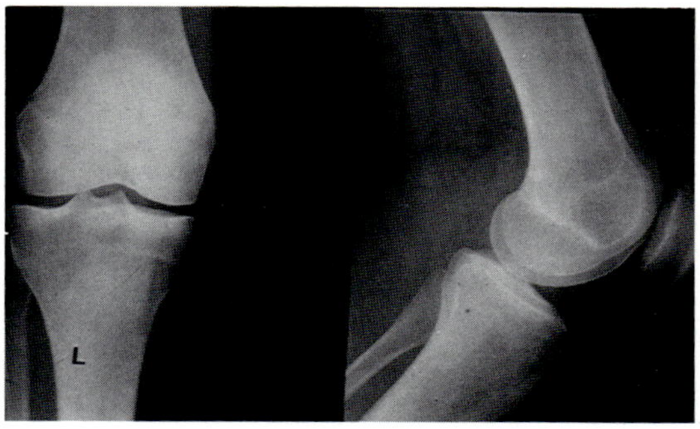

936 Synovial chondromatosis. The knees of a young man suffering from pain, swelling and repeated locking of the knee in which radiographs appear normal.

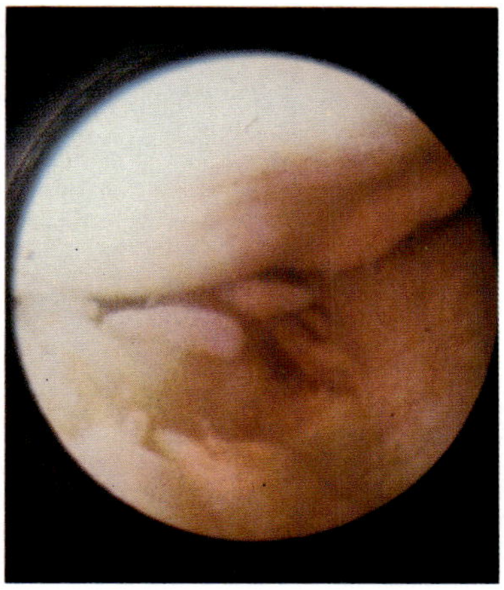

937 At arthroscopy multiple cartilaginous loose bodies can be seen.

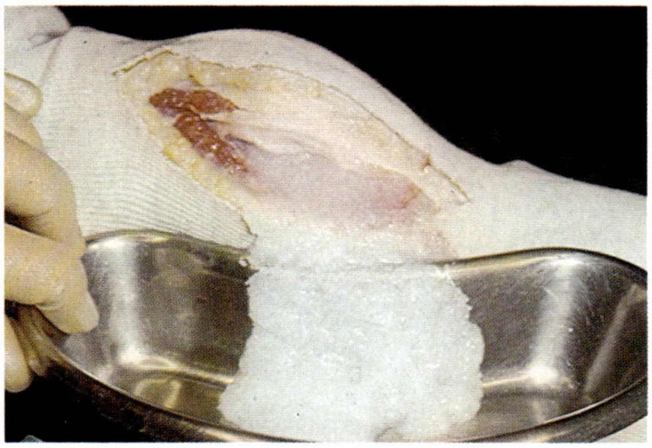

938 A large number of chondromata are removed at operation.

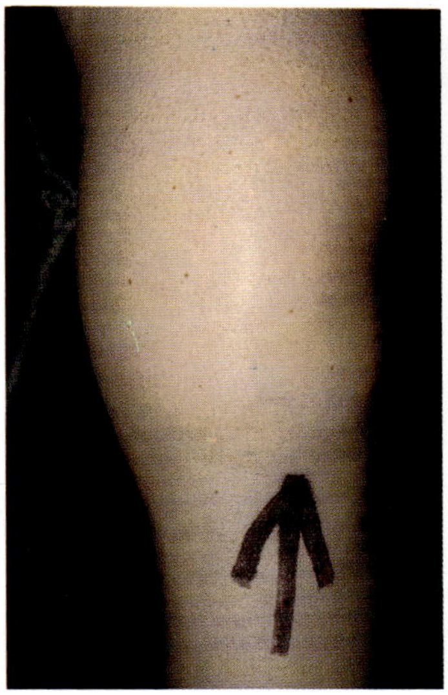

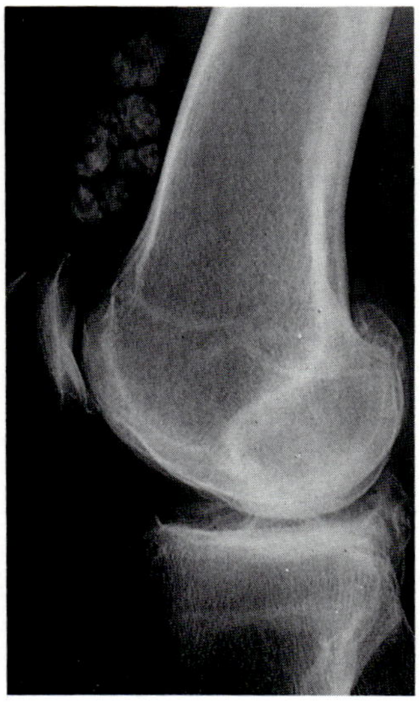

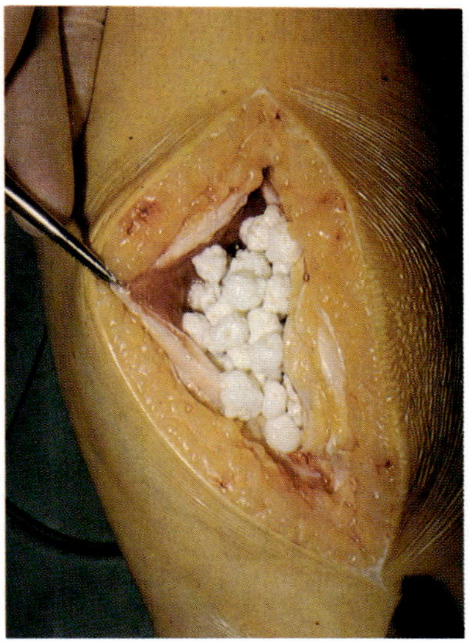

939–941 A gradual swelling of the knee developed in this patient. The radiograph revealed multiple chrondromata. This is probably the same condition at a later stage, when bone forms in several of the cartilage nodules.

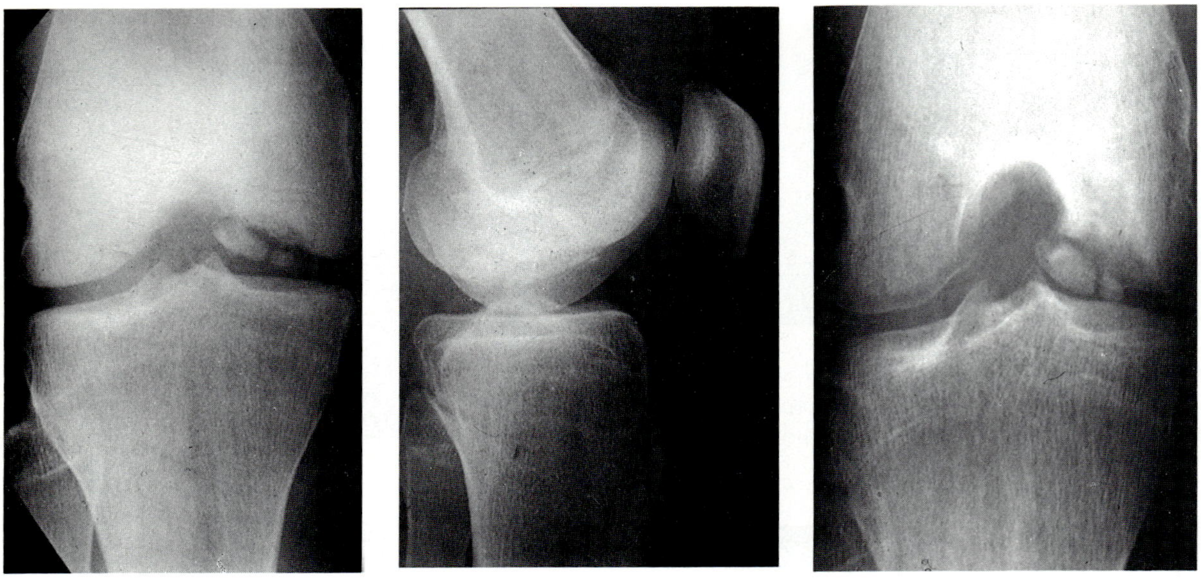

942–944 Osteochrondritis dissecans. This condition may occur in several joints, but by far the commonest site is the medial femoral condyle. Its aetiology is undefined. The lesion can be seen in the anteroposterior and lateral views but the extent of the lesion is best seen in the 'tunnel' view.

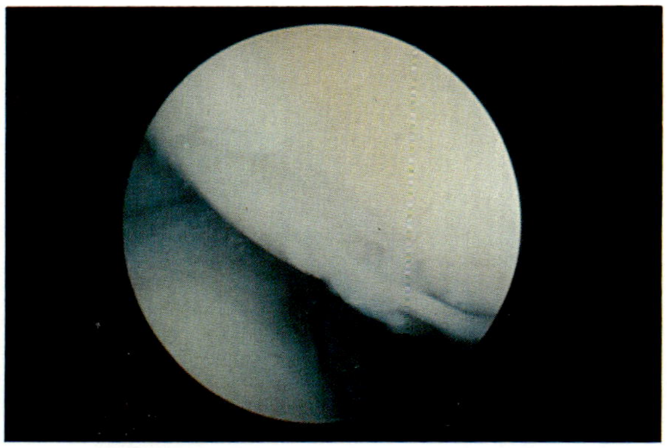

945 Osteochondritis dissecans seen through the arthroscope.

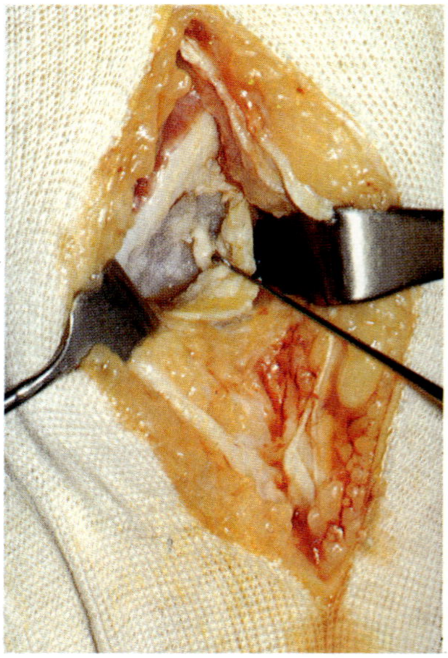

946 At operation the articular cartilage is seen to be separated with a minimal layer of subchondral bone and is eventually shed into the joint as a 'classical loose body'.

Ankle and foot

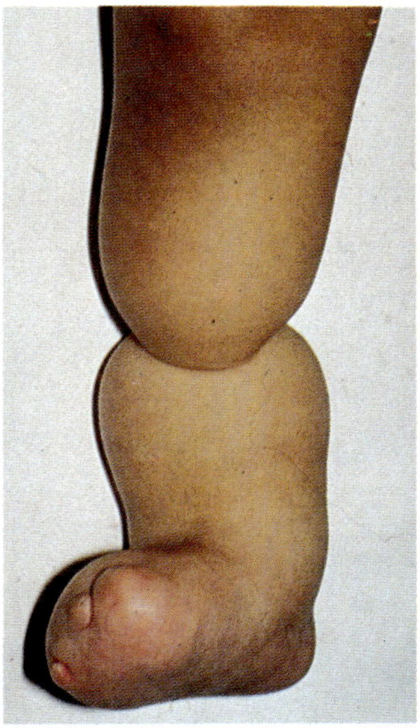

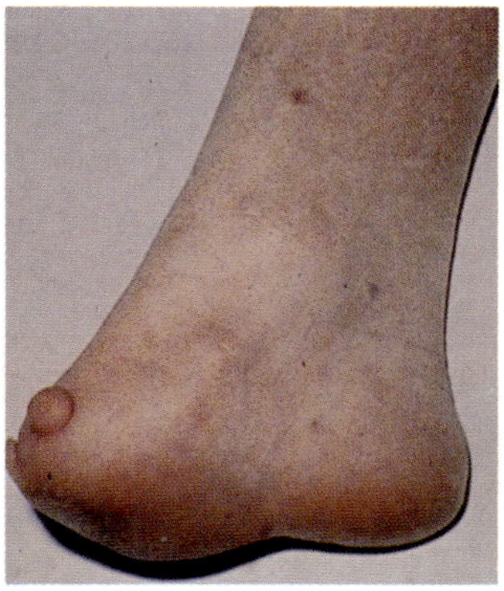

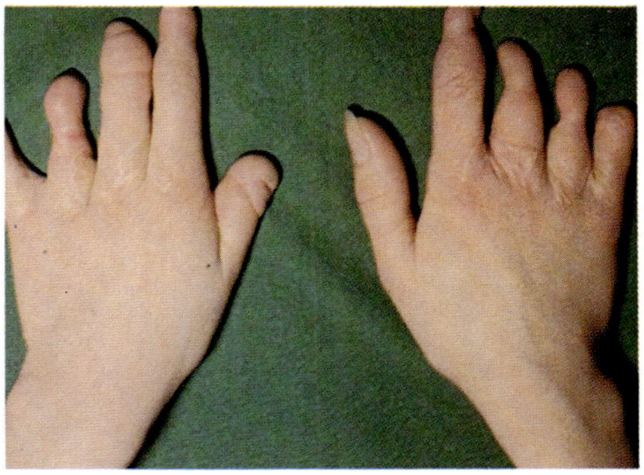

948 & **949** Congenital amputation of the forefoot. The fact this is not caused by a constriction ring is evidenced by the associated abnormalities of the hands. The aetiology is unknown.

947 Congenital constriction ring. Here constriction has prejudiced the normal development of the limb distal to it.

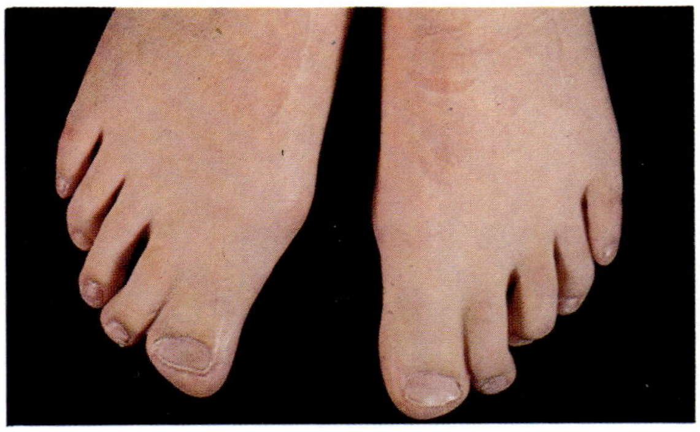

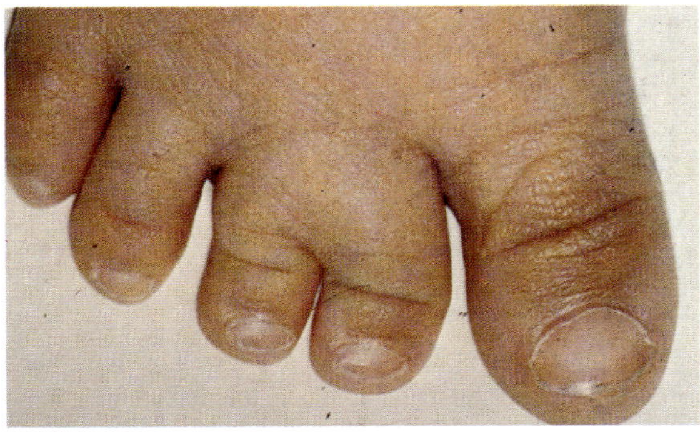

950 & **951** Syndactylism. Many varieties of syndactyly occur, varying from isolated fusion of two toes to widespread fusion of several digits of hand and foot.

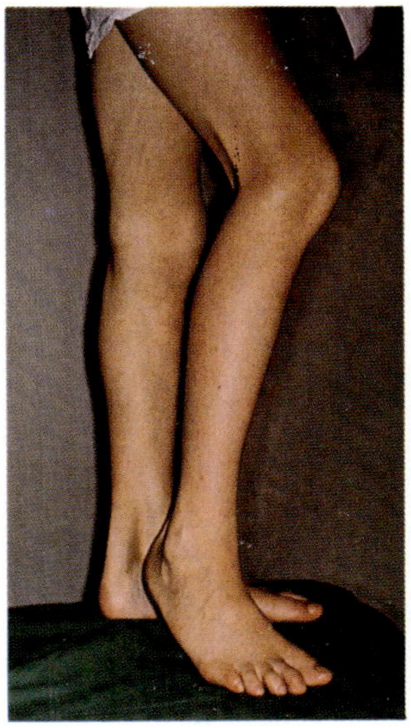

952 Congenital contracture of the calf. Of the many causes of calf muscle shortening, possibly the least common is a simple congenital contracture of the calf muscle which can be bilateral. There are no associated abnormalities, and no cause is discernible.

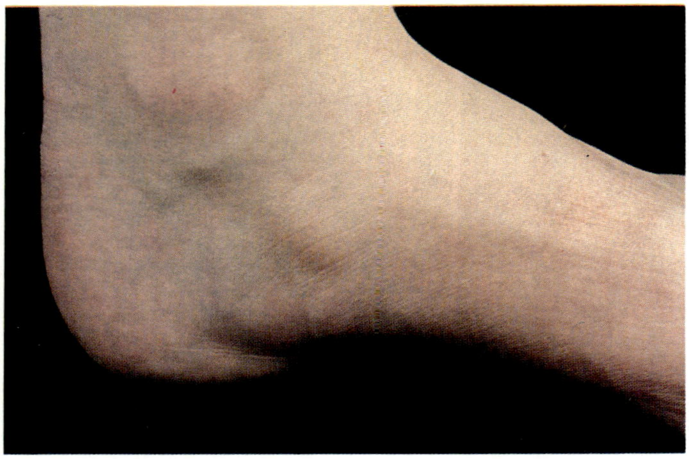
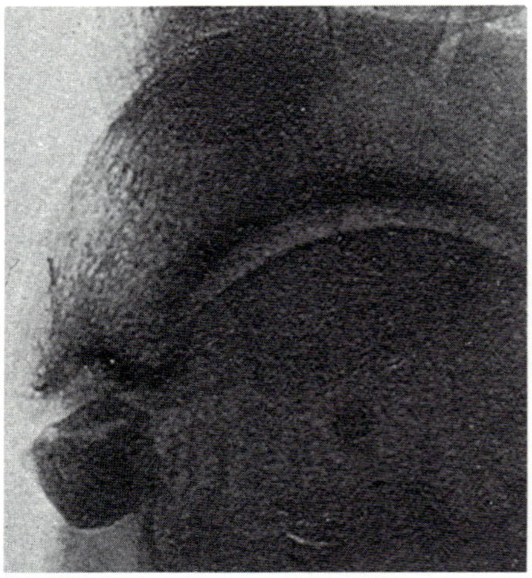

953 & **954** Os tibiale externum. This is one variety of several possible accessory tarsal ossicles. Although it is sited on the inner aspect of the foot, it derives its name from its position on the pre-axial border of the foetal limb bud.

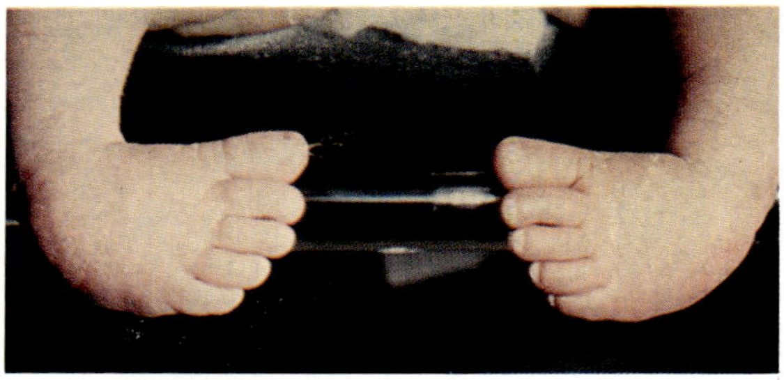

955 Congenital talipes equinovarus. The commonest variety of clubfoot, may be unilateral or bilateral; it may be postural or structural.

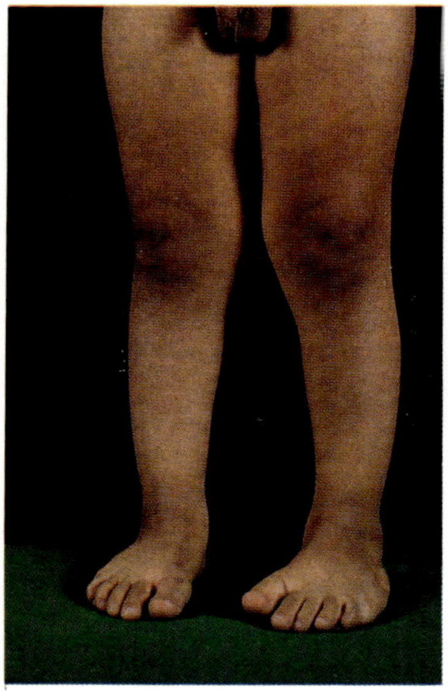
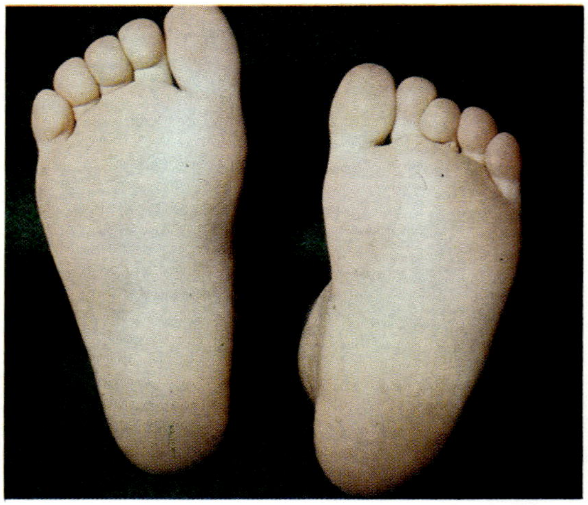

956 & **957** Talipes equinovarus: the residual deformity followed treatment that has not achieved full correction. The forefoot remains adducted. Note the shortening of the left foot and the inversion of the heel.

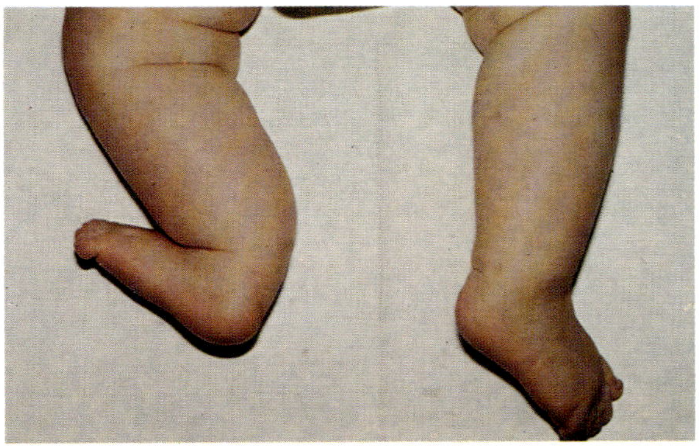

958 Congenital calcaneovalgus. This is the simplest variety of flatfoot. It is probably caused by abnormal intrauterine posture. The foot is fundamentally normal and therefore responds readily to conservative treatment.

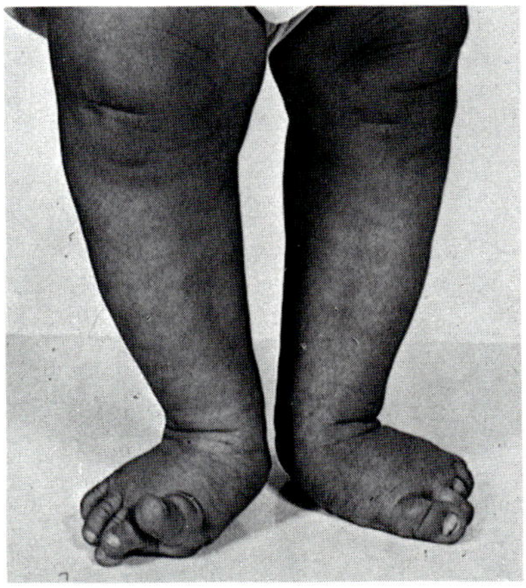

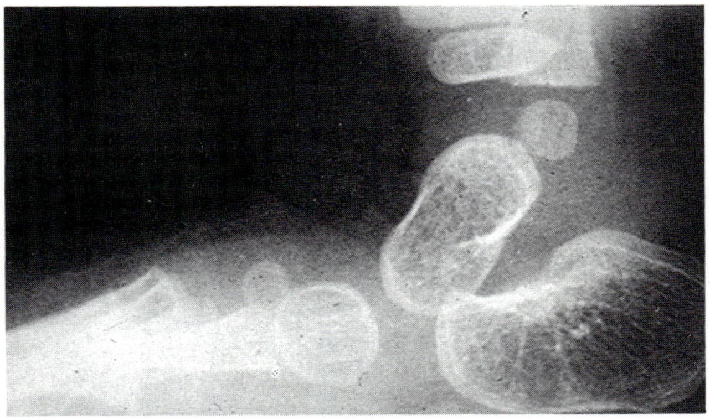

959 & **960** Congenital vertical talus. Extreme flatfoot position resulting from a structural abnormality. Treatment is difficult and often unrewarding. The vertical position of the talus distinguishes this from simple calcaneovalgus flatfoot.

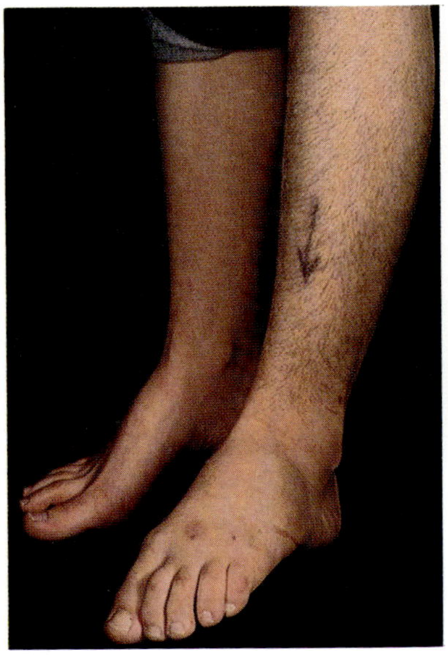

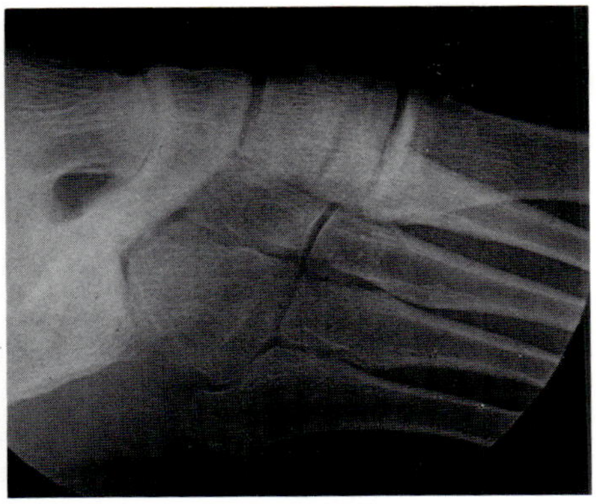

961 & **962** Spasmodic flatfoot. Also known as peroneal muscular spasm. A variety of flatfoot seen usually in adolescence. It may also be the presenting feature of any inflammatory disorder of the subtalar joint; in a healthy individual it is caused by a local structural abnormality. Radiograph shows a congenital bar of ossification between the calcaneus and navicular bones. Any variety of similar structural abnormality is the usual cause of spasmodic flatfoot in an otherwise healthy person.

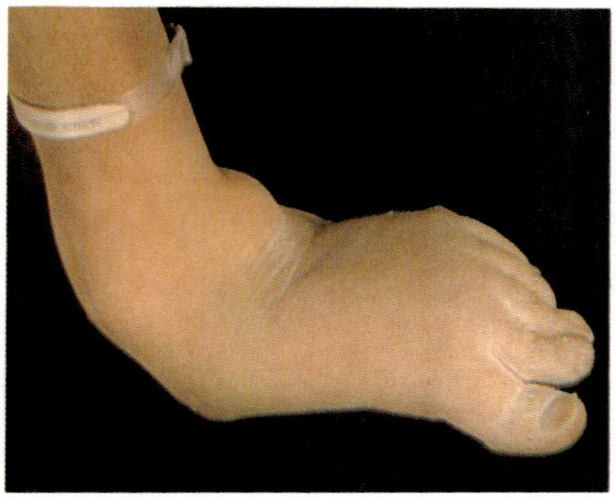

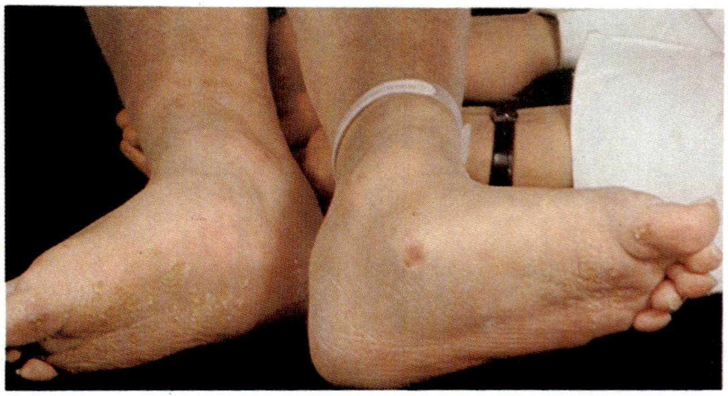

963 & **964** Pes planovalgus (flatfoot): an extreme example caused by rheumatoid arthritis leading to destructive arthropathy and collapse of the medial arch of the foot. Whereas pressure ulceration is common in pes cavus, it is rare in pes planus.

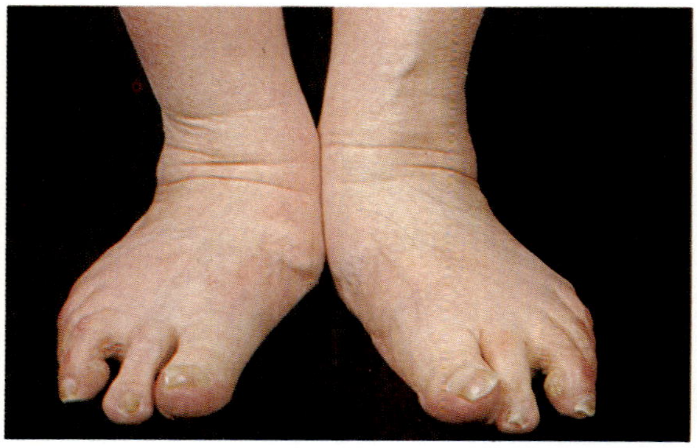

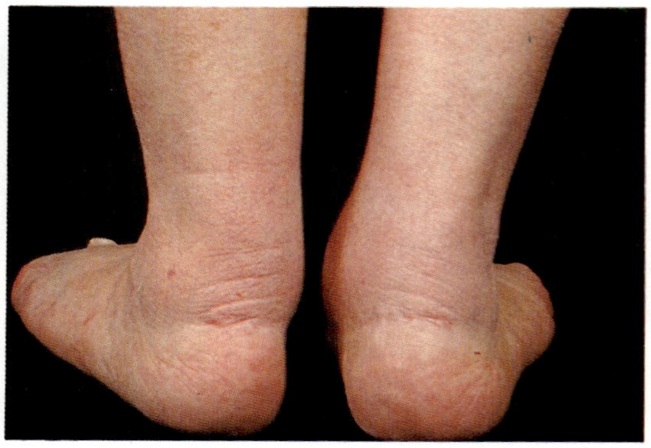

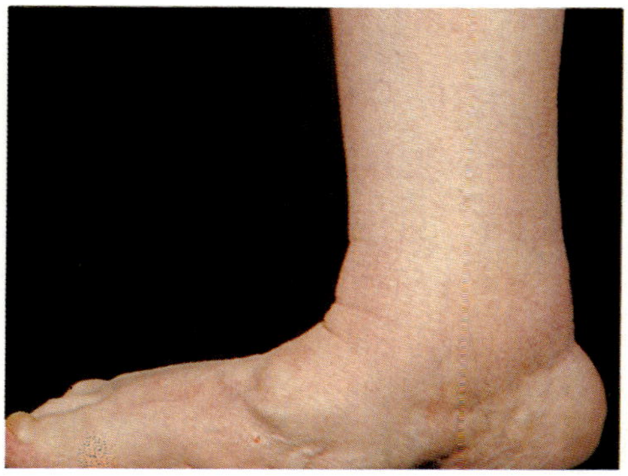

965–967 Postural flatfoot. The feet of an elderly and obese woman whose longitudinal arches have collapsed. These feet were fundamentally normal but have simply given way owing to increased body load and loss of muscle tone. From behind, the everted position of the heels can be seen. From the side the total collapse of the medial longitudinal arch is shown.

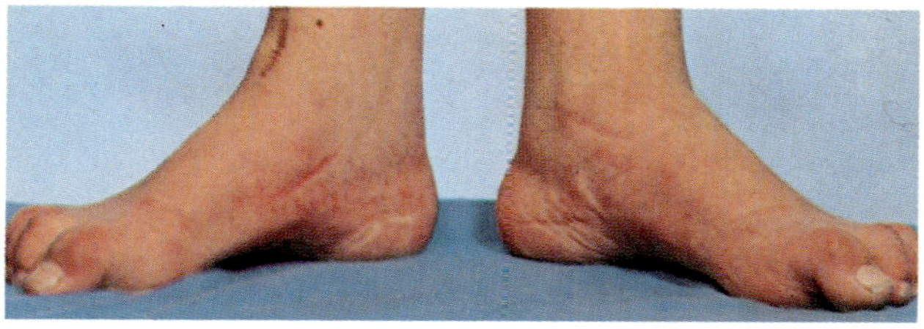

968 Pes cavus. The high-arched foot has a deformity that is the opposite to flatfoot and is clinically the more significant and more important deformity. Contrary to common belief, it is the more serious of the two extremes. Pes cavus is often the local expression of some other disorder.

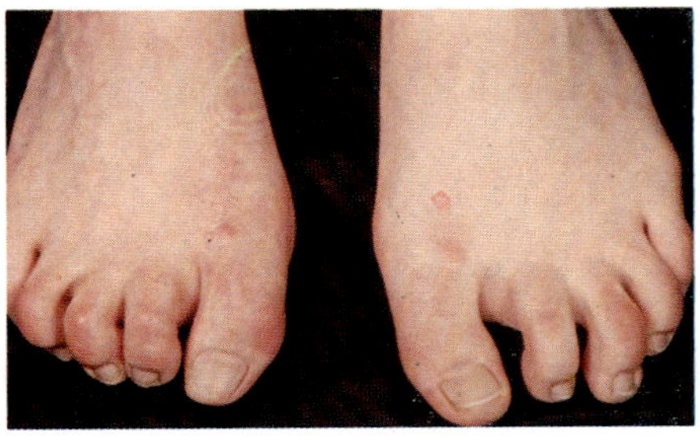

969 Clawing of the toes is usually associated with pes cavus.

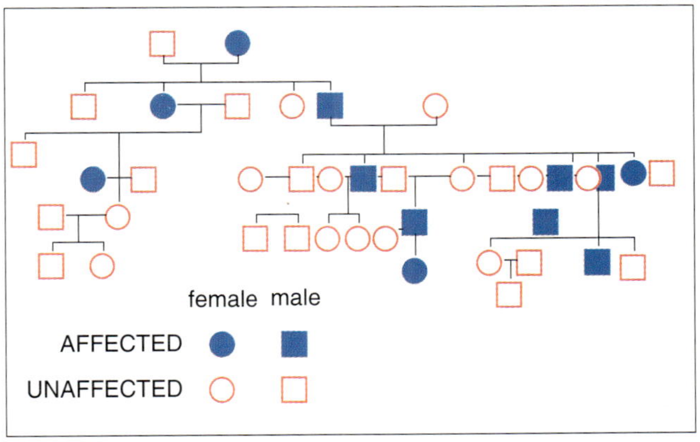

970 Familial pes cavus. There is a familial history in about 50% of patients with bilateral symmetrical pes cavus. The pattern shows that it is of autosomal dominant inheritance. It has been shown to be genetically linked to Friedreich's ataxia.

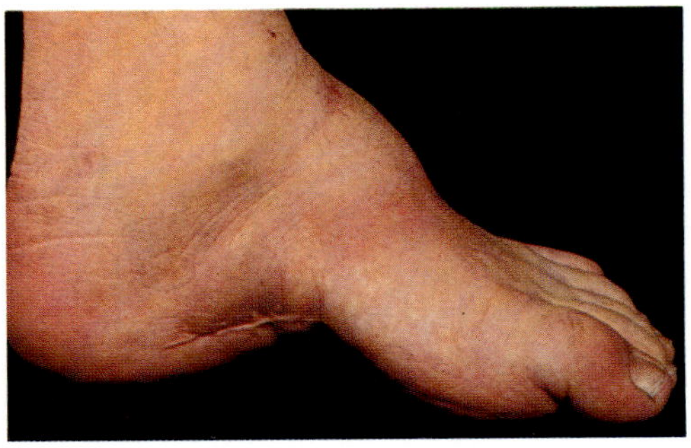

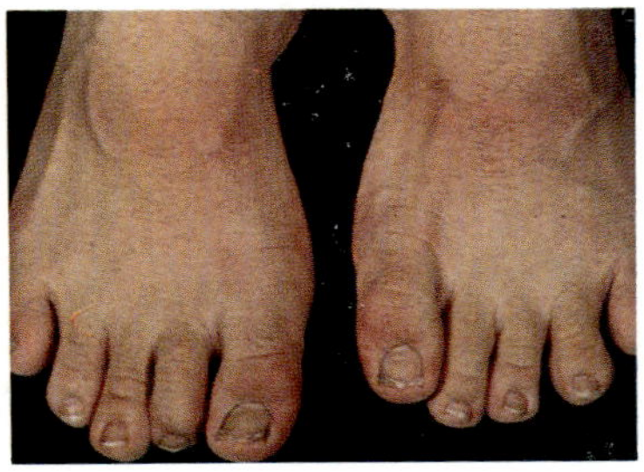

971 & **972** Friedreich's ataxia. The short stubby high-arched foot is characteristic in this disease. Both feet are affected more or less symmetrically.

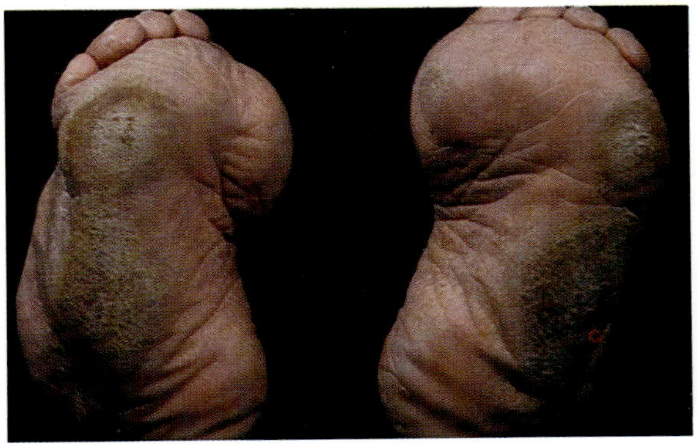

973 The feet of an older and more advanced case shows the very short foot, retracted toes, high medial arch and abnormal lateral weight-bearing callosities.

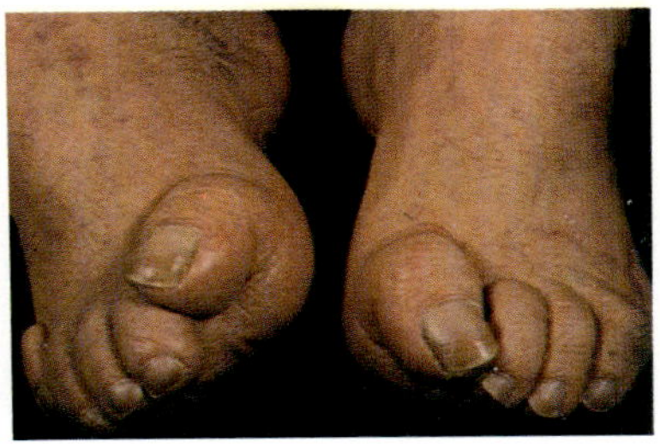

974 Peroneal muscular dystrophy. (HMSN type I). Pes cavus and retraction of the toes is often the earliest sign of a slowly progressive hereditary motor-neurone disease.

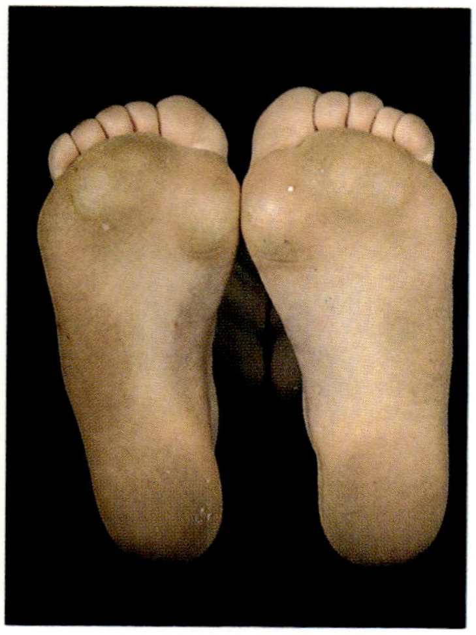
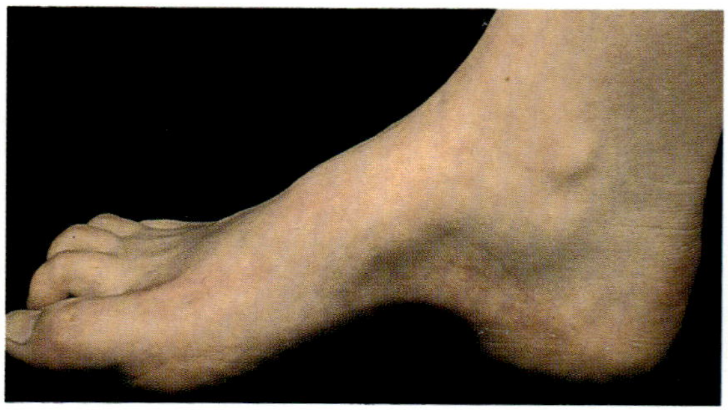

975 & **976** The feet of a young girl who complained of difficulty in obtaining comfortable shoes. Abnormal pressure points can be seen.

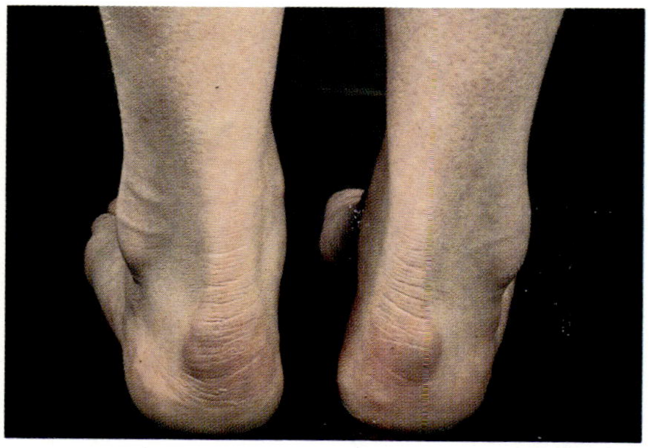

977 The back view of her feet show that the pes cavus is bilateral but not absolutely symmetrical, the right heel is more inverted.

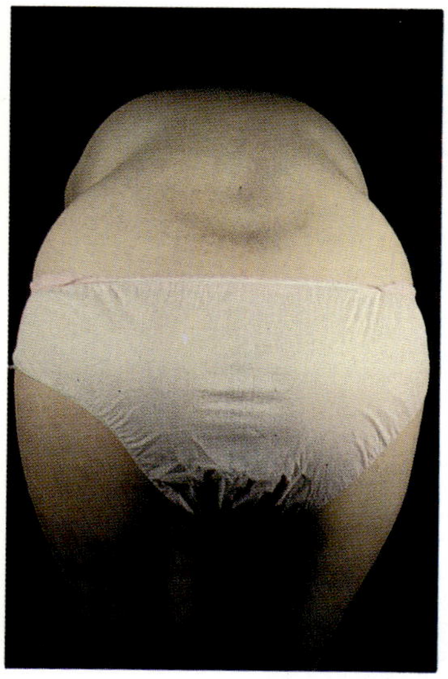
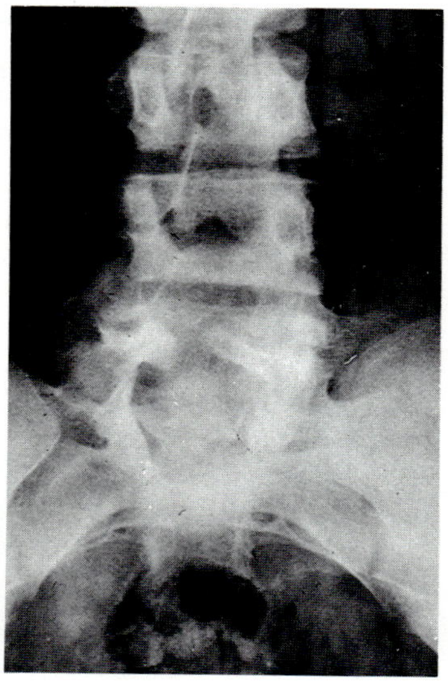
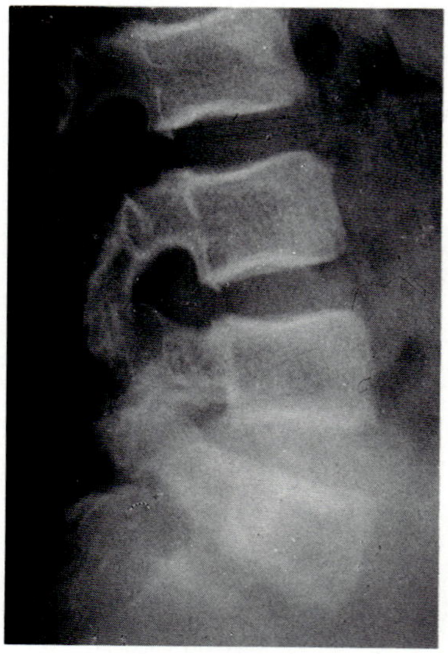

978–980 Examination of her spine revealed a depression at the lumbosacral region with some abnormal discolouration of the skin. Antero-posterior radiograph showed spina bifida of L5 and a defect of the posterior wall of the sacrum; lateral radiograph showed that in addition to the posterior defect, a mild degree of spondylolisthesis was present. After further studies she was classified as a case of congenital spinal dysraphism.

Poliomyelitis (see also 320–331*)*

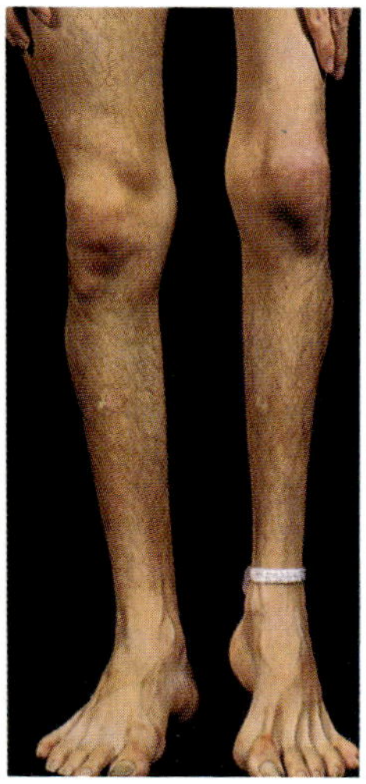

981 Post-paralytic equinovarus, following an attack of poliomyelitis in childhood. The patient's left leg is shortened and his calf is contracted, causing him to stand in equinus. The heel is in varus.

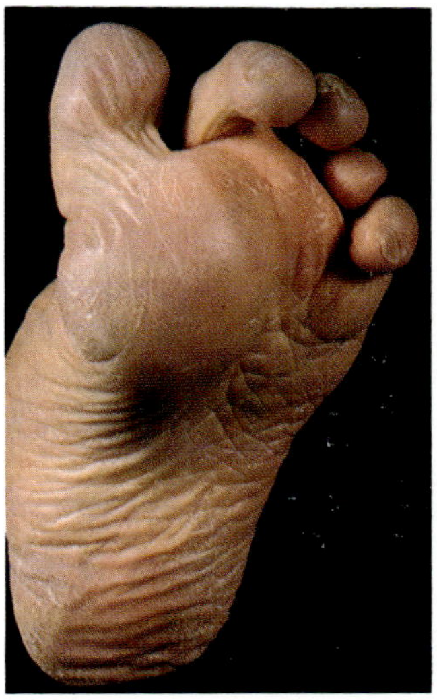

982 Deformity caused by muscle imbalance. The normally acting extensor hallucis longus in the presence of a paralysed tibialis anterior leads to imbalance in this patient's foot.

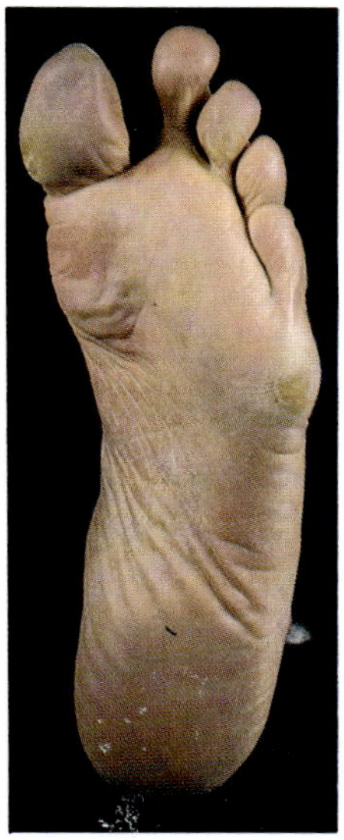

983 Pressure on the base of the 5th metatarsal bone is exerted by normally acting tibialis anterior and posterior muscles when the peroneal muscles have been paralysed.

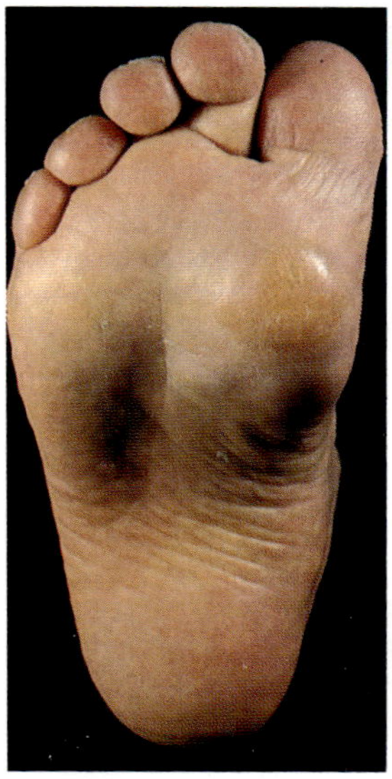

984 Excessive pressure on the head of the first metatarsal is exerted because of a strongly acting peroneus longus when its antagonist, tibialis anterior, is paralysed.

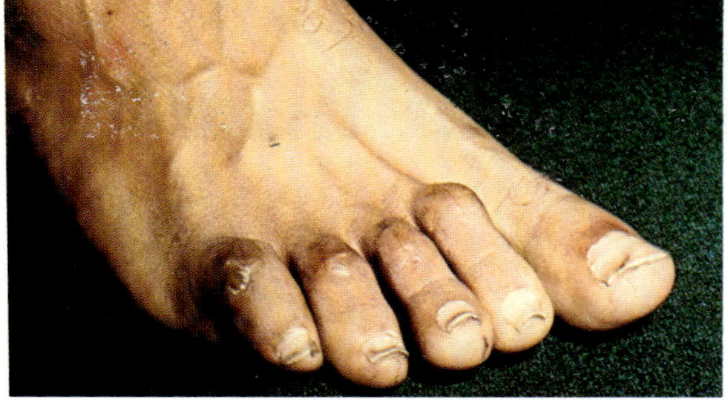

985 Clawing of the toes with secondary pressure on the PIP (proximal interphalangeal) joints is common. It is a result of imbalance between normally acting extensor tendons of the toes when the intrinsic muscles are paralysed.

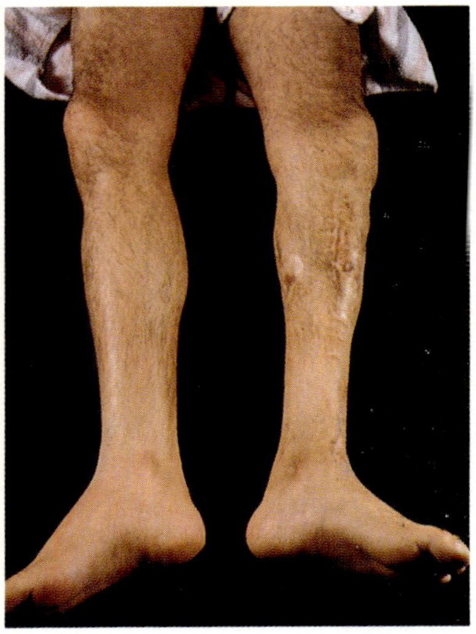

986 Volkmann's ischaemic contracture. This patient had a crush fracture of the left tibia and fibula. There is serious involvement of the posterior muscles which are wasted and contracted.

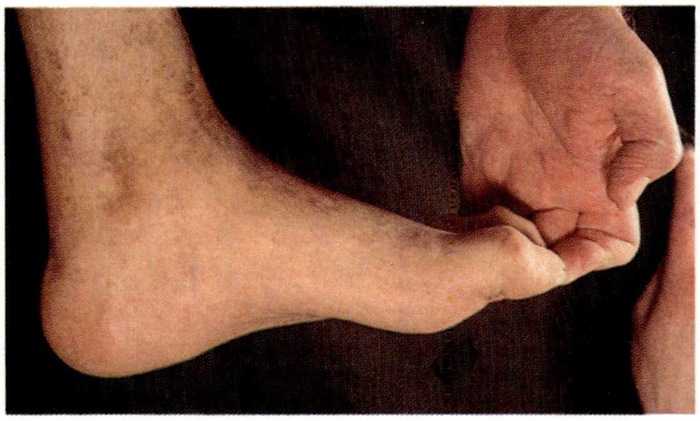

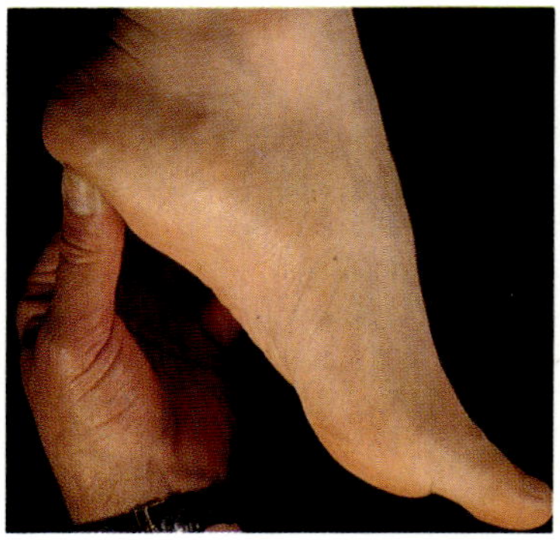

987 & **988** Ischaemic contracture of the long flexor muscles: when the ankle is passively dorsiflexed, the scarred long flexors force the toes into a fully flexed position; when the ankle is fully plantar flexed the toes can straighten.

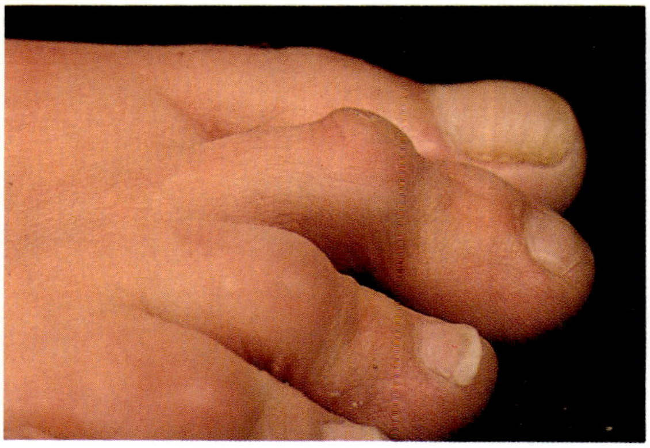

989 Hammer toe. Only one or two toes on each foot are affected. There are a variety of deformities of the toe, depending at which joint the principal deformity is sited. The deformity is fixed and often familial.

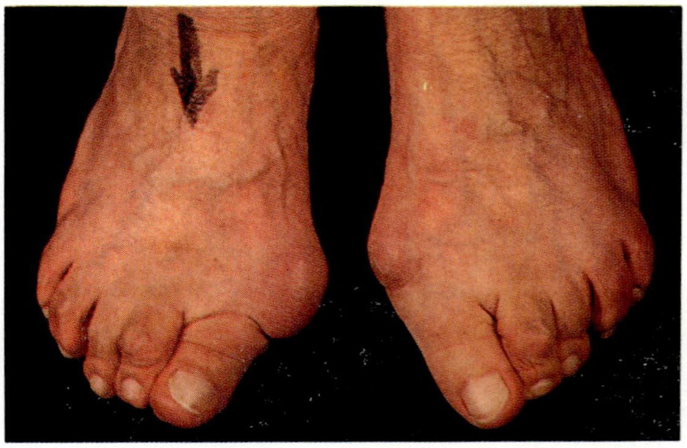

990 Hallux valgus. The angle subtended between the first metatarsal and the proximal phalanx is usually no more than about 10°. In this foot the angle is over 30°. The condition is often bilateral. An adventitious bursa over the prominent medial aspect of each metatarsal head has become enlarged and inflamed to form a bunion.

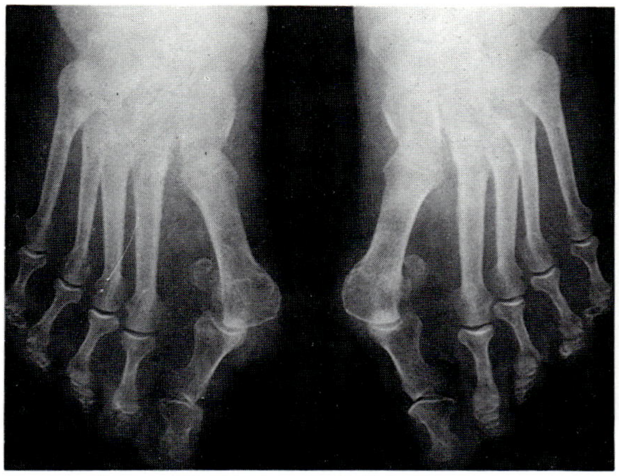

991 Metatarsus primus varus. The presumed cause of the hallux valgus shown in weight-bearing radiograph: it is a congenital abnormality of the first metatarsal bones which are in excessive varus (metatarsus primus varus). It is a condition of sex-linked autosomal inheritance.

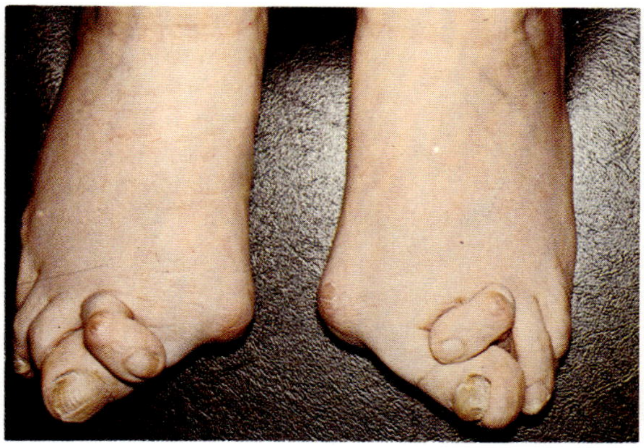

992 Hallux valgus: a more advanced case with bunions and overriding of the adjacent second toes. Note not only the severe valgus deformity, but also the considerable rotation of the big toes, the nails of which now face medially.

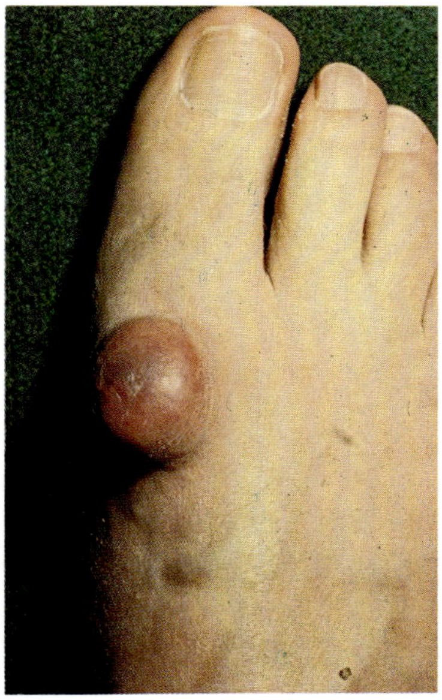

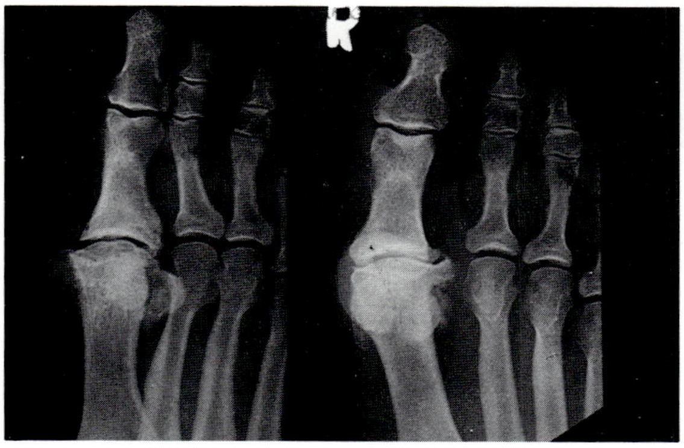

993 & **994** Hallux rigidus. The inflamed bunion in hallux rigidus occurs not on the medial but on the dorsal aspect of the head of the first metatarsal bone. Radiographs show arthritic changes of the first metatarsophalangeal joint and the dorsal exostosis.

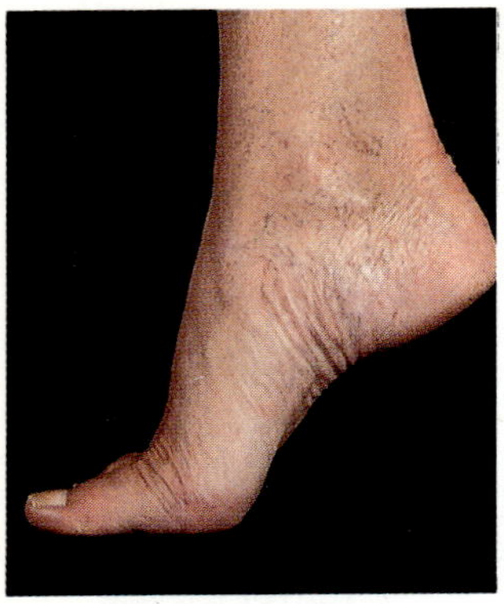

995 Hallux rigidus. In normal walking, the 'take-off' occurs at the metatarsophalangeal joint of the big toe which must therefore dorsiflex.

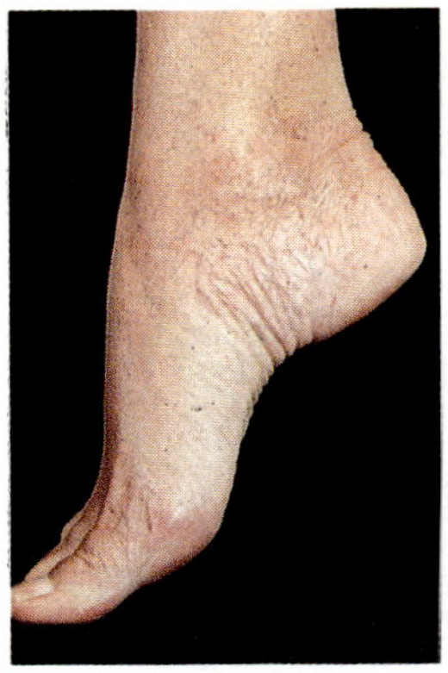

996 If it cannot do so the 'take-off' now occurs at the interphalangeal joint which is forced to hyperextend beyond the stiff metatarsophalangeal joint.

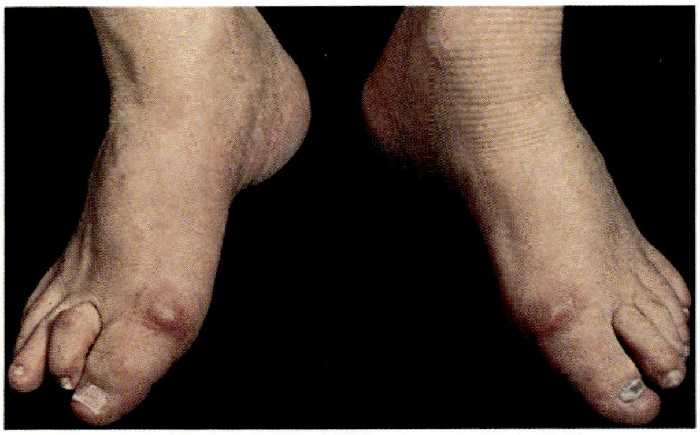

997 Bunion due to gout. This is the classical but by no means the commonest presentation of gout. Note the absence of any hallux valgus. The bunion is due to the deposition of uric acid crystals in the bursa.

Index